Carbohydrate-Addicted Kids

Carbohydrate-Addicted Kids

HELP YOUR CHILD OR TEEN BREAK FREE OF JUNK FOOD AND SUGAR CRAVINGS — FOR LIFE!

Richard F. Heller, M.S., Ph.D.

Rachael F. Heller, M.A., M.Ph., Ph.D.

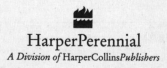

HarperPerennial

A Division of HarperCollins*Publishers*

*To the millions of carbohydrate-addicted children
and teens who struggle with a problem that
is not of their doing, and to their parents who
find themselves powerless to help*

A hardcover edition of this book was published in 1997 by HarperCollins Publishers.

HarperCollins books may be purchased for educational, business, or sales promotional use. For information please write Special Markets Department, HarperCollins Publishers, Inc., 10 East 53rd Street, New York, NY 10022.

First HarperPerennial edition published 1998.

The Library of Congress has catalogued the hardcover edition as follows:

Heller, Richard F. (Richard Ferdinand), 1936–
    Carbohydrate-addicted kids : help your child or teen break free of junk food and sugar cravings—for life! / by Richard F. Heller and Rachael F. Heller. — 1st ed.
        p.   cm.
    Includes bibliographical references and index.
    ISBN 0-06-018724-7
    1. Children—Nutrition—Psychological aspects. 2. Low-carbohydrate diet.
I. Heller, Rachael F. II. Title.
RJ206.H417   1997
613.2'083—dc21   97-16043

ISBN 0-06-092950-2 (pbk.)

99 00 01 02 ❖/RRD 10 9 8 7 6 5 4

Contents

PART III

The Sweet Taste of Success

PART IV

When Things Get Cookin'

APPENDICES

Acknowledgments

We wish to express our deep appreciation to the following people:

Mel Berger of the William Morris Agency—the best agent and counselor known to woman or man. His years of experience, thoughtful and incisive advice, common sense, creativity, patience, and hard work make him a man we both love and respect.

Claudia Cross, Mel Berger's intelligent, talented, and most excellent assistant.

Joëlle Delbourgo, Editorial Director of HarperCollins Publishers, for her understanding of the importance of this project as well as her invaluable insights and sage advice.

Leigh Ann Sackrider and Tim Duggan, Joëlle Delbourgo's intelligent, dedicated, sensitive, and encouraging assistants, for their very hard and essential work and superb editing.

Patricia Wolf, Linda Dingler, and Joseph Rutt of HarperCollins's excellent production and design teams, for their creativity, competence, and very hard work.

Laura Leonard, Senior Publicity Manager at HarperCollins, for her heart and smarts and wonderfully contagious enthusiasm.

Professor Paul Gilbert, M.D., Associate Professor and Acting Chairman of Medicine, Mount Sinai Medical Center, one of the finest minds and best hearts in medicine, for his insightful advice and recommendations, and for providing us with the best health care possible.

Professor Peter Dottino, M.D., Mount Sinai Medical Center, for his fine skill as a surgeon as well as for his clear thinking and sincere concern; for his conscientious and most competent care.

Leslie St. Louis, M.D., and Douglas E. Hertford, M.D., for their expert advice and sage wisdom and for their willingness to make available to us their well-earned and wide range of knowledge.

Norman Katz, Supervising Technologist of Electron Microscopy, Department of Pathology, Mount Sinai Medical Center, and his wife, Madeline—whose suggestions, comments, and encouragement were most important to this project.

Professor Alan L. Schiller, M.D., Chairman, Department of Pathology, Mount Sinai School of Medicine, for his insights, enthusiasm, and unswerving support.

Irwin Neus, D.D.S., his office coordinator, Adrienne Belanoff, and staff, whose interest, support, comments, and contributions to our research are welcome and valued.

Martin W. Weber, who asks the right questions at the right time and who has the right answers as well; one of those rare people whose professional and personal advice has been unerringly on target and who has been there whenever we needed him.

Ana Luisa Vazquez, Sharon Althea Smith, and Audrey Stedford, the finest of research assistants, whose industriousness, intelligence, commitment, and unending hours in the library made our research possible and our lives most enjoyable.

Deborah Heller DeLisa, Jonathan Heller, Caroline Heller, and Chris DeLisa (in order of appearance), the loves of our lives, for their encouragement, caring, insights, wonderful talks, and unfailing support.

Margaret Boulineau and her superb staff, for our wonderful home away from home.

Authors' Note

The information in this book reflects the authors' experiences and is not intended to replace medical advice. It is not the intent of the authors to diagnose or prescribe. The intent is only to offer information to help you cooperate with your youngster's doctor in your mutual quest for desirable health for your child. Please note that throughout this book, the term "child" may be used in the generic sense, to denote one's offspring, rather than to refer to an individual's early stage of development.

Only your youngster's doctor can determine whether this program is appropriate for him or her. Before any child or teen embarks on this or any other program, a physician should be consulted. In addition to regular checkups and supervision, any questions or symptoms should be addressed to your youngster's physician. In the event this information is used without your youngster's physician's approval, you are prescribing for your child, and the publisher and authors assume no responsibility.

There are many causes for eating, weight, behavioral, learning, and emotional problems in youngsters, as in adults. It is essential to rule out any other cause for your youngster's difficulties before embarking on this program. As with any eating or activity program, one size cannot fit all, and this program should be individualized in conjunction with a physician's recommendations. It is important that together you develop a specific program based on the physician's advice and your youngster's own particular requirements and preferences, so that your child may derive the most benefit.

Do not mix and match guidelines from this program with recommendations from other plans. At all times, you should be guided by your youngster's physician; let your child's doctor help you and make important suggestions. Bring this book to the doctor's office. Have your youngster's physician read it and understand the Program and advise you. As in all matters, the physician's recommendations should be primary. This program is not intended for those with medical problems or for pregnant or nursing young women or for the young child. Their needs are so specialized that they cannot be addressed here.

Note: As new scientific information becomes available, recommendations undergo changes. Print media do not allow the incorporation of such updates and changes. In addition, the author, editors, and publisher are not responsible for errors or omissions or for consequences from application of information in this book and make no warranty, expressed or implied, in regard to the contents of this book. Any practice described in this book should be applied by the reader in accordance with professional standards of care used in regard to the unique circumstances that may apply to each situation. The reader is advised always to confer with a physician.

The dialogue, quotes, biographical facts, and anecdotes recounted in this book are actual and true to life. They come from hundreds of interviews. No individual has been directly quoted, or described, unless specific written permission was obtained. All names used in this book, other than those of scientific researchers, have been changed to protect anonymity.

Notice: The terms "Reward Meal," "The Carbohydrate Addict's Program for Children and Teens (CAP-CAT)," "The (Carbohydrate Addict's) Step-By-Step Plan," "The (Carbohydrate Addict's) Jump-Start Plan," "The Carbohydrate Addict's Diet," and "The Carbohydrate Addict's Center" are registered and service trademarks owned by Drs. Richard and Rachael Heller and cannot be used without their written permission.

Car · bo · hy · drate Ad · dic · tion

A compelling hunger, craving or desire for carbohydrate-rich foods; an escalating, recurring need or drive for starches, snack foods, junk food, sweets.

Carbohydrate-rich foods include, but are not limited to: breads, bagels, cake, cereal, chocolate, cookies, crackers, danish, donuts, fruit and fruit juice, ice cream, potato chips, pasta, potatoes, pretzels, rice, pie, popcorn, and sugar-sweetened beverages.

In addition, many carbohydrate-addicted youngsters crave foods that contain sugar substitutes, including artificially sweetened sodas, sports drinks, candies, mints, gum, and other foods and beverages.

Introduction

A History of Success

The two of us have come to understand carbohydrate addiction from several very different perspectives. First, as carbohydrate-addicted kids ourselves we endured the pain, shame, and self-blame with which so many carbo-addicted kids struggle. Second, as adults we have dealt with the frustration, guilt, and family conflicts that raising a carbohydrate-addicted child can bring.

Though we hold the memories of our childhood experiences within us and continue to cope with parental concerns, we are also scientists. Now in the process of retiring, for almost a decade we have held two professorial appointments each and have conducted research at Mount Sinai School of Medicine in New York City and in the Department of Biomedical Sciences in the Graduate School of the City University of New York. In addition, Richard holds a third appointment as Professor Emeritus at the City University of New York.

**We truly understand the power that an addiction
to carbohydrates can have. We experienced it
as carbohydrate-addicted kids ourselves,
as parents, and today as research scientists.**

Over the years our professional duties have included the education of young medical students and physicians in the cause and treatment of carbohydrate addiction, the review and analysis of the work of other scientists in the field, and original investigation into the cause and correction of carbohydrate addiction itself. Basically our job has been to learn, to teach, and to share what we have discovered with others.

Based on more than a decade of research and more than six thousand personal stories, our first book, *The Carbohydrate Addict's Diet*, was written for the adult carbohydrate addict. It quickly proved to be an overwhelming success. Over three-quarters of a million readers sought the guidance we offered, and to date, the book has been published in three languages on four continents, and in Braille. It returned, over and over, to the *New York Times* bestseller list for a period of more than sixteen months.

**Our true success came in the responses
we received from our readers.**

But our true success came in the responses we received from our readers. More than twenty-two thousand calls and letters poured in, and virtually every letter or call reported the almost immediate elimination of carbohydrate cravings through our program. Weight losses varied from a too-rapid thirteen pounds in seventeen days to "a slow, steady, enjoyable weight loss." Grateful notes of appreciation let us know that "this is the answer to my prayers," "you have freed me for the first time in my life," and "I could do this for the rest of my life."

Readers reported higher energy levels, remarkable increases in the ability to concentrate, and elimination of mood swings, accompanied by improvements in blood pressure, blood fat, and blood sugar levels. Undesirable or "bad" cholesterol and triglyceride levels fell; "good" cholesterol levels rose. Our readers were not only feeling and looking better than they had in years, they were, they reported, getting better as well.

For many, it was not the weight but rather the recurring and compelling carbohydrate cravings that they had sought to eliminate, cravings that pushed them to eat unhealthily and to suffer the emotional and mental repercussions of the low blood sugar swings that often followed.

The reports of better health, energy, concentration, and attention continued to pour in. Again and again, letters confirmed that along with eliminating their cravings, our program was improving our readers' physical health and emotional and psychological well-being as well. Each letter confirmed our scientific findings and at the same time fed our souls—for we had personally experienced the power of this addiction as well as the joy of having it lifted.

> **We had experienced both the power
> of this addiction and the joy of having it lifted.**

Growing Concerns

Yet along with their stories of success, many of the readers wrote to us concerned for their children and grandchildren, asking how to adapt the diet to youngsters' needs. We answered, saying that the program had been designed for adults, and, moreover, children and teens had special requirements—nutritional, physical, psychological, and social—that had to be addressed. We added that although the original *Carbohydrate Addict's Diet* book had not been intended for children or teens, we would be happy to work with any youngster's pediatrician to modify appropriately the adult program for the young carbohydrate addict.

We soon learned that our readers' early requests for help for youngsters were only the first of many more to come. Successful adult participants in our research program continued to request help, not only for their own children and grandchildren, but for their nieces, nephews, and neighbors' children as well. We found ourselves overwhelmed with a growing demand for a program specifically designed to help the carbohydrate-addicted child and teen, which would, in addition, help the parent of the youngster as well.

> **We discovered that our own childhood problems
> may have had a greater purpose.**

We came to understand that our own childhood battles with carbohydrate cravings may have had a greater purpose—to help untold numbers of children escape the very difficulties we ourselves had endured. And so, with their parents' cooperation and their pediatricians' guidance, we opened our research to children and teens. The results were overwhelming.

Transformations

The Carbohydrate Addict's Program for Children and Teens worked—and worked well. The Step-By-Step Plan encouraged children as well as teens to make easy changes they were willing and able to make—and to keep making. On the Jump-Start Plan, older children and teens alike reported exciting turnarounds, many within a matter of days!

Parents excitedly related the changes for which they had hoped; physicians, teachers, and school counselors verified the transformations.

An intelligent fifteen-year-old boy had not been doing well in school; he was not yet failing but his teachers and school psychologist confirmed that he was far from living up to his potential. His parents reported that he was distracted, unmotivated, and unfocused. Getting him to do his homework, they explained, was an impossible battle. He moped around the house, interested in little except TV and snacking. He perked up, they said, when it came to sports—he enjoyed basketball and in-line skating—but when he returned to the house, his slow, distracted attitude and behavior returned.

He continually misplaced his possessions, forgot appointments, and broke promises. Punishment and the withdrawal of privileges had little or only temporary effect; yet within ten days on The Carbohydrate Addict's Program for Children and Teens, family and teachers alike saw a new young man emerge. His attitudes, manner, and behavior were "transformed." Apathy turned to energy, boredom to interest, and indifference to enthusiasm. His grades shot up—from low C's and D's to B's and B+'s— and the following semester he proudly presented his parents with a report card consisting of all B's and A's. His self-esteem and popularity grew. He became the bright, happy son his parents had seen as a child and had prayed for once again.

Apathy turned to energy, boredom to interest, and indifference to enthusiasm.
He became the bright, happy son his parents had seen as a child and had prayed for once again.

Other parents reported similar successes:

A pretty but overweight thirteen-year-old girl, whose precocious flirting and manner of dress had shocked and worried her parents, lost the cravings and weight that had ruled her young life and behavior. As the pounds dropped, and she felt and looked more like her normal-weight friends, she seemed to feel far more self-confident. As her rebellious and flamboyant behaviors dropped away, she began to act in ways more appropriate to a girl her age. Her grades and self-esteem shot up, her interests broadened to include school, her future education, dance, soccer, and other sports—all of which continued to be balanced, of course, by an appropriate interest in boys.

These reports, and others like them, confirmed our deepest hopes. Parents, teachers, and health professionals alike verified that learning problems, attitude problems, and mood swings all responded more quickly and completely than anyone had thought possible. Parents who brought their children to us because of concerns regarding the impact of their youngsters' weight on their future health found an unexpected bonus in transformations of attitude, mood, and ability, along with struggle-free weight loss. Self-esteem grew, and "difficult" children as well as "impossible" teens became the productive and happy youngsters their parents hoped they could be.

Too Far to Travel, Too Long to Wait

For research purposes, we defined "success" as a marked reduction in the number and the intensity of carbohydrate cravings along with a decrease in the consumption of carbohydrate-rich foods to the exclusion of other nutritious foods. In addition, our definition of success entailed the achievement of other goals appropriate to the individual child or teen.

**Success was defined in terms
of each individual youngster's needs.**

For one youngster, success might be defined as weight loss and the maintenance of an ideal weight level; for another, success manifested itself as the elimination of mood swings or the ability to control them. With these goals defined, our program was soon showing an unheard-of 70–80 percent success rate. While these numbers may seem high, they did not seem unusual to us. After all, we reasoned, our youngsters have been identified as carbo-addicted; all we were doing was correcting the underlying cause of the problem. One would not be surprised to find that an antibiotic had a similar success rate when given to those patients with an infection for which the antibiotic was developed. Why, we reasoned, should we expect any less? But word of our success spread and the response was enormous.

**Within only a few months, we had a waiting list
of two years and growing.**

Within only a few months of officially opening our research program to children and teens, we had a waiting list of over two years and growing. Before long, although we had helped over several hundred children, as well as their parents and other family members, to learn about carbohydrate addiction and its cause and correction, we had hundreds more waiting to join our program. With each day requests for our assistance poured in, doubling, tripling, or quadrupling the number of people to whom we had already offered help.

Fortunately, we had an answer for those who were unable to travel to Mount Sinai Medical Center or to wait years for an opening in our research program. We set to work, putting our Carbohydrate Addict's Program for Children and Teens into the book you now hold in your hands. We have added our own personal stories and the experiences of many of the youngsters and parents who shared this important time, then added many of the recommendations, strategies, meal plans, and recipes that have helped others to achieve and to maintain their success.

This program was designed to bring your family together around the common goal of helping your youngster, you, and all your family members feel good, whole, and healthy again—on many levels. It can, at the same time, be adapted to enable you to work one-on-one with your youngster despite the resistance and nonsupport you may encounter. The program is intelligent and based on solid scientific evidence. No matter what your youngster's preferences, no matter what time and financial limitations may present themselves, we will try to help you adapt the program to meet these needs. Though we have included a variety of choices, making the program appropriate for a wide range of ages and a whole host of different lifestyles and preferences, always check with your youngster's physician first.

This program was designed to help you, the parent, help your carbo-addicted youngster, but grandparents, other relatives, teachers, counselors, and physicians will find help here as well.

This program was designed to help you, the parent, help your carbohydrate-addicted youngster. Grandparents, other relatives, teachers, counselors, and physicians will find help here as well. The Carbohydrate Addict's Program for Children and Teens has been designed to cut your youngster's cravings, hunger, and excess weight; to reduce blood sugar swings; and to minimize or eliminate associated emotional, psychological, learning, and behavioral problems.

If you are tired of worrying about the physical, emotional, and psychological effects that your youngster's eating may have in the long run, if you are weary of fighting a "losing battle," if you are caught between nagging, fighting, and giving up—over and over again—please know that you are not alone; this book was written with you and your family in mind, and in the hope that it may provide the answers you have been seeking.

Carbohydrate-Addicted Kids

one

Tough Beginnings, Happy Endings

No One to Trust: Rachael's Story

I felt proud and pretty as I pulled on my new two-piece bathing suit. I turned and posed in front of the floor-length mirror. I was only nine years old, and although I wasn't sure exactly what it meant, I thought I looked very sexy. I looked over my perfect ensemble. My beach bag was the same yellow as my bathing suit, and my sandals were the same orange as its trim. I looked absolutely smashing!

It was only half a block to the beach. I had begged my parents to let me meet them there. I wanted to bask in the glory of strutting down the street alone, all grown-up and captivating.

The three boys who walked toward me must have been around sixteen or seventeen years old, but to me they were grown-up men. One of them did a double-take when he saw me coming. I was overwhelmed. This was incredible! They were looking me over! Coyly, I looked down at the pavement as they passed. I saw his feet stop. He was going to speak to me!

"Hey, fatso," he called. "Don't you know enough to cover up all that blubber?"

I looked up startled. One of the others joined in.

"That's right, piggy. Better be careful, someone might accidentally put you on a spit." He reached for my pigtails, held them above my head, and turned me around on my toes, forcing me to rotate like the pig he described. The top of my bathing suit slipped up under my armpits. My chest was bare, and I was vulnerable and helpless.

"Oink. Oink." My torturer laughed as he displayed me to his friends. "Look what I caught. A fat little piggy."

"Joe, come on. Leave the little lard-butt alone," one of the others called. My torturer gave one final tug and let me go, then, turning their backs to me, they walked away.

I couldn't breathe. I couldn't move. I didn't know what "lard-butt" meant but I knew it was something terrible. I was over-whelmed with shame. I didn't even notice that I was crying. I pulled my bathing suit top down over my naked chest and des-perately sought to make sense out of what had happened. I knew something was wrong and I knew that I must be to blame for it but I couldn't put it all together.

Me fat? I wasn't fat. My father told me I was beautiful!

Me fat? There must be some terrible mistake. I wasn't fat. My father told me all the time how beautiful I was. He had me model my new bathing suit for him just yesterday, and he told me I looked just like a movie star. Why were these guys calling me names? Why were they doing that to me?

I was crying so hard that I couldn't catch my breath, but with each tear, as I moved closer and closer to the beach, the truth sunk in. I *was* fat. I really *was*. That's what the kids at school were whispering about, that's why no one wanted to be my partner on class trips, and that's why my mother would stare back at the adults who stared at me.

My stomach tightened in fear. Why had my parents betrayed me? Why had they lied to me? These guys and the kids at school and all the people who stared, they were really telling the truth. I wasn't pretty. I wasn't. I was just . . . fat. And that meant that I was ugly.

I made my way to the beach and plodded through the sand to my parents' umbrella. "Hi, sweetheart. What's the matter? Have you been crying?" my father asked. The tears burst through anew.

"I stubbed my toe and it really hurts," I sobbed. It was the first of many lies to come.

*It would be thirty years before I would come to realize that my
intense craving for carbohydrates was not normal.*

Three decades passed before I learned that my intense
craving for carbohydrates was not normal and that the excess
weight that others found so objectionable was simply the mani-
festation of my addiction to junk food, snack foods, and sweets,
coupled with an unforgiving metabolism.

But at that time all I knew was the need—the hunger, the
cravings, the drive. Food was my focus and my joy. Breakfast was
a pleasure supreme. Cereal and milk with a banana, some warm
toast with butter, a tall glass of orange juice or, even better, some
chocolate milk. It was all so wonderful and I wanted more, and
more, and more. I felt so good when I ate, at least for a while.

But only two hours after breakfast, the warm feelings of satisfaction were replaced by a driving need for more food. I was
hungrier than I had been before I had any breakfast, and now I
needed something to eat with an immediacy that I could barely
communicate. All I knew was that I needed food—satisfying
food: cheeseburgers, hot dogs, fries, cake, cookies, candy—I
needed it right then and there. If I didn't get it, I felt bad, really
bad.

First I felt anxious; I would steal, plead for, or sneak the food I
needed. But if it was not forthcoming, in time my uneasiness
would turn to tiredness. I found myself unable to concentrate.
Sometimes I would get headaches, but more often than not, I
would feel as if I were walking in a fog. Even worse, at times I
would strike out without warning; my hunger seemed to make
me angry toward everything and everybody around me.

Eating always made me feel a great deal better, but almost
inevitably, by the middle of the afternoon, I would find myself
deep in my carbo cycle once again—hungry, irritable, unable to
concentrate, sleepy, and unmotivated. Food was the focus of my
life. I moved from fruit and cereal and toast for breakfast to
pizza, chips, cookies, cakes, and candy for lunch. I wanted no
part of regular meals. Snack foods and sweets were my staple. If
pushed I would eat sandwiches, but whole, well-balanced meals
held little interest for me.

> *Junk food, snack food and sweets were my staple.*
> *I wanted no part of regular meals.*

In the years that followed, my hunger and my weight grew. Though many carbohydrate-addicted children and teens are able to burn off the calories almost as fast as they take the food in, my metabolism was unforgiving and the pounds kept accumulating. Though some carbohydrate-addicted children and teens do not eat great quantities of food, but simply crave the wrong kinds of food for their growing bodies, at a very young age I could eat as much as, or at times even more than, a grown man.

> *Although I knew it was not normal, I never questioned why*
> *it was that the more that I ate, the hungrier I seemed to get.*

To make matters worse, the more I ate, the hungrier I seemed to get. Although I knew it wasn't normal, I never questioned why this was so. In a desperate effort to help me, my parents banned snack foods and sweets from the house. But, as they say, necessity is the mother of invention, and to feed my need, I became a young entrepreneur.

Within a short time I set up a black-market business in my elementary school. My classmates quickly learned to ask their parents to pack additional food in their lunch boxes, a request with which their parents happily complied. These children would then bring their extra sandwiches and desserts to me. I would pay my fellow elementary school classmates for the food they brought in (higher prices for peanut butter and jelly on white bread, lower prices for tuna or cheese). Other students would buy my low-cost contraband with part of the money they had been given to buy their lunches at school, and, given my wholesale prices, they in turn were free to spend of the remainder of their lunch money on pinball machine games and candy. I, of course, ate all the food that was left over and still had my profit to spend on additional goodies. It was an ideal setup, and everyone, it seemed, benefited. Still, my parents never understood how, with virtually no food or money, I managed to continue to gain weight by leaps and bounds.

*My parents never understood how I managed to gain
over fifty pounds in a few short years
though they gave me neither food nor money.*

By the time I was twelve years old, I weighed over two hundred pounds. I was already a veteran of diet doctors. Each week the newest in a parade of physicians would weigh me, yell at me, give me amphetamines and "water" pills, and take my parents' money. No one ever looked for a cause of my carbo cravings.

At twelve and a half I was hospitalized for stroke-level blood pressure. I was put on a low-calorie diet, and when I stopped losing weight, I was accused of cheating—which I was. I was summarily discharged. I felt like a convict. How many people get thrown out of a hospital before their thirteenth birthday?

As I left the hospital, a chubby, round-faced doctor told me that I was "killing myself" and that I had to get control of my weight. But he never told me how to do it. How I wish now that he had tried to discover what was causing my cravings in the first place. Without a cause there could be no cure, so my cravings and the weight gain simply continued.

*My diet solutions were themselves feeding my addiction.
Still, I blamed myself for every diet failure.*

At the ripe old age of thirteen, I failed again at yet another attempt to lose weight by calorie counting, and I failed in a subsequent attempt at age fifteen. I never suspected that the high-carbohydrate "healthy" breads, fruits, and juices I had been told to eat were making me hungrier with every bite. At sixteen I discovered powdered liquid fasts. Up and down went my weight as I moved from formula to formula, adding more and more powder to each drink or doubling the number of drinks in a day. I never realized that those "liquid meals" contained the same sugars I so desperately craved and that they were in fact feeding my carbohydrate addiction. In time I began to drink them like milk shakes along with a sandwich— or two.

With every new diet came time-limited success and then the inevitable failure. Each time my hunger and cravings would override my resolve, and I would be left feeling ashamed of my lack of willpower and hating myself even more.

My parents tried to help in any way they could.
I would lash out or steal and hide the food I needed.

My parents were themselves struggling unsuccessfully with their excess weight, and they vacillated between leaving me alone and hoping that I would "grow out of it," and trying to restrict my eating "for my own good." They would try one approach, then the other. But neither solution helped. Leaving me alone did absolutely no good; I was free to feed my every carbo impulse. Left to my own devices, I would eat virtually nothing but junk food and sweets. When they tried to restrict my eating, I would either lash out or go underground, stealing and hiding the food I needed.

My mood swings, irritability, secretiveness, and lack of interest in school only made matters worse. Each morning was a fight to get me out of the house and off to school. Some semesters I missed as many days as I attended. I knew that my parents were concerned for my health, my happiness, and my future, but to me they were the enemy—they stood between me and all that I wanted—to eat the food I craved, and to be left alone to watch TV, read, listen to my music, read a bit, and sleep. I had virtually no friends, and though my hunt for satisfaction filled many of my thoughts, deep within I was terribly lonely.

Even though I would have adamantly denied it,
I was heartbreakingly lonely.

Suddenly, in junior high school, the prettiest girl in the class befriended me. Her mother had great difficulty with her daughter's choice of me as her companion and told me so in no uncertain terms. At first I was devastated; humiliated and ashamed. Yet in the days that followed her candid conversation, I found comfort in her confirmation that my weight, as opposed to something else about me, was keeping me isolated and lonely.

My parents had repeatedly denied that my weight was as important an issue as my friend's mother suggested; they explained that anyone who was worth knowing would see past "a few extra pounds." Their magical thinking might have made them feel better, but it robbed me of the chance to deal directly with reality—to come to grips with the impact that my weight was having on my young life. Ironically, I found great peace in the clarity that my friend's mother's hurtful words offered, for she verified what I already knew.

I felt renewed in my commitment to lose weight, but once again, my body seemed bent on betraying me. Each new diet attempt was to fall to the cravings and intense hunger that invariably emerged.

By the time I was seventeen, my weight topped three hundred pounds.

By the time I was seventeen, my weight topped three hundred pounds. Actually, I probably weighed at least ten or twenty pounds more, but that was as high as our scale went. The pounds continued to mount. Strangers would stare or, even worse, look away so as to not appear impolite. My classmates' whispers had long ago turned to ridicule, then avoidance.

My desperate search for the "cure" for my weight problem continued into my twenties and thirties. From water fasts to hypnotism, Weight Watchers (six times), Pritikin, and Stillman, I tried them all. Behavioral modification, juice fasts, Atkins; up and down and up again. I even founded the Philadelphia chapter of Overeaters Anonymous. I once figured I must have lost and regained over six or seven hundred pounds, and always, in the end, my cravings overcame me and I would "cheat," then cheat again, then "take a day off." I would swear that I would start again on Monday. I lived an eternity of Mondays, but I could never lose the weight and keep it off. I felt as if my whole life was slipping through my hands like sand, and try as I might, I could not get hold of it.

I felt as if my whole life was slipping through my hands like sand, and try as I might, I could not get hold of it.

My health was suffering. I was hospitalized for petit mal seizures, periods of lost or reduced awareness, but when the neurological tests showed no cause, the doctors discharged me without a diagnosis. They had no clue that the tiredness and irritability that accompanied these periods of reduced awareness, and the reduced awareness itself, was an important indication that I was experiencing low blood sugar episodes.

I started to avoid seeing doctors. My high blood pressure, they would say, signaled impending doom, and my triglyceride and cholesterol levels were "through the ceiling." Long before I was old enough to vote, my body was revealing the wear and tear it was experiencing. By the time I was eighteen, I had developed a heart murmur and an irregular heartbeat, and the pain in my knees, feet, and back from the crushing weight made anything but minimal walking almost impossible.

I was desperate beyond words but I simply could not find a way out.

I could find no way out. I knew I was addicted to food, but there was no treatment program for my problem. I remember wishing that I were a drug addict or an alcoholic so that I could go someplace, away from all this pain, and be cured of my addiction.

I had no social life. The few boys I did date had problems of their own.

The years flew by; they were filled with pain, shame, and, most of all, the never-ending battle to gain control over my eating and my weight. The relationships I had were unhealthy at best; abusive and damaging, in reality. Still I never stopped searching for a way out—out of my addiction, out of my predicament, out of my life.

Finally, at thirty-six years of age, the answer came—not from someone else but from my own experiences and my own body.

At age thirty-six, the answer came from my own body.

It was a typical midsummer morning in New York, hot and humid. I was scheduled for an X-ray examination that morning and I had taken the day off from work. As per instructions, I had not had anything to eat or drink since the night before. I slept poorly; my air conditioner was acting up and I had trouble

falling asleep on an empty stomach. The early morning ringing
of the phone pulled me from my restless sleep; offering no
explanation, a technician from the X-ray laboratory informed
me that my appointment had been changed from morning to
late afternoon.

My bedroom was stifling and I was caught halfway between a
fitful sleep and a sweat-soaked consciousness. I confirmed the
time change, and as she quickly wrapped up the conversation,
the technician reminded me to eat and drink nothing other than
plain coffee or tea until my appointment later in the day.

As I dragged myself from my bed, my mind weighed the pros
and cons of going into work. As I considered whether to spend
the early part of the day at my air-conditioned job or to try to
enjoy a day off in my unpleasantly hot apartment, the reality of
the day ahead suddenly made its way into my consciousness. I was
not going to be able to eat anything until four in the afternoon—
nothing, nada, zip! I felt the panic rise. It might be even later, I
told myself, five or six o'clock by the time they were finished.

I tried to think of a way out of my predicament. I considered
rescheduling the appointment but realized that they might post-
pone it until later in the day once again. I considered spending
the day in bed, trying to sleep the day away, but I had too many
things to do, and until I could afford another air conditioner, I
knew I would find no relief at home. I even considered skipping
the X-ray exam altogether, but as I considered the alternatives, I
knew I would just have to tough it out—somehow.

Still feeling uneasy, I showered and, per my usual routine,
weighed myself. Two hundred and sixty-eight pounds. I am sure
I made some negative comment about my weight to myself at
the time, though I can't remember it now. I do recall that as I
headed for work, I counted the hours—the long hours without
food—that lay ahead of me. I reminded myself that I had done
it in the past, eating nothing, living on water and diet soda for
weeks at a time, that this brief fast was nothing compared to
what I had endured then. But the thought of a day without
food still loomed large and foreboding. I tried to tell myself
that others were able to handle this kind of situation all the
time. Still, something within me lay halfway between panic and
determination.

The most amazing thing happened: As the hours flew by,
my hunger and cravings never materialized.

In a halfhearted effort to distract myself, I headed off to work and dug into the tasks I had hoped to avoid. Then the most amazing thing happened: As the hours flew by, my hunger and cravings never materialized. Earlier I had purchased a cup of black coffee from the coffee cart but I barely touched it. The phone never stopped ringing and, before I realized it, I had worked right through lunch. I never noticed the time. It was not until two o'clock, when the coffee cart made its usual round, that I suddenly realized that I was less hungry than if I had eaten my usual breakfast and lunch. It didn't make sense; I wondered if I were getting sick. Amazingly, I had never felt better.

Not able to resist the coffee cart's call completely, I bought two French crullers for a special treat after my X-ray was completed. I figured that I could keep them in my pocketbook and enjoy them in the dressing room as a sort of reward for holding out all day. Feeling content with my plan, I faced the rest of the day's work and worked for another hour without another thought of food.

The X-ray appointment went smoothly, and at five o'clock I was once again on my own. Interestingly, I was not half as hungry as I thought I would be, so I headed for a nearby restaurant with a promise to myself that I would hold off and enjoy my crullers for dessert. And I was true to my word. I topped off my dinner of soup, salad, bread and butter, veal parmigiana, pasta, and coffee with my crullers—slowly relished in the back of the bus on the way home.

Although I had rewarded myself with all the foods I loved
the night before, I awoke weighing two pounds less.

By the time I made my way into my tiny studio apartment, the heat had lifted and I headed straight for bed. As I fell off to sleep, however, I remember thinking that I had blown my chances of losing weight by eating so huge a meal and wolfing down the crullers to boot. But when I awoke the next morning, another surprise awaited me. The scale testified that I was two pounds lighter than the day before. It was incredible! And it didn't make any sense at all—at the time.

I assumed the weight loss had to be "water weight" and I was certain that I would gain it back, yet the scientist in me literally saved my life that day, for instead of "assuming" it was water weight and letting it go at that, I found myself designing an experiment.

Why not eat what I had eaten yesterday again today, I thought, and see what happened. After all, it had not been that difficult—I hadn't been hungry all day and I really enjoyed eating all I wanted for dinner, guilt-free. It didn't sound that difficult, just unusual. What did I have to lose? I asked myself. So I decided to give it a try.

Skipping breakfast that day was easy; no problem at all—though this time I did drink the coffee I had "coming." Lunch was a little more difficult. Everyone was going out to eat or bringing food into the office and, though I was not really hungry, I still wanted something to eat. Still, the promise of a repeat of yesterday's dinner held more appeal than some mediocre lunch, and I managed to hold out through the afternoon. To add strength to my promise to myself, I bought another two crullers and packed them away again, as my after-dinner treat.

Dinnertime found me ready, willing, and more than able to enjoy my well-earned reward at my favorite local pizza place. I ordered a Greek salad, a cheese steak sandwich, and two giant slices of pizza with anchovies and pepperoni, to go. A diet soda completed the fare and, with my crullers secreted in my brief-case, I toted the whole meal home so that I might enjoy it in the privacy of my own apartment while watching the six o'clock news. I was in heaven!

After the meal, I turned to my crullers and found, much to my surprise, that I could eat only one. I was stuffed! The truth was that after the first half of the meal, I wasn't hungry anymore; still I refused to fail to finish "what I had coming." Now only one cruller remained, and as I put it aside, I promised myself I would have it before I went to bed.

The next morning, though the house still smelled of pizza,
I had dropped another pound.

But I never did eat the cruller. I went to sleep without the slightest desire for an evening snack. The next morning I found that I had lost another pound. I remember thinking, "Another pound and the house still smells of pizza! This is crazy."

And, crazy or not, this strategy worked, and continued to work. My days flew by; I skipped breakfast and lunch each day and ate whatever I wanted for dinner. I was less hungry and had fewer cravings than I had ever had in my life, and my weight continued to drop—day after day, then week after week.[1]

In time I began to experiment with foods—one by one, testing different foods and combinations to see which, when eaten at breakfast and lunch, would not trigger my cravings or weight gain. I found that breads, cereals, juice, and fruit at breakfast triggered hunger by eleven A.M., and that a lunch with bread or fruit led to a midafternoon drop in energy and rise in cravings. A midday snack of cookies, crackers, or fruit triggered an evening of snacking, followed by almost inevitable weight gain.

On the other hand, I found that breakfasts and lunches made of protein-rich meats, chicken, and fish; fiber-rich salads; and many vegetables left me craving-free and allowed my weight to continue to drop. Balanced evening meals that incorporated vegetables and salad helped keep my cravings and weight down.

For the first time in my life I was free.

I did not fully understand the underlying logic behind what I was doing—I did not understand *why* this way of eating was working. But I did know one thing: For the first time in my life I was free—free of the cravings, free to enjoy (yes, actually enjoy) losing weight, and most of all, free of the self-blame that had been my almost constant companion. It did not matter to me that no one understood what I was doing or why I was doing it, I knew that it was working, and I was determined to give it my best.

---

[1]This program will *not* require your youngster to skip lunch or breakfast; the skipping of these meals was only the first step in the development of what would become The Carbohydrate Addict's Diet, and helped Rachael to discover that the frequency of carbohydrate consumption triggered her addiction and to determine which foods initiated her cravings and weight gain.

And give it my best I did. I simply continued to do what I had been doing and, virtually without effort, I lost 150 pounds. For the first time in my life, I discovered what it was like to look like a normal person—and feel like one, too. My intense and recurring cravings were gone. I felt reasonably hungry when it was time to eat and I felt satisfied with normal-sized portions of a variety of foods. It might not seem like a very big thing to some people but, to me, it was almost too good to be true.

After nearly thirty years of struggle, trial, and defeat, I had stumbled upon the most important discovery of my life—that my cravings were "triggered" by certain foods: foods to which, it appeared, I was especially sensitive; foods that I craved but that, when I ate frequently—throughout the day—left me tired, irritable, unable to concentrate, and, most of all, craving more . . . and more . . . and more. Most amazing of all was the fact that these very foods were those that I had been told were "healthy" or "diet foods" and that I had been cautioned to include at all meals as the basis for any "sensible" weight-loss plan!

More importantly, I discovered that when I ate these same foods (breads, pasta, fruit), as well as some snack foods and sweets less frequently, or combined them with other foods, the overwhelming cravings that had literally ruled my life for over three decades simply disappeared. I had done it. I had found a way out. I no longer had the cravings and weight problem that had haunted me throughout my life. Yet I was still able to enjoy the foods I loved every day as long as I kept in mind *how* I ate them.

There was no doubt about it;
I found my personal miracle.

It was my personal miracle. In this simple discovery—how and when to eat which foods—lay the key to eliminating the physical imbalance that ruled my cravings, my feelings, my behavior, my moods—the very life of my addiction.

Today, my victory can be seen, in part, in my weight loss of 165 pounds (fifteen additional pounds dropped off without my even trying!) and the struggle-free maintenance of that weight loss for over thirteen years. My physician says my health recovery has been astounding. The irregular heartbeat and heart murmur have disappeared. My cholesterol and triglyceride levels are ideal. I have the blood pressure of an eighteen-year-old (one that is not carbo-addicted), and my blood tests place me in the lowest risk level for heart disease in the country. My energy is literally without bounds. I can concentrate when I have to and totally relax when I want to. My mind is clear and focused, and I am relaxed and happy.

Today I am truly free.

For I am truly free; free of being overweight and free of the fear of gaining the weight back. Yet even more important is another, less visible, victory—a freedom from my cravings and mood swings; from a deep and penetrating tiredness, self-blame, and shame; from states of semistupor, the feeling that life is passing me by; and most of all, from a lifelong battle with an addiction that I was able neither to understand nor to control.

In some ways my release from my addiction may have come too late: too late for me to experience the feeling of being young and attractive, surrounded by lots of friends and facing a lifetime ahead; too late to enjoy proms, dances, and days at the beach; too late to go steady or share secret talks with my friends about boys we wanted to date; and, even worse, too late to have children.

For, although with every fiber of my being I ached for a child of my own, I was at the same time terrified at the thought of bringing another soul into this world who might suffer as I had, and by the time my cure came, it was too late in my life to begin planning a family.

I will never take my freedom for granted.

Though I will never take my freedom for granted, though it is more precious than I can ever describe, I am still aware that my childhood and young adulthood can never be reclaimed and that my chance to hold and mold children of my own will never come to pass. My addiction has robbed me of these forever.

Still I am blessed, for sometimes in the quiet of the morning, a calmness comes over me and I know that even the loss of these gifts has had a purpose. If what I have learned can help others avoid the pain I endured in my youth, it will have been more than a fair trade after all.

The Human Garbage Can:
Richard's Story

I was a chubby baby and a stocky child; not really fat but certainly not slim, and though I grew to be a "big" boy, it was simply attributed to my "healthy appetite." By the time I was eleven or twelve, my bike provided all the freedom I needed. I had a few good buddies, and on Saturdays my parents would give me some money and send me off for the day. I was on my own and I owned the world!

My friends and I would ride over to the Bronx Zoo or the park to explore and find adventure; still, the highlight of my Saturdays was food. At home my choices were limited. I was forced to eat "well-balanced" meals that invariably included overcooked vegetables without taste and salads made of nothing but lettuce and sprinkled with lemon juice.

I lived for weekends, when my life was my own.

On Saturdays, however, my life was my own. I lived on candy, ice cream, and cookies. I knew every store and street vendor in the neighborhood and I knew where you could get the most for your money. Quality did not matter. Quantity was my goal.

The owner of the little store at the corner sold broken cookies for half price. He was a kind, grandfatherly man who never missed an opportunity to comment on my red hair and freckles. But his teasing was always gentle and sensitive, as if he just wanted to make me know that he liked me. He often had a bag or two of my favorite cookies behind the counter, specially priced because they contained broken contents.

When the weather permitted, my friends and I would bike over to the freight yards near the East River. At one of the factories, we were always made welcome to all the broken sugar cones we wanted. We would each bring a large shopping bag and something to drink, and then, carrying our booty to the shade of a boxcar on a rail siding, we would stretch out on the ground and pretend that we were hobos enjoying our loot.

I would wolf down sugar cone after sugar cone and guzzle my soda, only to find, each time, that the wonderful feeling of satisfaction was fleeting. An hour or two later, I was ravenous once again.

Alone in the dark, eating and being entertained at the same time.
Who could ask for more?

Rain, cold, or snow brought an adventure of a different sort. This was a purely solitary indulgence: the Saturday movie complete with cartoons, a short subject, a newsreel, a serial, a double feature, and all the food I could stuff into my mouth. What glory! Alone in the dark, eating and being entertained at the same time. Who could ask for more?

The money my parents gave me could not keep up with the demands of my cravings. I took to collecting bottles and trading them in for cash to buy candy, chips, and ice cream. Still I couldn't get enough. My metabolism burned up a great deal of the caloric overload but it was no match for my relentless appetite. By age twelve I was wearing "stocky" clothes, though it wasn't until a few years later, when girls entered the picture, that I would begin to care about the extra inches and unwanted pounds.

At fourteen, I learned the tricks of the trade.

At fourteen, I was given the job of my dreams. My brother found a place for me to work in the legitimate theater. In the evenings and on Saturdays I could be found at the Majestic Theater on Forty-fourth Street in New York, checking coats and, during intermission, selling candy and cold drinks. Finally I had money of my own to do with as I wanted. But, amazingly, I no longer needed the money for food. I had mastered a whole new set of tricks to satisfy my carbohydrate cravings. By lifting, from their tracks, the locked sliding doors at the back of the candy counter, I could get to the candy before the manager arrived on the scene. The chocolate-coated and pastel candy-coated almonds were my favorites.

Long before the days of cellophane wrap, the only thing that stood between me and my almonds was a neatly folded cardboard box flap. With a little practice, I became expert at prying open the flap without a trace. At first I removed only one almond from each box but, when no one noticed, my greed got the better of me. In the days that followed I had to force myself to remove no more than three or four almonds from each box. Fear of losing my job and my carbohydrate connection kept me from taking more, and miraculously, no one ever seemed to notice.

The excitement of the con and the power of my cravings pushed me further. Now chocolate-covered raisins and nonpareils became fair game, and virtually no one who bought candy at the theater ever got a full box. My cravings and my waistline grew. Orange drink sales provided a new benefit, with the added choice of profiting by either drink or money. By combining the leftovers in the cardboard containers discarded by the patrons, I was able to "reconstitute" full containers. A little water filled in when remainders were low. A carefully replaced paper cap completed the operation. If I were craving a sugary orange drink, I would drink my fill from a new orange juice container and replace it in stock with the "reconstituted" version. If money was my goal, I could place the "reconstituted" container among the unsold ones. When my boss asked for the money for the containers that had been sold, he would not expect payment for those that had been manufactured by this chubby redheaded kid from the Bronx.

The new flood of carbohydrates fed my addiction, and it was no wonder that my metabolism simply could not keep up with my eating. My weight continued to creep higher and higher and would normally have put me at a social disadvantage, but I worked every night and Saturdays from morning to evening, so as long as I continued to work at the candy counter, I did not have to face my nonexistent social life.

Without work to fill my time and food to fill my thoughts,
I found myself with a newly emerging longing—
an undeniable need for female companionship.

When I was sixteen, the candy concession was bought out by a national firm (I often wondered if my boss sold the business because I was literally eating up the profits), and with my weekends free, I found myself with a newly emerging longing—for female companionship.

It soon became evident that the slimmer boys got the prettiest girls, and suddenly the quality of my appearance had meaning. The extra tire of fat around my waist did nothing to add to my desirability and, in a vain attempt to hide it, I would cinch in a wide belt under my pants, then pull my slacks on over it. It probably looked pretty strange to everyone else but I thought it hid the fat. Before long, my vanity gave way to comfort, and one hot summer day I threw away the belt and gave up on the illusion that I was able to hide the extra pounds.

All through my youth, my weight made me the last pick for any team sport, but while I had learned to live with being an outcast when it came to sports, I was not as willing to face rejection when it came to the opposite sex. I dated a bit, for, thankfully, in those days a few extra pounds was not as critical in determining popularity as it is now. Even so, though my weight probably did not seriously interfere with my social life, I remember feeling self-conscious about my weight.

"I get the burger," laughed one of my friends. "Richie gets the rest."

Rather than making fun of my weight, the guys would tease me about my appetite. I remember going to a drive-in restaurant with three of my friends. The waitress returned with our orders saying, "Okay, I have three cheeseburgers, two fries, a side of onion rings and a plain burger." She waited for us to indicate who owned which order. "I get the burger," laughed one of my friends. "Richie gets the rest."

My carbohydrate craving was ever-present, and while my parents did not seem to think of it as a serious problem, I knew well the battle I was silently fighting. I wanted to eat little else but junk food, snack foods, and sweets, yet, at the same time, I also wanted to look good. Even in my naiveté I knew that my junk food cravings were getting in the way of my looking the way I privately imagined I could look.

I longed to do better at school, and though neither I nor anyone else recognized it at the time, the food I so craved and the low blood sugar levels that followed my junk food feasts were greatly affecting my schoolwork as well.

> *As carbohydrates became my primary source of nutrition,*
> *I became less and less able to concentrate.*
> *I just couldn't seem to retain what I had learned,*
> *and my grades dropped with each successive school year.*

Reading had always been a problem, but now, as snack food, junk food, and sweets became my primary source of nutrition, I found that the long school day loomed ahead, an unwarranted sentence to be served for a crime I had never committed.

After school I had great difficulty in concentrating on my homework (though at the time I only knew I hated it), and my grades dropped with each successive school year. I just could not seem to sit down and do what was expected of me. Though I lived in fear of being humiliated by my teachers and disappointing my parents, I simply could not force myself to buckle down and do the work that was required. When I did, I couldn't seem to retain what I had just learned.

I managed to do enough to barely get by, and I graduated from high school with a grade average only one point above passing. I joined the army reserve. Active duty involved boot camp and unrelenting physical demands, but I knew it would take off some of my weight. Or so I thought. Army food seemed designed with the carbohydrate addict in mind. Their fine array of limitless bread, pancakes, rice, biscuits, rich gravies, fruit, juices, pasta, corn, and desserts fed my already flourishing addiction. In a matter of weeks, extra-large portions and second helpings added fifteen pounds to my well-padded frame. No amount of rigorous activity could burn it up as fast as I was shoveling it in. I was the only recruit who left basic training weighing more than he did when he entered.

With boot camp over, my appetite had been primed to expect bigger and better things. So the weight I had gained in training not only remained, it continued to rise.

*My weight and my ability to concentrate were constant battles,
but I never put the two together.*

From time to time, when I simply could not stand being over-weight anymore, I would try to control my eating, but somehow, each successive year resulted in a net gain of two or three or four more pounds. Into my thirties, each larger size was a lost fight in a war on which I could not get a grip. My weight and my ability to concentrate were constant battles, but I never put the two together.

I fought to stay focused and to perform up to par. Though I tried to concentrate, I felt as if I were moving through thick syrup; I often thought it must be easier for others, but I simply did not know why it was so hard for me to retain what I had learned. I flunked out of college on the first try, but, when I went back, I noticed that a heavy morning breakfast resulted in hunger and my inability to focus by eleven A.M., and that my exhaustion in the midafternoon meant midday classes were doomed to failure. I noticed that my energy was fine in the morning if I had only a cup of coffee for breakfast or skipped breakfast altogether and that, after my midday tiredness, my energy would pick up again later in the day. By carefully sched-uling classes to coincide with times that I was best able to concen-trate, I succeeded in graduating. I used the same strategy in graduate school, and again succeeded, though at the time I never directly connected my eating with what seemed like my unique personal rhythm.

As a professor and researcher, I always tried to work my schedule around my ability to focus, never realizing that my ability to focus could be made constant by changing the way in which I took in my food.

*My ex-wife would never admit that she found my excess weight
unattractive but I knew the truth.*

My weight still continued to climb each year, and while my then-wife shrugged off my voiced concerns, saying that I was "a big guy" and fine just the way I was, she would always point to the slimmest man on the beach, it seemed, and comment on his physique. Or, even worse, furtively check him out when she thought I wasn't looking.

I became known as the "human garbage can."

Though my appetite continued to be a source of what seemed like good-intentioned humor to all who knew me, deep inside I often found myself resenting the teasing. As a child, when I cleared the table, my parents came to expect that I would eat up all the leftover food as well. It front of his friends, my brother would laugh at me and call me the "human garbage can," but I acted as if it never affected me. My then-wife and our children also came to expect me to eat anything that remained at the end of a meal. As the marriage deteriorated, this custom turned into a taunting family game, and my children would leave what amounted to garbage on their plates and try to get me to eat it.

Again and again I would take off some weight, though, more likely than not, a diet started in the morning met with lost resolve (and lost self-esteem) by nighttime. A bag of cookies and an entire pint of rich ice cream constituted my typical evening snack. I never understood what people meant when they said that they weren't hungry. I was always hungry.

Over the years I tried calorie counting and Weight Watchers (a couple of times). They worked for a while, but inevitably I would become tired of living by the numbers, of the limited portions, and of the lack of satisfaction, and would end up eating what I wanted, and all that I wanted.

In my early forties I tried a daily regimen of running and worked up to a total of over forty to fifty miles a week. I kept it up for two years but with zero effect on my thirty-eight-inch waist, which was, in fact, approaching forty inches.

Finally I just gave up, resigned to living with my love handles
and pot belly, until a casual comment from a colleague
led me to a life-changing discovery.

At that point I just gave up, resigned to living with my love handles and pot belly and watching them grow. In the back of my mind, however, I was concerned that I would continue to gain weight as I got older, and I worried about the effect of the weight gain on my health. The truth was, I was hungry most of the time, and sometimes I simply could not control my eating. I crossed my fingers and hoped that my metabolism would continue to burn up a good portion of my huge intake of calories.

My professional duties brought me to Mount Sinai School of Medicine, and when I joined the faculty, I met men and women at the forefront of new and exciting discoveries. But it was a casual personal statement from one of my colleagues that led me to the discovery that would change my life, freeing me of both my addiction to carbohydrates and my difficulties in concentration, at the same time.

At lunch one day my friend commented on the great amount of food, as well as the high proportion of carbohydrate-rich foods, I was consuming. "Oh, I always eat like that," I responded. "I always have." Without negative judgment, he pointed out that if he ate that way he would find himself "in a stupor by the middle of the afternoon." He added that he suffered from low blood sugar and congratulated me on my freedom to be able to eat as I wanted. His words rang in my ears, and the next day I pumped him for all the information he could provide on what hindered and helped his ability to concentrate.

In a matter of days I felt better than I ever thought I could.
It was like nothing I had ever imagined!

Growing concerns for my vascular health prompted me to try his methods, though they had been designed primarily for those with blood sugar problems. In a matter of *days* my mind was clearer and more focused than it had ever been. I felt as if someone had added 40 points to my I.Q. level. Late into the evenings, I stayed up for hours working on projects that had seemed, in the past, too much trouble to even begin. I was a different person!

His program, however, did not allow me to enjoy many of the foods I truly loved. There must be a way, I thought, to have the food I enjoy and still feel this good. And if there was, I was going to find it.

With my mind free and clear, I went to work discovering new ways to stabilize my blood sugar levels simply by changing *how* I ate the foods I wanted. I used every bit of scientific ability at my command; I searched the computer data bases, scoured the medical journals, and carefully and painstakingly kept detailed notes of the effects that food had on my hunger, my energy, and my ability to concentrate. Each personal discovery gave me a clearer understanding that what was important was not what was in the food, but, rather, how the food affected *my* body.

Friends began commenting on my weight loss, and I had indeed lost fifteen pounds, literally without trying. I was eating all the foods I loved every day but I was eating them in a different way. When I missed a lunchtime meeting because I had forgotten to eat, I suddenly realized that my ever-present cravings, my constant companion since childhood, were gone.

My physical exam showed that my blood pressure and blood fat levels had greatly improved. Whatever I was doing was working: I was getting thinner, healthier, and better. In time, easily, almost without effort, I went down to the weight (165 pounds) and body shape I had sought all my life.

> *I am forever free of the clouded thinking,*
> *the excess weight, the slowly deteriorating health, and*
> *the carbohydrate cravings that ruled so much of my life.*

As of the writing of these pages, I have remained at this weight for more than twelve years. Though looking good is satisfying in itself, more importantly, I am forever free of the clouded thinking, the slowly deteriorating health, and the carbohydrate cravings that ruled so much of my life. My discovery, indeed, was a dream come true, but one that lacked someone with whom to share it.

Two Minds, One Mission:
The Continuation of Richard's Dream

It was a truly magical meeting. It was my first weekend out after the collapse of my sixteen-year marriage, and it was Rachael's first desperate attempt to leave an abusive relationship of eleven years. I packed myself and my two daughters, then nine and twelve years of age, off for a weekend of folk music and the company of old acquaintances.

I was hoping to find someone to share my life, my love,
and my new body. In the past I might have spent the weekend
alone, allowing myself the right to eat my troubles away.

In the past I might have spent the weekend alone, allowing myself the right to eat my troubles away, but now food was no longer my comfort or my tormentor, so I sought other diversions and other company. Without my compelling cravings and with so much pain already filling me, I found myself strangely without appetite and soon left the community dinner table in favor of a quiet corner where I might make some music and share the company of others.

There I sat, playing my guitar for several hours as old friends and new acquaintances came, sat for a while and sang, and moved on.

I saw her from the corner of my eye. A dark-haired woman
with a bounce to her step and a sadness in her face.

Then I saw her from the corner of my eye. A dark-haired woman with a bounce to her step and a sadness in her face. It seemed as if she were trying to be happy but a deep sorrow was pulling her down. The discrepancy tugged at my soul, for it mirrored exactly what I was feeling.

Pulling a chair in behind the group, she joined the semicircle of people facing me. Her face was haunting; intelligent yet emotional, soft but powerful.

So there I sat, playing my guitar, singing to her and wanting everyone else to leave. And in time they did, and, miracle of miracles, she stayed. I put down the guitar and moved to her side and we talked—all through the late night and into the early hours of the morning. Real feelings, real fears, real hopes. It was magic.

We held nothing back—well, almost nothing.

We held nothing back—well, almost nothing—for as much as we shared, the one thing we did not talk about at first was our respective battles with weight and eating.

Finally Rachael broke through the unspoken wall. She told me of her struggle with her weight: the burden of weighing three hundred pounds for over twenty years of her life and the self-blame she carried for even longer.

Then, with some hesitation, she began to reveal what she had learned about her own body and her own addiction. I listened in stunned silence. This is impossible, I thought. It was as if she had been describing me; my own struggles, my own doubts, and finally, my own victory. I tried to explain that her experiences were reflections of my own, and though I knew my words sounded hollow, I hoped she would understand the impact her story had on me. I could see that she was not sure if she could believe this most amazing of coincidences, so I pressed her no further. Instead, as we said good night, I took her hands in mine and kissed her once. "I want to get to know you—very slowly and very well," I said. "How does that sound to you?" She nodded and smiled and I went off to sleep happier than I ever imagined a person could be.

We filled the next two days with each other. We wanted nothing more than to be together and talk. In some amazing way, within a matter of hours, the pain of the past healed in the sharing. We turned to exploring our mutual discovery regarding our eating and our weight. We compared what we had learned about our cravings: what triggered them, what stopped them once they started, and what kept them at bay. At the time, neither of us fully understood the underlying cause of the cravings, so we did not use the term "carbohydrate addiction," we simply talked about what we had learned and how we were able to be successful when there had been nothing but failure in the past.

Then Rachael revealed her life's dream: to bring this discovery to others who suffered as she had, to adults who might benefit from her struggles, and to children who might be spared the pain she had endured. I was transfixed. I, who had never wanted much more than to enjoy my own life with my own family and to do good in the world, saw a focused purpose and meaning beyond that which I had always imagined. I wanted to share her life, and her dream as well, and I asked her if we could work on the project together.

The weeks, months, and now years that have followed have been filled with the joy of making that dream—our shared mission—come true.

The principles that worked for us personally, as well as our own research and the scientific discoveries that already existed in the medical literature, led to the resounding success of our first book, *The Carbohydrate Addict's Diet.* The years of research that followed at Mount Sinai Medical Center in New York, coupled with the experiences of literally thousands of adults and youngsters, laid the groundwork for the two plans that make up The Carbohydrate Addict's Program for Children and Teens that we share now with you.

Today we have come to understand that our respective years of struggle were, in fact, years of learning—important and useful years—years that have allowed us to help adults, teens, and children alike to reach for and to achieve the self-respect, success, dignity, and ideal health that are theirs to claim as their birthright.

What Is "Carbohydrate Addiction"?

Americans of all ages are eating so many carbohydrate-rich snacks—three times as many as they consumed only a decade ago—that food addiction is becoming the rule rather than the exception. And so are the weight-related, psychological, physical, and emotional problems that go along with it.

Carbohydrate-rich snacks consist of starches, snack foods, junk food, and, most of all, sugar, sugar, sugar. It has been estimated that the average American consumes six hundred calories from sweets each day, *not* including fruits and other natural sources of sugar. If we adjust this estimate to take into account the immense consumption of juices, sugar-laden drinks, fruits, and snacks typical of youngsters' diets, we can probably expect that for most kids—carbohydrate-addicted or not—sugars constitute the major portion of their caloric intake. It is no coincidence that, at the same time, obesity in children has reached epidemic proportions and that mood, learning, and behavioral problems in youngsters have hit an all-time high. Our children are drowning in a flood of carbo-rich foods that are making them overweight, unfocused, undermotivated, hyperactive, and overly mood-responsive.

If you think your youngster may be addicted to carbohydrates, it is essential that you learn to separate fact from fiction when it comes to the powerful physical forces that may be driving your youngster's addiction to carbohydrate-rich foods.

Myth #1: It is "natural" for kids to want to eat only junk food, snack foods, and sweets.

While it is true that a preference for sweet foods seems to be an inborn part of our physical makeup, there is, at the same time, a complementary tendency that pushes both animals and humans to seek other foods as well. So while newborn babies have been shown to respond with smiles to sweet-tasting drinks, children whose bodies are in balance will naturally select a variety of protein-rich and high-fiber foods along with their carbohydrate-rich choices.

While a *preference* for sweets or starchy foods may be natural, an intense or repeating craving for these foods is not.

A youngster who experiences a recurring, compelling drive for carbohydrate-rich foods, often to the exclusion of other foods, is not necessarily showing a "natural" pull to these foods but, rather, may well be showing signs of an undiagnosed physical imbalance.

This physical imbalance feeds itself, literally. When carbohydrate-addicted youngsters eat the carbohydrate-rich foods they crave, and eat them frequently and without balance, they end up craving more of the same. And little else. The cycle, once started, is hard to stop—often almost impossible—until the physical cause of the addiction is understood and corrected.

Myth #2: If a youngster is not overweight, an addiction to carbohydrates is not a serious problem.

We often tell parents of overweight youngsters that they are very fortunate, for the visibility of their child's excess weight makes it easy to diagnose that their youngsters may be suffering from a silent but potentially destructive physical imbalance.

The child who eats little else but starches, snack foods, junk food, or sweets, but who is normal-weight or even somewhat underweight, may, on the other hand, appear to suffer no ill effects from an overly carbohydrate-rich diet. Nothing, however, could be further from the truth.

Normal-weight and overweight carbohydrate-addicted kids alike often exhibit learning, behavioral, social, and mood-related problems that most parents and health professionals fail to realize are actually diet-related.

If your carbo-craving youngster is overweight, be thankful that his or her body is showing you that it is out of balance and in need of help. If, on the other hand, your child or teen is normal-weight or underweight, it is essential that you do not allow yourself to be lulled into thinking that this addiction will have little or no effect on your youngster's current or future happiness and well-being.

Myth #3: Most kids will outgrow their carbohydrate cravings.

When most of us were growing up, the prevalent belief was that a fat baby was a healthy baby. In the same way, youngsters with unusually short attention spans or behavioral problems were tolerated or, if they were male, it was said that "boys will be boys." When behaviors became too extreme, a stern reprimand or a sterner hand was thought to be appropriate. At the same time, it was assumed that children "naturally" craved sweets and snack foods and that indulging them with goodies would do no long-term harm.

"They will grow out of it" was the byword, whether referring to children's poor eating habits, chubby bodies, behavioral problems, mood swings, or all of the above. But for the most part, these children did *not* grow out of it. Instead, as adults they continued to eat many of the same foods they craved as children. Although, as they entered adulthood, they may have traded their Kool-Aid for diet soda and their candy bars for chocolate mousse, they continued to rely on junk food, snack foods, and sweets as the mainstay of their diets.

Research shows that children who survive mainly on starches, junk food, snack foods, or sweets may never outgrow these eating habits.

Now long-term research studies have confirmed what many parents have feared: Children who survive mainly on starches, junk food, snack foods, or sweets may never outgrow these eating habits. Rather, as they enter adulthood, carbo-addicted kids may face physical, emotional, and interpersonal problems that may worsen with each decade.

Those who, as youngsters, had difficulty concentrating, had little motivation, acted out, or were hyperactive may grow up to become sullen or moody, achieving below their capabilities, and may continue to have social and personal difficulties. Others who struggled with weight problems in their youth may continue to gain weight or, after maintaining an ideal weight for several years, may put on unusual amounts of weight when faced with a first pregnancy or stressful situations. In time, overweight or not, young carbo addicts can become unhealthy, underachieving, and, in some cases, unhappy adults.

Whether you are looking at the cravings that drive your youngster's food choices, the foods themselves, or the weight, blood sugar, or other physical, psychological, or behavioral problems that result from these food choices, carbohydrate addiction and the physical imbalance that causes it do not go away with time. They only get worse.

Though periods of increased growth spurts may offer temporary reprieves, the overweight child will almost certainly get heavier with each passing year and will very likely suffer the emotional, social, and psychological scars that go along with weight problems, in addition to almost inevitable health problems.

The learning-challenged youngster may receive coaching, counseling, and special help, but without an understanding of the cause and a solution to the problem, this child may be robbed of essential skills, left with little but low self-esteem and a sense of hopelessness.

The moody teenager is likely to become the moody adult, taxing personal relationships and alienating potential employers.

The hyperactive youngster may calm down a bit as he or she grows into adulthood, but this youngster is likely to become the anxious and/or rebellious young adult.

A problem uncorrected usually grows worse.

We have seen it in ourselves and in the children and teens with whom we have worked over the years. Educational, career, relationship, and lifestyle choices of the carbohydrate-addicted young adult are often limited and dictated by a disability that is both preventable and reversible.

Pay no attention to the false promises that are meant to console or quiet you. Most carbohydrate-addicted youngsters do not grow out of the problem; at best they learn to live with it—often at great cost. At worst they suffer without reason or recourse and often go on to have carbohydrate-addicted youngsters of their own.

THE HIGH-CARBO LOWDOWN

Scientists define carbohydrates as chemical compounds containing carbon, oxygen, and hydrogen in a certain proportion. In terms of the food you eat, carbohydrate-rich foods can be defined as those that contain significant amounts of starch and/or sugar.[1]

The term "simple sugars" refers to carbohydrates usually derived from cane, beet sugar, fruits, or corn. You may recognize them as sucrose, glucose, fructose, or corn syrup. High fructose corn syrup is rarely, if ever, made up of fructose only. Contrary to its name, the sugar in high fructose corn syrup may be partially or mainly composed of the simple sugar glucose. Fructose (fruit sugar) is *not* a complex carbohydrate; it is a

---

[1]While some forms of fiber are made up of carbohydrates, these fibers are usually not absorbed by the body, and therefore are not one of the substances that would determine if a food is carbohydrate-rich.

simple sugar—simpler than sucrose, which contains two simple sugars, fructose and glucose. The fiber in fruits may be quite beneficial and may help in reducing the effects of the fructose it accompanies, but when manufacturers process the fruit, removing the fructose to use as a sweetener in other foods or by itself, the fiber benefit is lost, and it may be no better for your body than the table sugar, sucrose. Fruits and fruit juices, table sugar, and honey contain simple sugars. They, as well as foods that contain significant amounts of them, should be considered carbohydrate-rich.

In contrast to simple sugars, the term "complex carbohydrates" is used to described starchy foods. In chemical terms, starches are long chains of sugars that the body will usually digest more slowly, and to which it will often react less quickly and less strongly in terms of insulin release and blood-sugar swings. Foods rich in complex carbohydrates (or starches) include, among others, grain products and foods made from grain products, which includes rice, bread, cereals, crackers (without added simple sugars), and some vegetables, including peas, corn, potatoes, and legumes (starchy beans).

Carbohydrate-rich foods are an essential source of energy for the body. While the process of digestion is complex, in general, simple sugars cross the stomach lining and enter the bloodstream as glucose. Complex carbohydrates, on the other hand, are broken down into glucose later in the small intestine and released into the bloodstream more slowly. Glucose may be absorbed from the bloodstream and used as fuel by muscle cells or organs. It may also be absorbed by the liver, where it can be stored or turned into fat, and then released into bloodstream for storage in the fat cells.

Carbohydrate Addiction Defined

Some parents tell us that the moment they heard the term "carbohydrate addiction," they knew we were talking about their kids. Other parents tell us that they thought "addiction" might be too strong a term to describe their youngsters, or that they were not sure which foods were carbohydrates. In Chapter 4 you will be able to take a simple quiz to help determine if your youngster does indeed appear to be addicted to carbohydrates, but for now, let us define carbohydrate addiction as we have researched it for over a decade and lived with it for most of our lives.

Carbohydrate addiction is a compelling hunger, craving, or desire for carbohydrate-rich foods. It is often experienced as an escalating, recurring need or drive for starches, snack foods, junk food, sweets, and sugar-sweetened or artificially sweetened foods or drinks.

Carbohydrate-rich foods include, but are not limited to, breads, bagels, cake, candy, cereal, chocolate, cookies, crackers, danish, donuts, fruit and fruit juice, ice cream, potato chips, pasta, potatoes, pretzels, rice, pie, popcorn, and sugar-sweetened sodas and sports drinks.

Carbohydrate-addicted kids may also crave artificially sweetened foods, drinks, mints, candies, and gum.

While a simple desire or preference for carbohydrate-rich foods does not indicate an addiction to them, a youngster who craves these foods intensely, repeatedly, and to the exclusion of other foods is most likely suffering from a physical imbalance. In the pages that follow, you will learn about the causes of carbohydrate addiction, what makes it worse, and how to free your youngster from its grasp. For now, it's important to understand that the addicted youngster is not simply "indulging" a desire for these foods.

An "indulger" often enjoys a snack of carbohydrate-rich foods when he or she has not had an opportunity to do so for a while. Once finished with the snack or goodie, the youngster—now satisfied—moves on to other activities. Subsequent meals may or may not include additional carbohydrate-rich foods, but as a matter of course, nonaddicted youngsters will usually naturally choose to balance carbos with protein-rich foods (meat, chicken, fish) and a variety of vegetables.

Carbohydrate-addicted youngsters, on the other hand, feel as if they *need*—and they must have—these carbohydrate-rich foods, and the more they have, the more they need. When these foods are denied to them, or given to them in limited amounts, they may become extremely upset.

Some carbohydrate-addicted kids simply have no interest in foods that are not carbohydrate-rich. It may seem that these youngsters are simply being difficult or that they are "spoiled." More likely, their cravings are a sign of a physical imbalance. Other youngsters may use carbo-rich foods as their staple and add to them all the other foods they can gather and eat.

Signs and Symptoms

Carbohydrate-addicted parents of carbohydrate-addicted children and teens may understand why their children are "always hungry," "never seem to get enough," or "won't eat anything but junk food." Nonaddicted parents, on the other hand, may hold the silent belief that if the youngster really wanted to, he or she could "use a little willpower."

**Intense and recurrent cravings are themselves
signs that a physical imbalance may exist
and must be corrected.**

It is essential for carbohydrate-addicted and nonaddicted parents alike to understand that the craving for carbohydrate-rich foods is simply a sign, a signal that a physical imbalance exists and must be corrected.

Correcting this imbalance does *not* require eliminating the foods your youngster loves; it simply entails changing the way in which a child or teen takes in these foods, learning how to time the consumption of carbohydrate-rich foods and combine them with protein-rich and fiber-rich insulin-balancing foods. In this way, insulin levels are brought into balance, blood sugar levels are stabilized, and your youngster's carbohydrate-craving cycle can be broken without deprivation or denial.

CARBOHYDRATE ADDICTION: SIGNS AND SYMPTOMS

How many of these signs and symptoms describe your youngster?
- A focus on starchy foods, junk food, snack foods, or sweets (often to the exclusion of other foods).
- A desire to snack rather than eat whole, balanced meals.
- Swings in energy levels, moods, ability to concentrate, or motivation.
- Unexplained outbursts of anger or periods of withdrawal.
- Heightened emotionality, including sensitivity, crying, insecurity, or clinging.
- Weight problems or incidents of uncontrollable eating.

While there may be many reasons for one of these signs or symptoms, the youngster who displays two or more may well be suffering from an addiction to carbohydrates.

Carbohydrate-Addicted Kids Are Different

Though most parents are unaware of the research, scientific studies show that carbohydrate-addicted kids differ from their nonaddicted counterparts. The bodies of carbohydrate-addicted kids respond differently to the foods they eat, how often they eat them, and the nutritional balance of their meals. Their cravings, behavior, feelings, abilities, attitudes, weight, health, even their personalities, reflect differences that are related to differences in body chemistry.

Scientists have known about these differences for decades. Food addiction was first reported in the scientific literature in 1947, and carbohydrate addiction was described over thirty years ago! Although each year hundreds of research articles explore the underlying processes that contribute to the carbohydrate addiction cycle, it was not until recently that the physical cause for this imbalance was described in two articles we wrote in the journal *Medical Hypothesis*.

Before we discuss the cause of this imbalance, however, let's take a look at what it feels like to the youngster who is living within its clutches.

A Fighting Chance:
Jennifer's Story, Part 1

It was Saturday morning, and, though the research area of the hospital was pretty much closed, we had come in to catch up on paperwork. When the phone rang, we picked it up and heard a voice far more mature than that which we would usually associate with a fourteen-year-old girl.

"My name is Jennifer Payne,"[2] she began. "I am fourteen and a half and I would like to be part of your program." Before we could respond, she continued, "Do my parents have to come?"

We explained that, in addition to needing their consent, we preferred to have parents take part in the program and added that we required physician's approval as well. We asked Jennifer if having her parents come to see us with her presented a problem.

"I don't know," she said softly. "I'd rather just do it myself." After a moment of silence we heard someone call to her. Jennifer's manner changed.

Her voice became formal and loud. "Well, you know, I was just checking it out. It's not really for me. Thanks anyway. Bye."

Before we could respond, Jennifer hung up.

Two days later Jennifer's mother called and asked to speak to us directly. Like Jennifer, she got right to the point.

"Earlier in the week my daughter called to find out about your research program. I wonder if you could tell me a little about it and how we can join."

It had been a long two days for Jennifer and her family. Her mother, herself a carbohydrate addict, had for quite a while suspected that something was bothering her daughter.

---

[2]In all cases, names and identifying details have been changed.

After some prodding, she had convinced Jennifer to talk to her but, when they approached Jennifer's father, they "hit a brick wall."

"He doesn't want to hear it," her mother explained. "He says that it's my fault, that I overfeed her. He says that all she needs to do is to control herself. But I know she has a real problem. I have the same problem, and I don't want her to end up like me."

Jennifer's mother didn't offer any other details over the phone, and we decided to wait until we saw both mother and daughter in person before we delved any deeper.

The fourteen-year-old who entered the office two weeks later was clad in the biggest T-shirt we had ever seen. The shirt hung loosely, making it difficult to judge her weight (which we were pretty sure was her intention). On her hands, dimples marked the spots where knuckles would normally be and her round face indicated that there were a number of unwanted pounds hidden beneath her outfit.

Jennifer's mother was a short, pretty woman, about thirty-seven or thirty-eight, with dark curly hair and a wonderful smile. Except for the gray strands in her hair, she could almost have passed for Jennifer's older sister. Jennifer's mother carried approximately sixty extra pounds and seemed somewhat uncomfortable with her appearance. They both sat down in the office.

Jennifer's long dark hair hung half in her face, and she looked down at her hands when she spoke. Her voice was much quieter and less composed than it had been when she talked to us on the phone.

We asked what had brought her to the program. Her mother waited for her daughter to answer.

"You helped Ann Marie," Jennifer blurted out, "but when I followed the diet it didn't work for me. I did everything she did. I tried to follow it exactly but I don't know . . ." Her voice trailed off.

Ann Marie, Jennifer's friend, had been part of our research program for several months. Her carbohydrate cravings gone, she had lost fifteen pounds in less than three months and emerged like the proverbial butterfly.

We explained that each youngster was different and that following Ann Marie's program was as inappropriate. as trying to wear her eyeglasses.

"She said that," Jennifer admitted. "But I didn't believe her. I figured she was just trying to keep it for herself. But I had to try something and I guess I just didn't think my father would let me come."

Jennifer's mother's face softened. "I don't like to talk about him but he's just impossible," she said. We assumed she meant her husband. "He won't understand that she, we both, have a problem. It's not like we don't try. He thinks it's just a matter of willpower. It's not that he objects to her coming, he just thinks it's a waste of time. He thinks she would just lose weight if she really wanted to. I wish you would talk to him."

We explained that we would rather work on helping Jennifer as much as we could and let her father see the results as they emerged. Our experience had proven that success was the best persuader of all.

They agreed. With the thought of success alive in the room, Jennifer's manner changed. She sat up and began to talk about her feelings in relation to her weight and her food cravings. Her mother later told us that she learned things in that hour that she had never known about her daughter.

"It's not that I'm *fat* fat," Jennifer began. "I can still wear regular clothes and my legs aren't bad, so I look all right in shorts but my stomach sticks out and I'm . . ." Jennifer shrugged.

"You're just not as slim as you'd like?" we suggested.

"Exactly. Not like Anna, my best friend. Or even Ann Marie now."

"What does your doctor say?"

Jennifer's mother joined in. "He says that he's not happy with her weight. It's not that it will do her any real harm at the moment, he tells us, although with boys and everything . . ." Her voiced trailed off, then she continued, "But he's concerned about her health and how much weight she'll put on in the future. He's also worried by the fact that she never exercises. She tries to get out of gym whenever she can. It's the only trouble she's ever been in at school; she has absolutely no interest in sports. He would like to see her lose twenty, even twenty-five pounds. He says that she's been gaining slowly over the years and it's not good for her."

"What do you think?" we asked her mother.

"I think she's just like me. And I worry about her. I was okay until I became pregnant with her, then I gained about forty pounds. It's been uphill ever since. Now she's started gaining weight earlier than I did and I'm . . . worried.

"I know it's not her fault," her mother continued. "She eats like I do. She'll start off the day trying to 'be good,' she'll hold on for a while and try to control herself. I see her fighting to stay away from the junk food from the time she gets home from school but most of the time it's like something inside just breaks loose. If she had her way, she would do nothing but eat, sleep, talk on the phone, and watch TV. A part of me says she still needs to use more willpower and then I see what it's like for her. You can see how bad she feels but she just can't seem to control herself. I know, I'm the same way."

We turned to Jennifer. "Let's assume for a moment that you are carbohydrate-addicted and that your body pushes you to want the breads and the pasta, the snack food and junk food and sweets. How would things be different if you didn't feel like you wanted them so much or so often?"

"I don't know. It would just be so much easier. I could do my homework without thinking about eating all the time, or counting the hours until dinner, or feeling like I failed again, eating stuff I didn't want to. I wouldn't feel like I let myself down all the time. I got an A+ on my report on cholesterol in health class. I know what all that junk does to your body. I just don't know why I can't control myself."

Jennifer continued, "It's not like I don't try to control myself but I get so hungry. Ann Marie said she's not hungry anymore—not like she was before. If I could feel like that I would have, you know, a fighting chance. Now I just feel like I can never win." Her face clouded and some of the misery of her self-blame showed through.

"What else?" we asked, wanting to help her voice her frustration, as well as her hopes.

"If I were thin, I would be able to wear clothes that fit tight around here." She pointed toward her waist. "My mother says

I'm always hiding my body but when I put the clothes on that she picks out, I look like a pig." She stopped, her eyes filled with tears.

We asked for more specifics about Jennifer's eating habits and dieting history. We found that she had been hiding more than her figure. From her friends, she had been hiding her compulsion to eat. She had kept food hidden in her schoolbag, eating in the girls' bathroom stall. She admitted that she would often pass on chances to go over to friends' houses after school because she would have to abstain while she watched them snack or, if she gave in and enjoyed the food with them, she would be teased about not being able to stick to her diet. From her parents, she had been hiding her inability to control her eating, or so she thought; sneaking bits of food from the refrigerator and buying candy and cookies with her allowance or money she had borrowed from friends or earned by baby-sitting.

The impact of Jennifer's carbohydrate addiction was spreading; she had developed a secret world of eating and was learning to lie and isolate herself to protect that world. She had never told her mother about the cruel remarks or teasing she got from friends. She was too ashamed.

Like so many of our teens, Jennifer had already experimented with several diet regimens. "I tried calorie counting but that didn't last long. Then I went to Weight Watchers with my mother and after that to Jenny Craig, but I gained weight on them both! It's true. Ask my mother. And I really stuck to it. That exchange thing didn't work and I hated the food they gave you. I couldn't eat at school or go out with my friends for pizza. Even though they say it is, it just isn't made for a kid.

"And," she added, "I was still hungry all the time."

Jennifer admitted that she had tried over-the-counter diet pills without her parents' knowledge or consent. "Some of the kids at school got hold of them and I thought pills might help. They made me very nervous. I couldn't sleep, I hated the feeling. Some of the kids have even heavier stuff but I was afraid to take it."

Jennifer's eyes filled with tears. "I don't know what to do. I've tried everything and nothing works. I'm hungry all the time, and if somebody doesn't do something, I'm going to end up, you know, really fat."

We asked Jennifer's mother to give us more information about Jennifer by taking The Carbohydrate Addiction Quiz for Parents of Children and Teens. (You can take it too when you read Chapter 4.) We invited Jennifer to take the test as well. Their results were very similar, although Jennifer's answers revealed that her cravings were more powerful than her mother had ever suspected. The results confirmed our suspicions: Jennifer was indeed a carbohydrate addict, and a candidate for the program.

In easy-to-understand terms, we explained the scientific basis of Jennifer's addiction. We reiterated that the cravings were neither Jennifer's fault nor her mother's, and that, in combination, the changes that Jennifer would make in the weeks to come would help reduce or eliminate her cravings.

"Imagine that you were allergic to a particular food, let's say strawberries for instance, and that you broke out in hives whenever you ate them," we explained. "The hives would be a way that your body has of telling you that it didn't like the strawberries, that it couldn't handle them well. Now let's say you didn't want to avoid eating strawberries or that you needed them for good health, and then, let's suppose, you found that there was a special way of eating them that would make your body react to strawberries just like everyone else did."

We explained that in the same way, Jennifer's cravings and weight gain were her body's way of saying it could not handle the carbohydrates she was eating, in the way she was eating them. Jennifer did not have to avoid these foods, we added, if she simply ate them in a different way, a way that could correct her body's response to them.

"The changes you will be making on this program will help your body respond differently, more appropriately, to the carbohydrates you eat without requiring you to reduce the amount of carbohydrates you enjoy each day.

"When your body responds normally, the cravings—and the weight—fall away naturally," we added, then we turned to the Program that would help bring balance back to her body and her life.

You will learn more about Jennifer in the chapters to come, but for now, it is important to understand that Jennifer is not alone in her difficulties. She is just one of millions of youngsters who struggle with their cravings and their weight, who suffer the health, social, and self-esteem problems that often go along with being overweight, and whose parents may find themselves caught somewhere between frustration and powerlessness. It is a difficult situation for everyone involved . . . and it is getting worse.

In Chapter 5 you will learn more about the growing epidemic of juvenile weight problems, the cause, and, most importantly, what can be done to stop it. But weight gain is only one of the many ways in which carbohydrate addiction can wreak havoc in our youngsters' lives.

Alex in Charge:
A Special Story, Part 1

The eight-year-old boy who sat before us was slender and sinewy. There didn't appear to be an ounce of fat on his wiry body. Clad in big sneakers that didn't reach the floor and fashionably baggy pants, he sat silently and kept his eyes fixed on his swinging feet. Occasionally he sneaked a furtive glance at his parents, then looked down and silently waited for the unknown to unfold.

His vulnerability touched us and we tried to make him welcome. With each of our attempts, however, he seemed to retreat even more. When our greetings to Alex[3] met with no response, his mother began.

"We don't know if we're in the right place but we're not sure where else to go." She paused, then continued. "It's not like there are places or clinics we know of . . ." Her voice trailed off.

"We're not even sure if there *is* a problem or not," his father continued.

"I mean, 'addiction' is a really strong word, and I'm not sure that's how we would describe what's going on. I mean,

---

[3]In all cases, names and identifying details have been changed.

Alex eats only junk food like my wife says, but I'm not sure that it's not something he'll just grow out of."

"Alex was adopted," his mother explained, "and he's always been incredibly active. We got him first as a foster child, then we legally adopted him two years later. He was almost a year old when we first got him, but from the time he was able to walk, I swear he never sat down. I don't think I've ever seen him walk; it's as if he only knows how to run. As a toddler he would fall a hundred times a day but he'd get up and start running again. We could hardly ever get him to take a nap; he would just keep going until he collapsed. Then he would sleep like he was dead and wake up and start all over again."

"He doesn't stay with anything. He starts to play with something, then ten seconds later he's picking up something else. You sometimes get the feeling he doesn't even focus on things that are right in front of him. We've worked hard with him and he somehow is managing to sit still in class but just barely, and he hates it. His grades have never been great, he has a real problem with reading," Alex's father added. "It's not like he doesn't try, it's just really hard for him."

His mother leaned forward. "He's a wonderful artist," she added emphatically, "and he loves sports. I sometimes think if we had enough money to put him into private school . . ." His mother's face mirrored her pain and feelings of guilt.

"Anyway," his father continued a bit roughly, "last month we got a call from school that they wanted to test him and see if he had an attention deficit problem or some other problem."

"We weren't sure what to do," Alex's mother continued. "They haven't finished testing him yet and though we didn't want him labeled as having a psychological or learning problem that could follow him for the rest of his life, he really does have a very hard time concentrating. The problem is, in order to get the special help that he needs, they have to test him. We didn't know what else to do."

Alex's father shook his head. "The thing that got us concerned is when they began talking about putting him on medication for some kind of an attention disorder. They're still testing him but they told us that's what they're thinking of doing. We really don't want him to have to take drugs unless it's absolutely necessary. He's so young and . . . "

Alex's legs stopped swinging and he seemed even quieter. It seemed that tears might be welling up in his eyes. We generally tried to include kids in all consultations so that they did not feel that they were being left out or that decisions were being made without their input. In this case, Alex was not participating and seemed very uncomfortable. We tried again to speak directly to him but he remained distant and withdrawn.

Alex's mother picked up where her husband had stopped. "We've noticed that sometimes Alex is more in control than others. I mean, sometimes it seems like he just can't focus on anything, he runs from one thing to another, nonstop. Sometimes he'll lash out and yell at us or kick or throw things; it's like he simply has no control. At other times, though, he's much better.

"We have tried to figure out what makes the problem worse but we aren't sure. Sometimes we think that all the junk food and candy or soda he's been having is making him act out but he can get as hyper after he's been eating just plain fruit or noncaffeine diet soda, so we can't figure it out."

Alex's mother had a wonderful face, sweet and sensitive, but, as she described the episodes with her son, her features clouded over. Her husband, tall and square-jawed, sat across the room and his wide shoulders slumped as he, too, disclosed the concern and frustration they were experiencing. Alex continued to hang his head, and we thought he might be crying. This family was indeed in pain, and, though each wanted things to be better, clearly no one knew what to do.

We asked Alex's mother and father to describe a typical day's eating in the life of their son, from the time he awakened to the time he fell asleep. The list contained virtually nothing but carbohydrate-rich foods.

"He simply won't eat anything else," Alex's father explained. "The doctor said not to worry, but I think he was talking about Alex's weight, which is fine. I don't think his doctor really understands that although Alex doesn't eat a lot, that's *all* he eats—just junk food and sugary stuff. Occasionally he'll eat a sandwich or fruit but mainly it's junk, junk, and more junk."

We asked Alex's parents if there was any pattern to their son's mood swings or attention problems or what some might consider hyperactivity. They offered two important observations.

"He seems much better when he first gets up in the morning," Alex's mother explained. "I'm not sure if it's because he's rested or what but he seems much calmer, more centered, and less all-over-the-place when he wakes up. He sits down at the table in the morning and he's able to eat and talk to us. After that, for the rest of the day, he doesn't stop."

"And he seems to get worse as the day goes on," his father added.

"Yes, by the afternoon, he's impossible." She glanced guiltily down at her son and reworded her thoughts. "Whatever it is, by the time he gets home from school, he's . . . it's really hard for him to control himself. He's into everything, inside the house or out. There's almost no day that goes by without him hurting himself. I was supposed to take the first year off to be with Alex. Then we figured I would go back to work and put him in day care or leave him with my mother. But I still can't go back to work full-time. My mother can't handle him and when he gets older, I'm afraid of what will happen if I'm not there when he comes back from school . . ." Her words trailed off once again.

There was a great deal of pain, frustration, and worry in what Alex's parents reported but, in addition, there were the two key signs we were waiting to hear. In combination with an intensely carbohydrate-slanted diet, the fact that Alex seemed less hyperactive before eating his first meal of the day and the fact that he became more overly active, less able to concentrate, and more likely to experience mood swings as the day went on suggested a strong possible link between Alex's difficulties and a low blood sugar problem.

First, we corrected Alex's parents' assumption that "healthy" or "diet" foods, like fruit and diet soda, would not trigger blood sugar plunges, explaining that anything that tastes sweet—naturally sweet, sugar-sweetened, or sweetened with sugar substitutes—is likely to release insulin, and the more often these foods were eaten without the balance of other, stabilizing foods, the more likely their consumption would be followed by blood sugar swings.

We asked them to take The Carbohydrate Addict's Quiz for Parents of Children and Teens, and their answers, independently, confirmed that Alex was a moderate carbohydrate addict. Only Alex's weight and the lack of a family history based on his biological parents kept him from falling into the strong addiction category. But while his parents were taking the quiz an interesting situation developed.

Until that time, Alex had not eaten anything since rising in the morning. His parents had left the house in a hurry that morning, and when Alex refused any breakfast, his parents had not fought his resistance. Now it was eleven A.M. and Alex said that he was hungry. The only foods immediately available were those located in a nearby vending area—fruit juices, cookies, candy, and similar snack foods. Alex asked for orange juice and two boxes of plain raisins; what would normally be viewed as a "good healthy snack." But not for Alex.

Within a short time, a dramatic change came over him. He fidgeted without stop and his leg swinging became more intense and bordered on becoming destructive kicking. He rose and began exploring the room, first silently picking things up and putting them down. We offered drawing materials, and though he accepted, he moved from page to page making only a few meaningless marks on each page, then turning to another. His mother called to him, trying in vain to direct his behavior. Her words seemed to chase him around the room but he was faster than the speed of sound. When he did pause momentarily, her attempts to verbally catch his attention fell on deaf ears. He seemed absolutely impervious to any outside influence. Only physical contact, his father's hand placed strongly on his arm, brought any eye contact between Alex and his parents.

After a while Alex seemed to wind down and what had been solitary agitation turned into a demand for attention. Now Alex whined and goaded one parent, then the other. He seemed intent on soliciting any kind of reaction, positive or negative.

"That's what it's like," his mother blurted out. "Either he's off and running, oblivious to us, or he just won't leave us alone. It's always an extreme; one way or another," she added, disentangling herself from his probing fingers on her face. "It sometimes feels like he's tormenting me. I can't help it, it just does . . ." She began to cry openly.

We understood. We had seen it many times before. The situation was painful and frustrating for the youngster and the parents alike. Everyone involved felt alternately angry, helpless, or misunderstood, and then guilty. We also knew that a change in diet that could stabilize Alex's blood sugar levels might well bring some surprising results for everyone involved.

In the chapters to come we will tell you more about Alex, his challenges, and his most treasured victory, but for now, it is important to keep in mind that although a youngster's difficulties may not be measured in pounds or inches, that child, too, may be one of millions of youngsters who struggle with the powerful effects of an addiction to carbohydrates.

three

What Causes Carbohydrate Addiction?

A parent is usually the first to know. Although scientists have devised elaborate ways to measure the physical imbalance that leads to an addiction to carbohydrates, in most cases it is the parent who is first to recognize the powerful cravings that drive the carbohydrate-addicted youngster. Long before the physician ever makes more than a casual comment about a child's weight or growth or nutrition, long before learning, behavioral, or mood difficulties begin to surface, it is often the parent who has tried, usually in vain, to bring balance and good nutrition to a youngster's eating.

> **Although parents are usually the first to identify
> the problem, they may feel powerless
> to do anything about it.**

All too often, parents live with the concern that their youngsters may be doing harm to their health, well-being, and happiness, yet parents may find, at the same time, that they are all but powerless to help their children. While carbohydrate addiction is often easily recognized by those who live with it, scientists and physicians require specific measurements with which to define, diagnose, and treat this all-too-prevalent problem.

The Science Behind the Addiction

From conferences at Harvard's Medical School to respected textbooks in the field, food addiction has been classified as a "true" addiction in keeping with the rigorous criteria set by the World Health Organization and the American Psychiatric Association. In 1994, in an article we authored in the journal *Medical Hypotheses,* carbohydrate addiction itself was shown to fit the classification of a "true" addiction by these same criteria.

> **Carbohydrate addiction was first described in the medical literature over three decades ago.**

Though many may act as if this were a new or radical idea, in scientific terms the concept is far from new. Researchers have been exploring the cause and treatment of food addiction since 1947 and have been examining and writing about carbohydrate addiction since 1963. Yet, until recently, no effective treatment for the problem, no real help, has been available.

Fortunately, over the last ten years or so, a proliferation of scientific findings in the field has enhanced and widened our level of understanding. A review of the guide that scientists have used to conduct research for decades, *Index Medicus,* along with a review of the nation's top medical computer search programs, reveal that in the past two years over two thousand research articles have appeared in which a variety of aspects of the processes involved in carbohydrate addiction have been examined. Moreover, fortunately for our youngsters, much of the research specifically focuses on the impact that these processes have on children and adolescents.

Reports in the *New England Journal of Medicine,* the *Lancet,* the *Journal of Clinical Investigation,* and other respected medical journals conclude that:

- A key to understanding the cause of carbohydrate cravings, excess weight gain, and low blood sugar swings in young-sters and adults alike appears to be an imbalance in the hormone insulin.
- An increased risk for many of this country's top killer dis-eases and health risk factors, including undesirable blood pressure and blood fat levels, heart disease and circulation problems, stroke, and adult-onset diabetes, all appear to have their origins in childhood and adolescence and emerge in early or middle adulthood as a result of an often-undiagnosed insulin imbalance.
- Many of the mood, attitude, behavioral, and learning prob-lems that so frequently plague our children and teens may be tied, in whole or in part, to the low blood sugar levels that likewise are linked to these insulin imbalances.

Even the former Surgeon General, Dr. C. Everett Koop, in his *Surgeon General's Report on Nutrition and Health,* points to the fact that insulin is a hormone that "modifies energy balance and may contribute to obesity." He goes on to add that excess levels of insulin and the body's resistance to insulin "can occur in all types of obesity and may be a link between high blood pressure, obe-sity, and the body's inability to handle carbohydrates."[1]

The scientific name for this imbalance in body chemistry (specifically in terms of insulin levels) that leads to an addiction to carbohydrates is hyperinsulinemia (meaning too much insulin). This physical imbalance often goes undiagnosed, espe-cially in children and teens, and when it remains uncorrected it can lead to the intense or recurring carbohydrate cravings that give carbohydrate addiction its name, as well as to the mood, behavioral, and learning difficulties, health problems, and weight gain that often go along with it.

In general, children and teens (as well as adults) who intensely crave carbohydrate-rich foods are *not* responding to some sort of character flaw, overindulgence, or set of emotional or family problems, but rather are simply exhibiting the early

---

[1]Medical terminology within or outside quoted statements are translated for ease of comprehension.

signs of this imbalance in their body's chemistry. This excess of insulin is brought on and made worse by how they are eating the very foods they crave. Though this insulin imbalance appears to be genetic in origin, in the pages to come you will learn that there is much that can be done to halt its powerful impact.

When All Goes As It Should— and When It Does Not

To understand how carbohydrate addiction can overpower your youngster, compare the ways in which the hormone insulin works in the normal (nonaddicted) youngster versus your carbohydrate-addicted child or teen.

When the *nonaddicted* youngster consumes carbohydrate-rich foods, the body releases insulin. Insulin, which has been called the "hunger hormone," stimulates the youngster to continue eating. Simple carbohydrates in the meal or snack (such as the sugars found in candy, cookies, cake, fruit, and juice) are quickly changed into blood sugar. Insulin then ushers some of this newly made blood sugar to muscles and organs (including the brain and the rest of the nervous system), where the blood sugar provides much-needed energy.

Insulin acts like a "doorman," opening the "doors" (or *sites*) to many kinds of cells so that energy, in the form of blood sugar, can enter and fuel their activities. With that job completed, in the nonaddicted youngster, insulin signals the liver to put some of the remaining blood sugar into short-term storage for quick energy. Any extra energy that still remains is turned into fat and put into long-term storage in the fat cells. Blood sugar depends on insulin to open cell "doors" and help maintain an ideal balance between blood sugar available to cells for immediate use, and blood sugar stored away for future use.

In the *nonaddicted* youngster, just the right amount of insulin is released and insulin levels remain in balance, ushering just enough blood sugar into the cells that need it. Over time, as blood sugar levels slowly decrease or when the demands of activity or other stresses signal the need for more energy, the liver's energy reserves—along with the continuing digestion of proteins and fats, the breakdown of complex carbohydrates, and energy released from the fat cells—will continue to fuel the body for many more hours.

**When nonaddicted youngsters eat carbo-rich food,
their blood sugar levels remain balanced.**

When *nonaddicted* youngsters eat a carbohydrate-rich meal, the brain chemical serotonin is released, and with it a "stop eating" signal is given. Upon finishing the meal, nonaddicted youngsters feel satisfied and complete, and will remain so for several hours.

In the carbohydrate-addicted youngster, however, things can go wrong. When carbohydrate-addicted children and teens eat junk food, snack food, or sweets, their sensitive bodies can overreact and overrelease insulin. Excess insulin levels can throw off the vital blood sugar balance; cells may be inundated with an unneeded excess of blood sugar or left starving for their critical share of food energy, or, alternately, first one then the other.

**The overrelease of insulin sets up a series of
inappropriate (abnormal) physical responses in a child
or teen that can lead to many physical,
psychological, and behavioral problems.**

In carbohydrate-addicted youngsters, the excess insulin that is released can sweep too much blood sugar out of the bloodstream, too quickly. *Where* the excess blood sugar is channeled will help determine what next happens to the youngster.

If the muscles and organs allow insulin and blood sugar to enter, they enter quickly, and blood sugar levels may plummet. Sensing low blood sugar levels, the body may release a second hormone, adrenaline. Adrenaline might be referred to as the "excitement" hormone because it can bring about what is called the "fight or flight" response. In prehistoric times this release of adrenaline and the response it can cause probably gave "cavekids" an extra chance at survival by providing them with a burst of energy to keep on going to secure food. Today many carbohydrate-addicted kids, responding to this release of adrenaline, may be viewed as frenzied, unfocused, hyperactive. We call these youngsters Carbo Burners because their bodies tend to quickly burn, rather than store, the carbohydrates they have just taken in.

Other carbohydrate-addicted youngsters' bodies, however, respond in a different way to the high level of insulin their bodies release. In these youngsters, organ and muscle cells close down (*down regulate*), probably as a way of protecting themselves against what we call an "insulin insult" (damage from excess levels of the hormone). In an attempt to protect themselves, the "doors" to these cells, through which insulin and sugar would normally enter, now literally disappear for the time being. The cells, and the youngsters as well, are said to have become "insulin resistant."

Blood sugar, unable to enter these cells and no longer able to be burned as fuel, must now be channeled elsewhere, for storage. The bodies of these youngsters provide the most expandable of storage facilities, the fat cells. In time, these young carbo addicts are almost bound to gain weight, while at the same time their muscles and nervous systems (and other organs) may be starving for the very food energy that is being channeled into storage. We call these youngsters Carbo Collectors, for their young bodies seem intent on saving, rather than spending, the food energy they take in.

But whether they are Carbo Burners or Carbo Collectors, most carbohydrate-addicted youngsters fail to achieve a feeling of simple satisfaction that nonaddicted youngsters experience after the completion of a meal. Though there is still some speculation as to the exact physical mechanism responsible, it appears that the excessively high insulin levels these youngsters release interfere with an appropriate rise in the neurotransmitter serotonin—the brain chemical that should make them feel satisfied after eating.

> **Not enough serotonin means
> no "stop eating" message from the brain.**

Not enough serotonin means no "stop eating" message from the brain. At the same time, some of the excess insulin that remains in their bloodstream continues to signal carbohydrate addicts to keep on eating. These youngsters will seek the very foods that would make nonaddicted youngsters feel satisfied, but for carbohydrate addicts, these foods simply put them on the insulin merry-go-round once again.

Within an hour or two after eating, many carbohydrate addicts show some of the telltale signs of low blood sugar, reactive hypoglycemia,[2] including recurring cravings, tiredness, inability to concentrate, confusion, disorientation, demotivation, mood swings, headache, or irritability.

Whether blood sugar levels have dropped from heightened activity or from being stored in the fat cells, low levels of blood sugar will also push your youngster to seek out carbohydrate-rich food once again.

> **When carbohydrate-addicted youngsters eat carbo-rich
> foods, their blood sugar levels may spike then drop—
> changes in their behavior, moods, and cravings
> may simply reflect their bodies' imbalance.**

Though Carbo Collectors are most often overweight and Carbo Burners are normal-weight or underweight, the distinctions are not always clear-cut. Each youngster is unique, with his or her own special body, a body in need of help and balance. So whether your youngster is a Burner, a Collector, or a bit of both, understand that you and your youngster are facing a problem of balance, not one of discipline or blame.

---

[2]For a more detailed discussion of hypoglycemia, see page 118.

A New Perspective

A parent watching a youngster's renewed cravings may protest, "You can't be hungry again! You just ate!" or may feel helpless when a child or teen refuses to eat anything except junk food or sweets. It is vital to remember, however, that within only two hours after eating, low blood sugar levels and high insulin levels may indeed be sending your youngster a message that he or she is "starving" for a quick sugar "fix."

If it feels as if the more junk food your youngster eats, the more he or she wants, you may not be wrong. Scientists have documented the eating-craving-eating-craving cycle that so many carbohydrate-addicted youngsters (and adults) experience. Many of these scientists conclude, as did Dr. Paula J. Geiselman and Dr. Donald Novin in the scientific journal *Appetite*, that an excess in the release of insulin brings on low blood sugar levels that are, in turn, part of a "sequence of responses" that lead to hunger and "sugar-induced" overeating.

In the carbohydrate-addicted youngster, exercise and strenuous activity can also intensify low blood sugar swings. In an attempt to refuel before or after physical exertion, the carbohydrate-addicted youngster who is active in sports may crave great quantities of dense carbohydrates (sugar-loaded snacks, sweet drinks, fruit juice, and junk food, in particular). These intense and often undeniable cravings are easily understood once you comprehend the way your youngster's body handles, and mishandles, food.

It is important that parents are aware that the false sweetness of artificially sweetened drinks and foods may likewise trigger the same carbohydrate cravings and low blood sugar swings as do "real" carbohydrate-rich foods. In this case, the body is not responding to the "reality" of sugar but rather to the perception of sweet taste. It releases excess insulin but, in this case, the artificially sweetened food contains no carbohydrates for conversion into blood sugar. The insulin, looking for blood sugar to move into cells, will most likely usher what little blood sugar is present in the bloodstream to the muscles and organs or fat cells that will accept it. Again, blood sugar levels drop and youngsters may move into a hypoglycemic (low blood sugar) state. While the artificially sweetened food or drink may "hit the spot" at first, within a short period of time, youngsters will be reaching for more of the same or for some snack food, junk food or sweets.

To make matters worse, *some* carbohydrate-addicted youngsters respond to artificially sweetened foods and drinks and sugar-sweetened foods and drinks in similar ways. This may cause parents (and doctors and scientists) to question whether their cravings and behavior problems are "really" sugar-related. When we recommend that parents stop focusing on what is in the food but rather what the food (or drink) does when it is in their youngster's body, many find the similarity of the effects of carbohydrate-rich foods and those containing artificial sweeteners easier to see.

**Remember that excess levels of insulin
affect far more than just hunger or weight
in the carbohydrate-addicted child or teen.**

Remember: Excess levels of insulin affect far more than just hunger or weight in the carbohydrate-addicted kid. Any parent, witnessing the inexplicable lack of motivation or unpredictable moods that are the earmark of the low blood sugar levels, may wonder, "What's the matter with you? How can you be tired? You haven't done anything!" But no youngster can explain that even though he or she may be eating plenty of food, the body is simply not getting the food energy that it needs.

Mood swings are rampant and may be unpredictable. "It's like living with Dr. Jekyll and Mr. Hyde," some parents tell us. "I never know who is going to emerge from the bedroom." Little do they realize that they are describing a classic sign of low blood sugar swings.

**For many kids, lack of attention or motivation,
learning problems, and mood swings
are powerful, vital signs of low blood sugar levels.**

In recent years society has come to accept laziness, moodiness, and lack of motivation as generally acceptable behaviors in many children and most teens. We, who have experienced the problems firsthand, totally disagree. Lack of attention and lack of motivation as well as learning problems and mood swings may be powerful, vital signs of low blood sugar swings.

These symptoms may be, in reality, calls for help that parents need to recognize and understand, and to which they *must* respond. Just as you would not tolerate an unexplained fever, infection, or any other physical disorder that might keep your child from being productive, happy, and healthy, it is important to consider a new perspective—one that calls into account a physical cause—when you are confronted with your child's mood swings, lack of motivation, or learning difficulties.

High Carbo, High Impact: Scientists Document the Diet-Behavior Connection

Each year scientists document new aspects of the impact carbohydrates may have on our children. Dr. B. Spring and her colleagues noted in the *Journal of Clinical Psychiatry* that "Behavioral change after intake of carbohydrate-rich foods has been documented . . . "; "Fatigue and impaired performance on tests of concentration and speed occur approximately 2 hours after carbohydrate consumption." In children and teens, especially those who are carbo-addicted, we, too, have found that blood sugar highs hit much sooner than two hours, and swings to low blood sugar levels (hypoglycemia) can occur far more quickly as well.

In their research published in the medical journal *Circulation*, scientists such as Drs. Weihang, Srinivasan, and Berenson, after observing children and teens for more than a decade, have documented that in many youngsters, particularly those with high insulin levels, high-sugar meals overly excite the nervous system through the overrelease of adrenaline. In the end, whether through low blood sugar levels or activation of the "fight or flight" response, problems in attention, behavior, and mood are almost bound to occur.

Other scientists have documented that high levels of insulin and, in turn, low blood sugar levels, in the bloodstream can lead to anxiety or irritability. These low blood sugar levels can lead to a feeling of discomfort that propels the child or teen to reach for more and more food. Many of these youngsters, like their adult counterparts, crave carbos even when they are not hungry, as a way of staving off unpleasant feelings related to blood sugar swings. In a sense, their cravings are a type of withdrawal feeling, an experience youngsters soon learn they can stop temporarily with a high-carbohydrate "fix."

It is not hard to imagine the anxious youngster reaching for goodies to feel better. Like a shipwrecked person growing increasingly thirsty and trying to quell the desire to drink by swallowing more and more salty sea water, the carbohydrate-addicted youngster returns again and again to the carbohydrate-rich foods that are the source of hyperactivity and irritability, anxiety, and discomfort.

And the more often carbohydrate-addicted youngsters eat the very foods they crave most, and the less these foods are balanced by protein-rich and high-fiber foods, the greater their insulin imbalance grows—leading to even more intense or more frequent cravings. From a practical standpoint, carbohydrate addiction literally feeds itself. The more carbos are eaten, the more they are craved. The more they are craved, the more they are eaten. (See pages 72–73 for information on the power of timing and combining.)

Carbohydrate addiction literally feeds itself.

So whether your youngster is overweight or normal-weight, whether mood, attitude, behavioral, or learning problems are impacting on your child's life (and yours), the scientific findings point to the same physical culprit—excess levels of insulin—and the carbohydrate craving cycle that keeps kids addicted.

When the powerful physical impact of carbohydrate addiction is seen in its entirety, it is easy to understand why parents' pleas, reprimands, and warnings have little effect on breaking a youngster's carbohydrate connection, for only when the basic cause—the insulin imbalance itself—is corrected can the carbohydrate addiction cycle be broken.

IT'S NOT WHAT'S EATING YOUR KID, IT'S WHAT YOUR KID IS EATING!

THE INSULIN-CARBOHYDRATE CONNECTION

WHEN A NON-ADDICTED YOUNGSTER EATS CARBOHYDRATE-RICH FOODS*:

An appropriate amount of insulin is released.

Insulin takes blood sugar to muscles, brain, and other organs and liver for short-term storage. Any excess blood sugar is stored in fat cells.

Appropriate amount of blood sugar remains. Child feels fueled and pleasantly energized.

Serotonin levels rise appropriately; youngster feels satisfied and complete.

Two hours later:
As blood sugar levels naturally decline, liver and fat cells give up their energy to continue to fuel youngster's body, or youngster desires any of a wide variety of foods.

With each repeat of cycle, youngster receives experience of satisfaction and body is nourished.

*Based on frequent consumption of carbohydrate-rich foods, particularly those that are high in simple sugars, particularly without appropriate balance of high-fiber and protein-rich foods.

Biological processes are simplified for ease of comprehension. Children differ and may show differences in processes and symptoms.

WHEN A CARBO-ADDICTED YOUNGSTER EATS CARBOHYDRATE-RICH FOODS*:

Excess insulin is released.

Insulin *tries* to bring food energy (blood sugar) to muscles, brain, etc.
In "Carbo Burners" excess insulin makes blood sugar drop too quickly. Adrenalin may be released, causing hyperactivity or mood swings.
In "Carbo Collectors" muscle and organ cells become insulin resistant and a large proportion of blood sugar may be channeled into fat cells (child gains weight).

Too little of blood sugar remains and some youngsters may feel weak, shaky, tired, confused, inattentive, irritable or experience headache and report difficulty in concentration.

In response to low-blood-sugar levels, Carbo Burners, in particular, may release adrenalin which can lead to hyperactive behavior.

Serotonin levels do not appear to rise appropriately. Youngster does not feel satisfied.

Two hours later (or less):
With blood sugar and insulin levels out of balance, youngster experiences intense and recurring cravings for carbohydrate-rich foods often to the exclusion of other foods.

With each repeat of cycle, insulin and blood sugar levels may move increasingly beyond normal limits, negative responses and behaviors may become more extreme, and/or weight gain may increase. The cycle is likely to continue unless some outside action is taken to stop it.

THE POWER OF TIMING AND COMBINING

The insulin imbalance that drives your youngster's cravings may stem from the power of "timing" and "combining" carbohydrate-rich foods.

TIMING: WHAT'S YOUR YOUNGSTER'S FREQUENCY FACTOR?

The number of times each day that your youngster eats carbohydrate-rich foods will help determine how much insulin his/her body keeps in reserve and releases at the next carbo-rich meal or snack. We refer to the number of times each day a youngster eats carbos as "the frequency factor."

The more often your youngster consumes carbo-rich foods, the more insulin his/her body releases. The more insulin his/her body releases, the more often your youngster will crave carbo-rich food. It becomes a vicious cycle.

It is essential that parents understand that when it comes to rising insulin levels, the *amount* of carbohydrate-rich food needed to cause a jump in insulin is very small. One cookie or one piece of candy or a stick of gum (sugar-sweetened or artificially-sweetened) can cause repeated insulin jumps.

In deciding how much insulin it will prepare for the next meal, your youngster's body looks, not only, at the quantity of carbos that have been eaten recently but at how often carbos have been eaten as well. The carbo addict's body will release far more insulin if one cookie is eaten four times a day than if your youngster ate four cookies at one sitting. And less extreme insulin levels mean fewer blood sugar swings and for many youngsters, fewer behavioral, mood, motivationation, weight and learning problems, as well.

Hold-On Choices in The Step-By-Step Plan and Phase One of The Jump-Start Plan will reduce those all-too- frequent carbo snacks and meals and the insulin impact they can have.

A TIMELY EXAMPLE:
COMPARE THE IMPACT OF TIMING

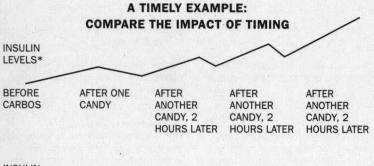

INSULIN LEVELS*				
BEFORE CARBOS	AFTER ONE CANDY	AFTER ANOTHER CANDY, 2 HOURS LATER	AFTER ANOTHER CANDY, 2 HOURS LATER	AFTER ANOTHER CANDY, 2 HOURS LATER

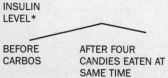

INSULIN LEVEL*	
BEFORE CARBOS	AFTER FOUR CANDIES EATEN AT SAME TIME

When high-carbo foods are eaten frequently (top graph), insulin levels rise and stay higher than after a single high-carbo load (bottom graph).

*Quantities indicated for illustrative purposes only.

COMBINING: THE COMPANY CARBOS KEEP

In addition to how often your youngster eats carbohydrate-rich foods, his/her insulin level will be determined by what other foods are eaten with the carbos at a meal or snack. This combination or balance can make the difference between normal blood sugar levels and blood sugar levels that spike, then fall.

A snack of just candy, for instance, will cause a much faster and greater blood sugar rise and be more likely to be followed by a blood sugar drop than a full meal which included high-fiber and protein-rich foods along with the same amount of candy for dessert. Fiber and protein slow and reduce insulin and blood sugar swings and help reduce many of the problems that can go along with them.

Perhaps our grandmothers were right when they said that we could have our dessert if we finished our dinners (including our meat and vegetables) first!

A POWERFUL BALANCE:
COMPARE THE IMPACT OF COMBINING

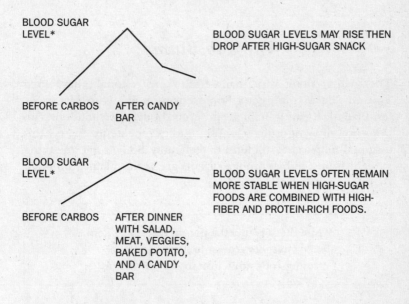

When high-carbo foods are eaten in combination with high-fiber and/or protein - rich foods, blood sugar levels are more stable.

Food Add-On Choices in The Step-By-Step Plan and Phase One of The Jump-Start Plan will balance out those carbo-only snacks and meals and the insulin impact they can have.

*Quantities indicated for illustrative purposes only.

In Its Own Time

Although for many youngsters, the intense and recurring carbo-hydrate cravings that are the earmark of this addiction begin in early childhood, for others these signs first appear during adoles-cence, triggered by the hormonal stresses of puberty, by peer pressure-related demands, by the emotional impact of family problems or divorce, or by other, less easily identified stressors. Carbohydrate addiction can appear for a while, seem to resolve itself, then reappear.

The definition of carbohydrate addiction does not lie in the time of its appearance, but rather in how it affects the minds, bodies, and even the very souls of our youngsters.

Who's to Blame?

The media, along with many health professionals, have long *assumed* that a youngster's home environment is to blame for less-than-ideal eating habits, and even though personal observa-tions as well as rigorous scientific studies repeatedly *disprove* this assumption, parents still tend to feel guilty. So let's get one thing straight from the beginning: Parents are *not* to blame, although there is now much they can do to help!

**While there is much a parent can do to help,
parents are *not* to blame for a
youngster's addiction to carbohydrates!**

Traditional attempts at self-control simply do not work with the carbohydrate-addicted child or teen. These youngsters are driven by cravings that are both intense and compelling. Unless the phys-ical cause of the addiction is removed, threats or bribes or similar tactics to gain control over a youngster's eating are simply useless.

Anyone who has ever raised kids knows that two children raised in the same environment may have vastly different eating habits. Children have their own personalities and needs, literally from birth, and very few of their parents' demands or strategies seems to have any impact on a youngster's own basic food preferences and tendencies.

We all know that the child who does not want to eat cannot be pleaded with, threatened, or persuaded to do so. In the same way, a child who craves only starches, junk food, snack foods, or sweets cannot be coaxed or intimidated into giving up these foods.

**The child who does not want to eat
cannot be forced to eat.
The child who wants to eat
cannot be kept away from food.**

At Yale University, distinct differences in food preferences have been observed in infancy, at one day of age. These early differences clearly indicate that biology, rather than a parent's influence, has a profound effect on what a child chooses to eat.

Youngsters who show clear signs of an insulin imbalance usually experience a strong biological drive that pushes them to seek starches, junk food, snack foods, or sweets, above all other foods. Though they may not understand that their bodies are not responding appropriately to the very foods they crave, these youngsters need a program that has been designed to correct their biology and, in doing so, relieve their parents of the futile struggle of trying to control the uncontrollable child.

Carbohydrate-addicted kids come from many different kinds of families. Some have been raised in restrictive environments, some in indulgent environments, some in homes that have found a healthy balance. No single environment, no single approach, produces carbohydrate-addicted kids. The genetics of carbo-addicted youngsters, rather than the dynamics of the family, seem to be most crucial in determining the cravings that drive carbo-addicted youngsters. Still, parents stuck in a "no win" situation naturally seek some explanation for their youngster's eating habits and, in doing so, parents tend to blame themselves.

> **Everything a parent does, or doesn't do, seems wrong.**

If parents withhold food, they fear they will force the child to rebel later; if they indulge the youngster's demands, they fear they are contributing to or perpetuating the problem. Everything they do, or don't do, seems wrong.

If you find yourself stuck in the middle of a "no win" situation, it is essential that you remember that children are far more than the sum total of their environment. They are living biological beings with strong and persistent drives. If these drives happen to be influenced by a physical (insulin) imbalance, children may literally not know what is good for them.

> **As a parent, you must correct the biological *cause* of your youngster's addiction to carbohydrates, just as you would correct the cause of any other physical problem.**

While a good family environment can help reinforce a healthy lifestyle, to succeed with a carbohydrate-addicted child, a parent must first get help in correcting the biological cause of the youngster's addiction to carbohydrates. The good news is that, in the pages that follow, you will come to understand what causes your youngster's addiction to carbohydrates and, most importantly, what you can do to help correct it.

An Addiction Ahead of Its Time

It is vital for parents to understand that, although the media has not yet discovered the power and prevalence of hyperinsulinemia (too much insulin in the blood), scientists have. In the lag time between when scientists discover and explore the devastating impact of a new health problem and the public is made aware of the problem, years—even decades—can pass in which a whole generation or two may needlessly suffer its effects. Just because you may not have heard of hyperinsulinemia until now, do not be fooled into thinking that it is uncommon. As researchers such as Dr. D. C. Simonson of Harvard Medical School found, "it is apparent that a substantial proportion of the population may be exposed to unrecognized chronic hyperinsulinemia." And, we would add, to insulin's destructive power as well.

Good Genes, Wrong Time

Carbohydrate-addicted kids seem to have the right genes at the wrong time. In a prehistoric world, carbohydrate-addicted children and teens would have fared quite well; in times of famine, they might have been the only ones to survive. However, in today's world of frequent snacks and limitless food opportunities, the very gift of survival turns against our children and can put them at a psychological, emotional, or physical disadvantage. Through no fault of their own, their self-esteem, well-being, and health can be compromised.

Often carbohydrate addiction is a family affair; in other cases it may "skip" many family members.

In many cases carbohydrate addiction is a family affair. Parents inherit a predisposition for carbohydrate addiction and pass it on to their children; and they in turn pass it to their children. *Parents may never suspect* that they themselves carry the genetic potential for this powerful biological imbalance.

Just as the gene for blue eyes may be hidden in a family of brown-eyed people, two parents may never exhibit an addiction for carbohydrates but still carry the hidden genes that will cause it to emerge suddenly in their offspring. In the same way, one child may be carbohydrate-addicted while a sibling may not be. In some cases carbohydrate addiction's power to influence weight gain may be passed along female lines, with girls showing weight-related problems while their brothers seem immune to weight gain, at least until later in life. Others may gain weight easily from early childhood. As in everything, no one size (or sign) fits all.

Parents who struggle with their own carbohydrate cravings may find that their toddlers perfectly mimic their own eating drives and preferences—reaching for sweets and junk food before they are barely able to speak. These children may not be modeling their parents' behavior, but rather exhibiting the same physical cravings and drives that are dictated by the underlying insulin imbalance. Other parents, who have never had to think about their own eating or weight, may suddenly find themselves with children whose eating patterns shock and concern them. In either case, parents often vacillate between blaming themselves and blaming their children. In fact, though much can be done, neither is to blame.

Carbohydrate addiction is brought out and made worse by the densely carbohydrate-rich foods that today's kids eat—and eat often.

In most cases today's youngsters tend to experience the drive for starches, snack foods, junk food, and sweets more strongly than did their parents, for although carbohydrate addiction is basically an inherited trait, it is brought out and made worse by an environment that constantly promotes and encourages the frequent consumption of the very foods that trigger the carbohydrate addict's cravings.

In the coming chapters, we will provide you with a simple quiz that has been scientifically tested and verified and that will help you to evaluate if your youngster is addicted to carbohydrates and the level of addiction.

Our Carbohydrate Addict's Program for Children and Teens will provide you with a choice of one of two plans, each of which has been designed to correct the underlying physical cause of your youngster's addiction to carbohydrates. Other chapters will arm you with strategies to help keep your youngster on track, recipes and quick-fix ideas to help make meals fun and tasty for the whole family, and motivation to help keep you going when you need it most.

Most of all, take heart. The worst part of this addiction is over, that is, not knowing what was causing it and not knowing what to do about it. We have been there ourselves. So have almost a million others who have found the answers they needed in the guidelines that follow.

First, let's determine if your youngster is, indeed, addicted to carbohydrates, let's look at the level of the addiction and see what that means, and then let's get on with solving the problem.

four

Is Your Youngster Addicted to Carbohydrates?

Chances are, when you picked up this book, you already suspected that your child or teen might be addicted to starches, snack foods, junk food, or sweets (or all of these). You have seen the behavior, you have had your concerns, and the term "carbohydrate addict" may have seemed to fit—but you may not have been absolutely sure. Before a corrective program can be started, let's determine whether your youngster does indeed appear to be carbohydrate-addicted.

Over a decade ago when we began our research, we were struck by the fact that although carbohydrate addiction was both prevalent and potentially harmful to health and well-being, no medical evaluation procedures and standards had been established to test for its presence. At that time (and to this day), blood sugar levels were tested by the use of a long, difficult, unpleasant, and expensive glucose tolerance test. Even after these exhaustive and invasive blood tests, gathered with difficulty and sacrifice, were analyzed, the results they yielded were inconclusive. Normal levels of insulin following the intake of food and low blood sugar cutoff points had not been standardized for children and teens. Without a standard defining "normal" levels, it was virtually impossible to establish whether the children and adolescents we were seeing were experiencing abnormal insulin and blood sugar responses to carbohydrate-rich foods.

> **At the time, no medical test existed that would let us evaluate whether a youngster's body was handling carbohydrate-rich foods normally or abnormally.**

It was essential for us to establish a test that would ascertain whether a youngster was responding normally or abnormally to carbohydrate-rich foods, so we set about the task of designing a test of our own. We needed a simple pen-and-paper quiz that could be used by parents to help them identify whether their youngsters showed many of the typical signs and symptoms of carbohydrate addiction as well as the insulin and blood sugar imbalances that often went along with it.

With the help of those first willing parents, we found an ideal way to determine if a child or teen was carbohydrate-addicted—and we did it without the expense, demands, discomfort, and inconvenience of lengthy blood testing that is still inconclusive to this day.

> **Our quiz will help you determine if your youngster has "normal" carbohydrate cravings and responses or is indeed carbohydrate-addicted.**

The test that follows contains questions that we have found can accurately determine a youngster's addiction to carbohydrates. It will help separate the carbohydrate addict (the youngster who experiences a physical imbalance) from the "indulger" (the youngster who just likes to snack, more out of habit than in response to a physical drive).

We have found that you do not need to incur the expense of, nor force your child unnecessarily to submit to, hours of blood testing. Along with your own observations, our quiz will help you determine if you may have a young carbohydrate addict on your hands. If your youngster is, indeed, carbohydrate-addicted, the chapters that follow will then help you understand what you can do to cut your youngster's cravings "naturally," by changing the child's physical responses to carbohydrate-rich foods.

For those children whose scores indicate that they are *not* carbohydrate-addicted but who consume too many snacks or too much junk food or sweets on a regular basis (as a matter of habit rather than biology), the Step-By-Step Plan of this program may still be appropriate. Although carbohydrate-addicted youngsters tend to reap the most dramatic physical benefits from this plan (because their problems are most extreme), carbohydrate "indulgers" can also derive the benefit of decreases in cravings and blood sugar swings. (See pages 44–46 for a distinction between the "indulger" and the "addict.")

As always, before making any changes in your youngster's activity level or diet, with this program as with any other, you should consult your child's physician.

Equal But Not Always Similar

No two carbohydrate-addicted youngsters are the same. Though we have generally found patterns of behavior that are common to almost all carbohydrate-addicted youngsters, differences in age, physical makeup, personality, levels of maturity, independence, and social pressures cause great variations.

For example, if allowed, some carbohydrate-addicted children or teens will eat junk food, snack foods, or sweets solely, to the exclusion of other foods; some will eat regular meals but crave carbohydrate-rich foods like snack foods or sweets an hour or two after finishing their meals, so it appears that they are "always eating"; others eat sporadically, but when they do eat, they consume great quantities of carbohydrate-rich food; while still others desire smaller portions of food while refusing to eat anything but snack foods, junk food, or sweets. As in all things, each youngster is unique.

> **We will provide you with easy-to-follow**
> **guidelines designed specifically to help your child**
> **break the addiction cycle—starting now.**

Determining if your child or teen is carbohydrate-addicted and the level of addiction—mild, moderate, or strong—is an important step in putting an end to the addiction itself. Once you answer the questions that follow and have the score in hand, we will provide you with easy-to-follow guidelines designed specifically to help your youngster break the addiction cycle—starting now.

THE CARBOHYDRATE ADDICTION QUIZ FOR PARENTS OF CHILDREN AND TEENS

INSTRUCTIONS

1. This quiz may be taken by one or both parents. Each parent should take the test alone and keep score on a separate copy of the answer sheet that follows. This quiz can also be taken by an exceptionally mature child or teen. (If a child or teen takes the quiz, all the questions that follow should be considered in the first person, that is, substitute the word "I" for "my child," and so forth). Again, a separate answer sheet should be used.
2. Take the quiz when you are alone. It should be done at one sitting. Until you have scored the test, do not discuss the questions or your responses with anyone else.
3. For each question, answer yes if the question is usually true and no if it is usually not true. If at all possible, answer every question.
4. This quiz is designed to compensate for "guesses." In the long run, any one answer will not influence the accuracy of the test and there are, of course, no right or wrong answers.
5. Answer each question as if it stands by itself—not linked to any other question.
6. This quiz is for the good of your youngster. Do not be concerned about how your child and your spouse might respond if they saw your answers. It is not unusual for a parent to be aware of a behavior or preference of which others are unaware.

Trust yourself and your own perceptions. Do not discuss answers with anyone else until after you have scored the quiz, and then, if you do discuss the answers, do not go back and change your responses.

Important Note: In the following questions, the term "child" refers to your youngster, either your child or your teen.

Answer yes or no to each question:

1. _____ My child consumes a substantial portion of his or her daily food in the form of snacks.

2. _____ Within two hours of eating a full meal that includes dessert, my child sometimes wants a snack or another dessert.

3. _____ If my child has a full breakfast, he or she is usually hungry again *before* lunchtime.

4. _____ Once my child begins to eat bread and other starches, junk food, snack foods, or sweets, he or she has a difficult time stopping until the food is gone or I put my foot down.

5. _____ At dinner my child will eat more bread, stuffing, potatoes, pasta, rice, and dessert than all other foods that are served.

6. _____ If my child had his or her way, most of the food that the child would choose would be starches, sandwiches, snack foods, junk food, or sweets.

7. _____ Fruit is one of my child's regular snacks.

8. _____ My child hits a "low" period and often feels tired and sleepy by midafternoon.

9. _____ At times my child has become quite upset when junk food, snack foods, or sweets have been denied.

10. _____ My child gets extremely tired after eating a large meal that contains bread, pasta, potatoes, or dessert.

11. _____ If my child is feeling "out of sorts," a snack makes him or her feel or act better.

12. _____ My child has a hard time going to sleep without a bed-time snack.

13. _____ My child frequently consumes sugar-sweetened or artificially-sweetened drinks, including sports drinks, powdered mixed drinks, fruit juices, fruit-flavored drinks, or sodas.

14. _____ My child tends to snack more when stressed, bored, anxious, tired, or angry.

15. _____ I think my child may, at times, hide food or wait to eat food when other people are not around.

16. _____ My child is, or may be, overweight or hyperactive, or experiences extremes in moodiness, lack of motivation, or an inability to concentrate.[1]

17. _____ I think that one or more of my child's blood relatives may be carbohydrate-addicted.

---

[1] With physician's counsel, non-diet-related reasons for these conditions must first be ruled out.

Scoring the Carbohydrate Addiction Quiz

As you may have noticed, some of the questions in the Carbohydrate Addiction Quiz for Parents of Children and Teens are likely to be answered yes by many people, while other questions are less likely to get an affirmative answer. For that reason, each question has been assigned a different value (number of points).

The higher the number of points assigned to a question, the more likely it is that a yes answer to that question indicates a youngster's probability of being carbohydrate-addicted.

Your youngster's score will help you determine the severity of the addiction. It will give you a perspective to determine where your youngster's level of addiction falls along the continuum of other scores. In addition, the description of your youngster's addiction range may sharpen and confirm your experiences and help you focus on critical points of change that may be vital to your youngster's health and well-being.

1. Using the answer sheet below, circle only those questions to which you answered yes.
2. Move across the dotted line and circle the value (the number of points) for that question.
3. Add up all the values, then read what the score indicates on the pages that follow.

Two parents of the same child may disagree when they evaluate their youngster's addiction to carbohydrates. One parent may see a child under unique circumstances; in the case of divorce, only when the child visits on weekends, for instance. In some circumstances, one parent may be more aware of a youngster's habits, feelings, or drives, or a youngster may be more open with one parent than with the other.

If your opinion differs from that of your spouse or ex-spouse, trust that your score reflects your awareness of your child's addiction to carbohydrates.

THE CARBOHYDRATE ADDICTION QUIZ FOR PARENTS OF CHILDREN AND TEENS

Answer Sheet

QUESTION NUMBER	VALUE
1	4 points
2	5 points
3	3 points
4	4 points
5	3 points
6	5 points
7	4 points
8	2 points
9	3 points
10	3 points
11	3 points
12	3 points
13	3 points
14	3 points
15	3 points
16	5 points
17	4 points

Total _____ (Total Possible Score: 60 points)

WHAT YOUR
YOUNGSTER'S SCORE INDICATES

Doubtful Addiction   (0—21 points)
Mild Carbohydrate Addiction   (22—28 points)
Moderate Carbohydrate Addiction   (29—44 points)
Strong Carbohydrate Addiction   (45—60 points)

Doubtful Addiction

A score of 21 or less suggests that, if your child or teen has periodic mood swings, behavioral or learning problems, or difficulty in controlling weight or eating, the problem does not appear to be related to carbohydrate addiction. Parents should look elsewhere to determine a cause of these problems.

Youngsters who score 21 or less and experience *no* weight, behavioral, mood, or learning problems but who need help in balancing their intake of junk food, snack food, and sweets (with more protein-rich and high-fiber food) may get the help they need by following The Step-By-Step Plan of the Program in the chapters to come.

Mild Addiction

Before taking this quiz, parents of mildly addicted youngsters often assume that their children are eating out of "habit" or boredom, in response to stress or anxiety, or to meet the increased caloric demands of sports or other activities. It is easy to dismiss the mildly addicted youngster's less-than-ideal eating patterns as "normal." Parents, however, must be aware that mildly addicted youngsters are often showing early signs of a progressive problem, one that will, in all likelihood, get worse, far worse, as the youngster gets older.

The mildly addicted young carbohydrate addict may not yet have a weight problem as such, though he or she may want to slim down a bit. Again, the lack of a strong weight problem in the mildly addicted youngster does *not* mean that the child is safe from the silent imbalance that can later lead to weight gain, particularly over time, as the child experiences some of the challenges of adulthood such as work-related or college-related stresses, or the demands of marriage, pregnancy, or adult family life.

Parents often voice concerns about the mildly addicted youngster's poor eating habits and their effects on learning, attention, and mood. These concerns are well founded, for even mildly addicted youngsters may show difficult-to-diagnose learning, attention, and motivational problems, as well as diffi-cult-to-live-with mood swings that, again, may only get worse as the youngster gets older. It is exceedingly rare that an addiction to carbohydrates, even one that is mild, goes away "by itself." Though your child is "only" mildly addicted, this program has been designed to balance your youngster's physical response to carbohydrates and can help you and your youngster correct the cause of health, learning, psychological, and weight-related prob-lems—for life.

Moderate Addiction

The young carbohydrate addict who appears to be in the mod-erate range may sometimes show early signs of future weight problems, though clearly this is not always the case, especially in the active or rapidly growing youngster. Each child is different. In some, a struggle to avoid gaining excess weight is only one of the signs of an active addiction to carbohydrates. So, while a ten-dency to gain weight easily is often an indication that your youngster may be carbohydrate-addicted, being slim most cer-tainly does not indicate that your child is addiction-free.

**Being slim does *not* indicate that
a youngster is addiction-free.**

At times, moderately addicted youngsters experience recurring hunger or food cravings that vary in intensity. Impulses to eat junk food, snack foods, or sweets may shift from being controllable at times to being overpowering but, since they vary so widely, the sporadic drive for carbohydrates makes consistent, good eating habits almost impossible.

Sometimes the moderately addicted young carbohydrate addict may be able to control impulses to snack or may experience a lessening of a desire for carbohydrate-rich foods—but other times this control may simply slip away. Parent and child alike may not understand why a youngster, at times, is able to maintain control over eating and, at other times, exhibits the inability (or what appears to be the unwillingness) to handle appropriately the drive to eat.

The parent of the moderately addicted child or teen may think that this kind of eating is normal while still harboring concern about the youngster's psychological, emotional, and physical health. Two parents of the same child may often disagree when it comes to evaluating their moderately addicted youngster, for these children can show widely varying and inconsistent behaviors.

It is essential to remember, however, that like the mildly addicted child, the moderately addicted youngster will not, in all likelihood, "grow out of it." In almost all instances addictions grow along with the child, setting up almost insurmountable problems in adulthood that could have, and should have, been prevented.

Strong Addiction

Many strongly carbohydrate-addicted youngsters are not happy with their weight, and parents often don't know how to help them. *With or without weight problems*, however, periodic difficulties in concentration, anxiety, hyperactivity or depression, lack of motivation, and regular and powerful mood swings often accompany a strong carbohydrate addiction.

The youngster with a strong carbohydrate addiction often finds that even the best efforts to try to control eating habits are undermined by recurring feelings of intense hunger and food cravings. The youngster, however, may have no way to express the feeling of being "driven" to eat. Any period of "healthy eating" is usually doomed to be short-lived and followed by failure.

Parents of strongly addicted youngsters often live with feelings of both frustration and concern. When strongly addicted youngsters are kept from the foods they crave, they blame their parents and sometimes rebel in anger. If parents then "indulge" the child, they may feel that they are failing in their responsibilities. Sometimes the need to survive takes over and parents may just give up.

The strongly addicted youngster likewise feels frustrated and guilty. These youngsters often feel isolated or abandoned or alienated and, though they may not admit it to anyone else, they may feel that they themselves are to blame for their own problems with weight or concentration, impulse control, motivation, or other behavioral and learning-related challenges.

Whom Is This Program For?

The Carbohydrate Addict's Program for Children and Teens was designed for mildly, moderately, and strongly addicted youngsters. If your child or teen is carbohydrate-addicted, the program offers you the means to correct the cause of your youngster's cravings for junk food, snack foods, or sweets; low blood sugar–related mood swings, learning, emotional, or attitudinal difficulties; or the weight problems with which your child or teen may be struggling.

**This program can offer your youngster
a healthier way of life and, for both you and your child,
a happier one as well.**

The parents of many carbohydrate-addicted youngsters have found that The Step-By-Step Plan of the Program (detailed in coming chapters) is also an easy way to incorporate a balance of protein-rich and high-fiber foods into the eating regimen of their nonaddicted youngsters. In addition, this program has been designed to reduce the excess insulin release that can, in adulthood, increase your child's risk for high blood pressure, adult-onset diabetes, and cardiovascular illness. It can offer your youngster the prospect of a healthier life and, for both you and your child, a happier one as well.

The Question of Weight

It is important to remember that there is no absolute correlation between how much a youngster weighs and the degree of carbohydrate addiction; although more strongly addicted youngsters tend to be overweight, this is *not* always the case.

If your score indicates that your youngster is strongly addicted and if your youngster's weight falls within a normal-weight range, it is quite likely that your child's metabolism is, at this time, "burning" excess calories at a very fast rate. If the addiction itself is not corrected, however, in adulthood the strongly addicted normal-weight child or teen is in danger of becoming overweight. Many slim or slightly overweight teenage girls fall into this category, gaining a great deal of weight as they enter adulthood—often with their first or second pregnancy—then finding themselves unable to lose the weight after giving birth. Still slim carbo-addicted young men often find that middle age brings unwanted pounds and serious health concerns.

**For the carbohydrate-addicted youngster,
slenderness does not equal health.**

Even though the slim carbohydrate-addicted youngster does not yet carry the burden of extra pounds, this child is likely to suffer increased health risks similar to those of an overweight youngster as both approach adulthood.

Even those carbohydrate-addicted children and teens who are destined to stay slim for life show an increased risk for health-related problems in adulthood if their addiction remains uncorrected, for they may still carry the underlying insulin imbalance that has been linked to nine of this country's top killer diseases and health risk factors.

If your child is greatly overweight, this may indicate an unusually slow metabolic rate, even for a carbohydrate-addicted youngster. There may be other factors, in addition to carbohydrate addiction, contributing to your youngster's excess weight. While this program will, in all likelihood, reduce or eliminate your youngster's carbohydrate cravings and help your child to lose weight more easily, you should work with your child's physician.

Every Step of the Way

You have already taken two of the three essential steps to helping your child or teen break free of carbohydrate addiction. First, by picking up this book you have acknowledged that you have a concern about your youngster's eating habits.

Second, by taking the Carbohydrate Addiction Quiz for Parents of Children and Teens, you have determined your child's level of addiction to carbohydrates—an important step in recognizing carbohydrate addiction's powerful impact on your youngster's feelings, thoughts, moods, behavior, weight, and health.

Now, in the chapters to come, we will guide you through a program of choice that has been designed specifically to help your youngster break free of carbohydrate addiction for life. And we will, of course, stay with you every step of the way.

five

The Many Faces of Carbohydrate Addiction,

Part 1: Lifting the Weight

A VERY PERSONAL NOTE TO PARENTS

We all know that eye color, hair color and texture, height, even the shape of a youngster's face, nose, lips, and earlobes are simple reflections of the genetics a child inherits. Why then does society have so much difficulty in accepting that the same influences exist in determining a youngster's weight and metabolism?

There is a completely erroneous belief that if we accept that a youngster's tendency to gain weight is inherited, it naturally follows that there is nothing that can be done to change "what's in the genes." This assumption is totally untrue. Just as many inherited disorders can be prevented, corrected, or eliminated, so a youngster's tendency to gain weight easily can be reversed by simple changes in diet and lifestyle. However, these changes *must* be aimed at correcting the underlying physical imbalance that is inherited in the first place.

We all know that two children raised in the same household may show clear differences in appetite and food interest. Still, when a child is overweight, instead of attributing this problem to a physical difference, society tends to blame the home environment, in particular, the parents. Assertions that blame parents for a child's battle with weight may cite a typical scenario: If one parent (or both parents) and the child are overweight, the assumption is that the parent has passed on "bad eating habits." This illogical argument denies the multitude of scientific research that has revealed the undeniable power of genetics in determining a youngster's weight.

Likewise, the lone overweight youngster born to two normal-weight parents is also demonstrating the genetic laws that influence so many other physical traits. For just as a blue-eyed youngster can suddenly emerge in a family of brown-eyed parents—the result of hidden genetic messages that are not observable—an overweight youngster can be born into a family of slim individuals, who may carry a silent "obesity gene." In the same way, an overweight child may be born into a family in which only one parent shares his or her weight struggles. And two siblings may differ in metabolism just as they would in eye or hair color.

Though society might choose to ignore these biological facts, it is unconscionable to assume that all overweight parents who have overweight children provide their youngsters with environments that encourage poor eating habits. In the same way, it is both cruel and completely unwarranted to assume that the overweight youngster born to normal-weight parents is particularly gluttonous, indulging in the most base of desires with no regard for ultimate outcome. If one follows this logic through to its natural outcome, one would have to assume that all normal-weight parents who have normal-weight youngsters must have provided optimally healthful eating environments. While we know that this is not the case, far too many are willing to condemn the overweight child and parent alike. One would not ascribe any physical attribute other than weight to poor parenting or simple indulgence yet, when it comes to excess weight, the placing of the blame holds no logic.

Ironically, almost without exception, it has been our repeated experience that overweight parents do a great deal more to provide healthful food and instruction for their children, along with positive role model behavior, than do many "naturally

slim" parents. They go out of their way to provide a more positive environment, in hopes that their children will escape the
weight problems with which they themselves have been bur-
dened. Likewise, the overweight youngster in a normal-weight
family is usually tormented by the problem and has tried virtually everything humanly possible to control both eating and
weight to no avail.

It is time to stop blaming the victim—all the victims, parents
and youngsters alike.

The pages that follow will offer you support and help, but first
we will give you the facts to help you let go of the wrongful accusations you might have heard—from yourself or from others.

Growing Concerns:
The Epidemic of
Juvenile Weight Problems

"Not only are adult Americans getting fatter, the bad news is that
children are catching up. According to a recent study over a
period of two decades, the proportion of overweight children in
the United States has increased by 50%. The nation appears to
be facing an epidemic of obesity."[1] Since 1988, when these star-
tling observations were first made by the PBS program *Innova-
tions*, the epidemic of juvenile obesity has snowballed.

In October 1995 the National Center for Health Statistics,
having studied children aged six to seventeen years, reported
that the number of kids who are overweight has almost doubled
in the last twenty-five years. According to the U.S. Department of
Health and Human Services, as of 1996, "Overweight affects a
third of the American adult population and a quarter of Amer-

---

[1] For adults, obesity is defined as being 20 percent or more over ideal weight. To
our knowledge, no absolute definition for obesity in children has been agreed
upon though many researchers use percentiles based on BMI (body-mass
index), based on age, height, and weight. There are many causes for eating and
weight problems in youngsters and in adults. It is essential to rule out any other
cause for your youngster's difficulties before embarking on this program.

ican children." And the problem is getting worse, with no end in sight.

While being overweight often affects a youngster's self-esteem and social life, the impact on a youngster's health may be worse. Only a few years ago, the U.S. Department of Agriculture's Human Nutrition Research Center on Aging issued a warning to parents that "one out of every of every four teens carries around enough excess weight to put him at high risk for suffering fatal heart attacks, strokes, colon cancer, gout, and other health problems, later in life." To make matters worse, there is little chance that a child or adolescent will "naturally" outgrow a weight problem. According to the well-respected obesity expert Dr. Albert J. Stunkard of the University of Pennsylvania, "if [weight] reduction has not occurred by the teenage years, the chances the adolescent can avoid becoming an overweight adult can be over 28:1."

If a youngster remains overweight into adolescence, the chances are 28:1 that he or she will become an overweight adult.

Without help, the overweight child becomes the unhappy, overweight adolescent, and the unhappy, overweight adolescent becomes the unhappy, unhealthy, overweight adult. Moreover, while scientists are still determining the exact incidence of the problem, up to 74 percent of overweight children have been found to suffer from an insulin imbalance that causes them to be addicted to carbohydrates.

Up to 74 percent of overweight children have an insulin imbalance that could be causing them to be addicted to carbohydrates.

The Insulin Link

On one hand, everyone acts as if ideal weight levels are simply a matter of using common sense and willpower; however, on the other hand, almost everyone recognizes that common sense and willpower approaches do not explain:

Why some youngsters seem destined to be heavier than others.
Why some youngsters cannot seem to get enough food, while other kids have little desire to eat at all.
Why weight that is lost through dieting is almost always gained back, often with a few extra pounds as a bonus.
Why so many kids gain weight easily while others can't seem to gain an ounce.

Most people will say that these differences can be explained by variations in a youngster's metabolism without realizing that the term "metabolism" denotes an impossibly complex concept that can be neither accurately described nor measured. So to say that a youngster has a "slow" metabolism has almost no meaning unless what you really mean is that the child or teen seems to burn calories poorly, that is, the youngster puts on weight easily. If this is what is meant by metabolism, in this instance, the metabolic rate is, in great part, the net result of a youngster's insulin levels.

Remember, if your youngster is carbo-addicted, it is very likely that he or she has inherited a tendency to release too much insulin after eating foods that are rich in carbohydrates. Metabolically speaking, excess insulin does two jobs too well. First, as you know, an excess amount of this "hunger hormone" drives your youngster to seek more food, more often, or in greater quantities.

With each new carbo meal or snack, more insulin is released and the cycle repeats; more carbo leads to more cravings, more cravings to more carbo, and so on. In response to insulin's erroneous messages that signal the body to take in more energy, your youngster naturally seeks more food. Signals to eat may be unusually strong and insistent because the food energy from the last meal remains trapped in the liver and fat cells, locked in place by excess levels of insulin. The food energy that may have been eaten only hours ago has become unavailable, as if it had been stored behind a large impenetrable door.

Second, extra insulin means that more of the food energy will be directed for storage in the fat cells (and less is likely to be burned). If insulin levels stay high, fat cells rarely get a chance to release the stored energy and the extra calories move along a one-way street headed straight to the fat cells.

Almost every researcher studying metabolism knows that eating carbohydrate-rich foods results in a rise in insulin levels, but in 1982 Dr. Paula Geiselman and Dr. David Novin discovered that some people actually release insulin just by seeing or smelling carbohydrate-rich foods. These subjects' carbohydrate-sensitive bodies respond to just the sight or smell of carbos in the same way that others would respond to a high-carbo meal and they are driven to eat and gain weight easily, not because of some character flaw or lack of willpower, but because of an inborn tendency for a trigger-quick and intense insulin release. In addition, excess insulin makes their bodies better fat-making machines as well. This unusually sensitive hunger-weight gain cycle has been confirmed by some of the most respected researchers in the field, including Dr. D. C. Simonson of Harvard Medical School, Dr. Judith Rodin of Yale University, Dr. T. Silverstone and Dr. E. Goodall of the Medical College of St. Bartholemew's Hospital, London, U.K., as well as many, many others.

> **Blood insulin levels in overweight teens has been found to be *four times* that of normal-weight teenagers.**

Dr. Allan Drash of the Children's Hospital of Pittsburgh carefully studied overweight adolescents and reported in the medical journal *Metabolism* that "it is clear that being overweight is associated with marked hyperinsulinism [excess levels of insulin]," and he added that excess levels of insulin were "characteristic" of all the overweight teenage patients he studied. How great were the differences? Blood insulin levels in overweight teens were found to be *four times* that of normal-weight teenagers. Dr. Guiseppe Chiumello and his colleagues in the Department of Pediatrics and Child Health at the renowned University of Milano reported in the journal *Diabetes* that overweight youngsters from two and one-half to thirteen years of age had blood insulin levels (again) over four times that of their normal-weight counterparts.

What is amazing to us is that, although scientists continue to document the powerful role that excess levels of insulin play in determining a youngster's weight and eating preferences, the media continue to give parents the message that youngsters are overweight because of "poor" eating habits, without adding that the same "poor" eating habits they describe may be brought on by an excess of insulin that drives these youngsters' cravings. Without this added and essential piece of information, without being told that their youngster's addiction to carbohydrates may be caused by an insulin imbalance, parents are subtly given the message that their youngster's eating and weight problems are the simple result of a less-than-helpful and not-so-healthy environment.

Dr. Albert Stunkard, in his landmark study on adopted children, demonstrated that, contrary to the media's message, a child's environment alone has little influence on whether the youngster will become overweight. Dr. Stunkard used a unique register in Denmark in which a great deal of information about adopted infants and their biological and adoptive parents is open to the public. Measuring the youngsters' "fatness" by calculating their body-mass index, Dr. Stunkard found a "strong relation" between the body mass of the adoptees as adults and that of their natural parents. He found no such link between the body mass of the adoptees and their adoptive parents, however, indicating that inherited traits played a much stronger role than the environment in determining a youngster's weight.

**Heredity is most certainly not destiny.
You can help your youngster change
his or her genetic "destiny."**

But heredity is most certainly not destiny. While the children of overweight parents may be genetically predisposed to becoming overweight, they are not doomed to it. Genes alone do not cause a youngster to become overweight although they can help fuel the cravings and the hunger that do. In the case of the carbohydrate-addicted overweight youngster, environmental/ behavioral influences, which include choices regarding the types of carbohydrates youngsters eat, how often they eat them, and which other foods are included, can influence your youngster's genetic destiny.

Insulin's Energy-Saving Response

The body of the young carbohydrate addict is intent on saving energy. To conserve the calories that might otherwise be burned during activity, it can cause your youngster to find activity and exercise unpleasant or, at least, not very rewarding. Your youngster may not be able to explain why he or she does not feel like being active. What you or others may label as "lazy" may be nothing more than the body's signal to conserve energy.

In the prestigious *New England Journal of Medicine*, Dr. Susan Roberts and her colleagues reported on a study that began looking at infants at seven days of age. These researchers found that by the time they were only three months of age, infants who were most likely destined to become overweight showed significantly less energy expenditure than those babies destined to become normal-weight. It is hard to imagine that these infants were guilty of being "lazy" or "unmotivated" or, even worse, that they "didn't want to be thin." Rather, it appears obvious that their bodies were bent on conserving energy, storing it away in their fat cells. The scientists who studied these babies did not test their blood levels, but we would bet that if they had, they would have seen abnormally high levels of insulin and low blood sugar swings as well, like those of overweight teenagers who likewise may be falsely accused of being lazy.

The newest version of blaming the victim comes from a study that connected television time with excess weight in youngsters. These researchers found that the heavier youngsters were those who spent the greatest number of hours in front of the television. From these findings came a simplistic explanation that truly surprised us. Based on their findings, the researchers concluded that the hours spent in front of the television decreased energy output so as to make these children fat.

We strongly believe this is only part of the story. While decreased activity levels in the hours spent watching TV may, in fact, decrease energy output, physical activity accounts for only 20 percent of the calories burned; the rest comes simply from the metabolic processes involved in living and growing. Surely extra time spent in front of the television cannot explain why some youngsters weigh 50 percent or more over their ideal weight. Besides, many youngsters who might be described as "couch potatoes" are thin.

While the TV-weight hypothesis may reflect some undefined degree of truth, we have found that it is being used as the newest of blame games that tells only part (a small part) of the story and that can be used to further negative attitudes toward overweight youngsters.

From our experience, we have found that it is just as likely that some of the overweight youngsters these researchers studied preferred watching television rather than spending time with peers who might ostracize or tease them. In addition, they may have preferred TV to sports and activities that were more difficult for them, given their overweight condition. When looking at studies such as these, it is essential to consider the possibility that the overweight youngster may not have the usual array of friendships and opportunities from which to choose. Add to these limited social opportunities and the burden of excess weight, the body's tendency to conserve energy, and a youngster's embarrassment at looking "fat" or "unattractive," as well as the fear of being ridiculed or teased, and it may very well be that being fat puts the youngster in front of the television, rather than the other way around.

Once a youngster is overweight, long hours in front of the television may well lessen his or her chances of burning calories and, since activity lowers insulin levels, of losing weight, but TV alone cannot be assumed to be the primary culprit. Furthermore, just as there are certainly a great many slim youngsters who watch TV, there are many overweight youngsters who are surprisingly active.

The Power of Prejudice:
Beyond the Facts

In this society, excess weight in youngsters can carry a devastating social stigma. The *American Psychological Review* asked ten- and eleven-year-old girls and boys to rank drawings of children with various physical handicaps. Pictures of overweight youngsters were ranked lower in preference than those of youngsters with crutches and leg braces, those in wheelchairs, those with a hand missing, and those with facial disfigurements, most likely because the children considered all the physical handicaps pictured, other than excess weight, as nonvolitional, that is, not the "fault" of the youngster involved.

Being overweight, on the other hand, is almost always considered to be caused by a child's gluttony, though scientific study after study, such as those mentioned in the appendix of this book, indicate that strong physical drives may impel the youngster to eat, even against his or her will.

Still, the prejudice persists and trickles down its influence at a remarkably young age. Children as young as three years of age may voice disgust or anger by adding the word "fat" to name-calling (as in, "Shut your big fat mouth") and elementary school children have demonstrated that they would prefer to have a friend who has been shown to lie, cheat, or steal rather than one who is overweight.

Year after year, researchers continue to confirm what the parents of many overweight youngsters already know—that the effects of prejudice toward overweight kids may affect their self-esteem and lead them to develop very unfavorable views of their bodies, and that these same youngsters may to go on to experience a myriad of discriminations and rejections as adults. Even worse, negative attitudes and prejudice toward overweight youngsters can influence not only personal opinions but professional attitudes as well. While many of us tell ourselves that we don't care how the average person judges us and we want our children to learn not to care as well, one would expect most health professionals to treat all youngsters equally. Parents of overweight kids often report quite a different experience.

> **The medical profession does not treat excess weight
> in the same way as any other medical problem.**

The medical profession does not treat excess weight in the same way as any other medical problem. To get a clear perspective on how your youngster's weight may influence his or her medical care, consider the following scenario: Imagine, for a moment, that instead of being overweight, your youngster were underweight and you were seeking help with this problem. On taking your child to the doctor you would report that your child had little or no interest in food, had lost his or her appetite, and seemed to be losing weight. Chances are, your doctor would show great concern. With compassion and patience, your doctor would seek the cause of this "problem"; looking for a *physical* reason that might explain the loss of weight and that might be corrected. Your youngster would not, of course, be blamed, nor would you; it would probably never occur to the doctor to tell you simply to force your child to eat to make him or her gain weight. Rather, using the available medical resources, your doctor would seek to identify the source of the problem and to correct it.

Now contrast this scene with what so many parents experience when taking an overweight youngster to the doctor for help with a weight problem. The parent of an overweight child or teen, reporting a youngster's excess interest in food, carbohydrate cravings, or weight gain, is usually told to put the youngster on a diet.

> **Youngsters may be accused of not *wanting* to lose weight
> or the mental health of the entire family may be questioned.**

In some cases the overweight youngster's willpower and motivation are assumed to be at fault. It may be assumed that the child or teen doesn't *want* to lose weight, or is using weight as a weapon to hurt other family members. Depending on the health professional's specialty, the psychological health of the entire family may be questioned. In the case of the *over*weight youngster, in contrast with the treatment of the *under*weight youngster, typically no cause for the cravings and weight gain is ever sought. Rather, it is usually assumed that parent or child or both are clearly to blame for the situation and that it is not the responsibility of the health professional to do anything but admonish parents to get the youngster "back on track." The typical attitude of far too many medical professionals toward the overweight youngster (and adult) is: "You wouldn't be fat if you didn't eat so much, so just don't eat so much."

This treatment is unfair and illogical, to say the least. We liken it to taking an asthmatic youngster to the doctor and having the physician say, "Well, you wouldn't have asthma if you would just stop wheezing." No help, no hope; just blame.

When it comes to the problem of excess weight, we have come to accept the blaming of the victim.

Too many of us who are overweight or who have been overweight have unfortunately come to accept that we are to blame for our own condition and therefore assume that we deserve what we get. Ironically, science shows that nothing could be further from the truth.

The Silenced Truth

Scientists have known for a long time that, contrary to all the advertising and media misrepresentations, in general the overweight do *not* eat more than the normal-weight; in fact, in many cases they may eat much less. Certainly some overweight youngsters and adults consume great amounts of food, but, likewise, some slender youngsters and adults eat comparable amounts and remain slim. Even more challenging to the "fat people eat too much" myth is the fact that many overweight youngsters and adults simply don't eat enough to make them "that much" heavier than their thinner same-age counterparts.

But the myth of gluttony persists and big business continues to make big money by perpetuating the belief that the overweight are to blame for their condition and then offering the public the newest solution to the problem, over and over again. Indeed, the weight-loss "industry" (and that is what it has become) continues to grow fat on the failure of those who seek help. No other medical problem is treated by nonprofessionals in weight-loss centers or groups that carry no licensing and are made to answer to no one for their lack of training and lack of success. The very fact that the overweight return again and again to these facilities is testimony to these centers' long-term failure rates.

Year after year after year, these same commercial weight-loss programs continue to hand out the same old one-size-fits-all approaches, occasionally advertised with the newest fashionable diet twist. Yet underneath it all, their programs are based on the singular assumption that their clientele eat too much of the wrong foods because they don't have enough willpower or simply haven't been motivated enough to control themselves.

No wonder these centers offer only short-term success at best. Their basic assumption, that the overweight eat more than those who are not overweight, is simply not true. As far back as 1967, scientists found that what you ate did not necessarily determine what you weighed. "Naturally thin" people, they found, have the ability to overeat without gaining weight. Though we have all witnessed this same truth with our own eyes, we tend to continue to view slim overeaters as the exception and the overweight overeaters as the rule. Scientists say that is not so.

For over three decades, scientists have known that what you eat does *not* necessarily determine what you weigh.

Over thirty years ago, in the journal *American Clinical Nutrition*, Drs. D. S. Miller and P. Mumford documented that some people are able to consume a great many extra calories, as much as an additional eight thousand to ten thousand calories more per week, than they would eat normally, and still lose weight. At about the same time, the renowned researcher Dr. E.

A. H. Sims and his colleagues overfed subjects by up to three thousand calories *per day* and, although their intent was to increase these subjects' weight by 25 percent, in normal subjects they could not bring about this weight gain. These subjects' healthy, balanced bodies just seemed to "burn off" the extra calories they took in. Indeed, given the ways in which the number of calories we consume varies from day to day, it would be virtually impossible to believe that we ourselves are controlling our weight solely by controlling our caloric intake.

The belief that caloric intake alone determines our weight and that thirty-five hundred calories equals a pound of fat does not make sense when we see, with our very eyes, that one person can seem to eat from morning to night and stay slim, while another appears to gain weight just by watching!

> **Scientists have known for decades that
> something else, other than food intake alone,
> determines how much a person weighs.**

In 1982, to explore the "you are what you eat" idea, Dr. J. B. Morgan and his fellow researchers studied "large eaters" and "small eaters" and found, ironically, that large eaters weighed less and had a lower percentage of body fat than did small eaters. In fact, Dr. Morgan's research revealed that these large eaters, who weighed less than the small eaters, consumed almost *double* the number of calories as the small eaters. It is obvious, from personal experience as well as from scientific research, that something else other than food intake alone determines how much a person weighs.

While your youngster may indeed consume a great deal of carbohydrate-rich food, it is also possible that, at the same time, your youngster may *not* be eating a greater number of calories than that consumed by slimmer kids of the same age and height. A large part of our perception of any process is influenced by the end result. In other words, much of our judgment of whether a youngster is eating "too" much is influenced by how much the youngster weighs. It's a funny kind of thinking that a great many of us share; we tend to think backwards, so that extra pounds can make your youngster's eating appear more pronounced and negative while if the same food was consumed by a slimmer youngster, that youngster might not be seen as overeating.

Food restriction is not the answer.

Wrong Answers

Food restriction is almost never the answer—neither for youngsters nor for adults. First, food restriction simply doesn't work. At least 95 percent of people of all ages who are put on food-restricting diets fail to lose weight and keep it off. In fact, the real statistics may be even more dismal. Most importantly, food restriction does not bring about permanent weight loss because it does not correct the cause of the weight gain.

In 1978 Dr. J. V. Durnin discovered that even when subjects suffered severe caloric restriction, those who were overweight tended to maintain their excess weight levels, and over ten years ago, Dr. R. Leibel of the Rockefeller Institute reported that when normal-weight and overweight patients took in the same number of calories, each group maintained its original weight status; in other words, on the same number of calories, the overweight stayed overweight and the normal-weight stayed normal-weight. Eating the *same food* as did normal-weight subjects, the overweight failed to lose their average excess weight of one hundred pounds per patient. Even worse, for the overweight to make any progress in their weight-losing goals, they had to eat far *less* than those patients who were normal weight. Clearly, while excess weight may, *in some*, be the result of too great an intake of food, others become overweight without eating much more, if at all, than those who are normal-weight.

**On the same number of calories,
eating the same food, the overweight stay overweight
and the normal-weight remain normal-weight.**

Why then, when scientists have repeatedly proven that there is a metabolic difference in those who are overweight—a difference that does not respond to food-restricting diets—do our medical professionals, media, and commercial programs continue to prescribe the same, almost bound-to-fail, food-restricting regimens over and over again? And why are those who fail blamed for their failure?

Weight-ism, intolerance for those who struggle with their eating or weight, seems to have become the last bastion of prejudice. Those who have never experienced the powerful drives that an addiction to carbohydrates can initiate usually assume that a carbo addiction is nothing more than an excuse for giving in to the same desires that nonaddicted individuals experience. Ironically, those who are carbohydrate addicts, and have been carbo addicts all their lives, also fail to recognize that their cravings are both qualitatively and quantitatively different from those who are nonaddicted. Carbohydrate addicts and nonaddicts alike assume, wrongly, that what they experience is the same as what others experience.

Young carbo addicts can't "just use a little willpower" and control their eating, anymore than they could see or hear better if they "just tried harder."

Though no one would ever expect two children to have the same accuracy of vision or hearing or be able to exhibit the same level of physical strength, many people assume that all youngsters experience the same drives for food and that their bodies use food in the same way. Intellectually, people may say they recognize that there must be differences but, when they come face to face with an overweight youngster or watch a child driven by carbo cravings, they almost automatically wonder why the young carbohydrate addict doesn't "just use a little willpower." In that question, they betray their expectation, their assumption, their demand—that carbohydrate-addicted youngsters be "like other kids" or, even worse, that they could be slim if they "just tried harder."

Sweeping generalities about youngsters who struggle with their weight simply do not apply. Some youngsters may crave carbos and have trouble controlling their eating. Others may deprive themselves in a vain attempt to keep themselves under control. Others may tell you that they "just love food." Some may swear that they do not eat enough to be as overweight as they are. All these youngsters are right because they are all different.

For your carbohydrate-addicted youngster, it is not what is in the food that matters, it is what that food does when it enters your youngster's body—how *your* youngster's body reacts and what can be done to help your youngster reach and maintain the right carbohydrate balance for his or her weight, health, and well-being—for life.

Silent Signals

Many parents ask us how they can tell how a youngster *really* feels about his or her weight. It's an important question and does not come with an easy answer.

Seventy-five percent of America's teenage girls, by one estimate, resort to diets presumably because they are dissatisfied about their weight though some may not be overweight. Others, overweight or not, may be unhappy with their weight and feel badly about themselves but can't or don't do anything about it. While girls are more likely to suffer the pains of negative self-image, boys are certainly not immune. Some clear signs that your youngster is troubled about weight include:

1. Avoidance of meals, social situations, gym class, or school, or avoidance of buying new clothes.
2. Exercising obsessively, to the point of negatively impacting on grades, social life, or continued good health.
3. Hidden use of over-the-counter "diet aids" or of cigarettes or illicit drugs.

Other danger signs that often indicate your youngster's concern about weight include talking about food all the time, stashing away food or stealing money, clowning or joking about his or her weight, physical aggression toward other youngsters or adults, increased need for approval or affection, or, in some, a distancing or avoidance of any meaningful communication.

Remember that weight concerns do not affect only teenagers; youngsters as young as three or four years of age are aware of weight differences, of the negative view this society holds of the overweight, and of the fact that some foods are "fattening."

How can you get an unwilling youngster to talk about weight concerns? Many youngsters will respond if you speak with "I" statements, revealing your own feelings, now and in the past, in relation to your weight and appearance. You might add some social experiences you have encountered. Don't make these experiences too difficult to hear and don't expect an immediate response; many youngsters will mull what you have talked about and, as you know, express their feelings when you least expect it. Listen for questions that may contain hidden statements; listen to what your youngster is not saying as well as to what the child is willing to talk about.

A Fighting Chance: Jennifer's Story, Part 2

Jennifer wanted to make changes as quickly as possible. "Please," she asked, tears filling her eyes. "Isn't there something I could do that would help me lose weight faster. The kids at school have been . . ." She started to sob and, though she did not finish the sentence, we knew only too well what she was going to say.

We explained what would be required for her to begin the quick entry form of the Carbohydrate Addict's Program for Children and Teens. We call it The Jump-Start Plan, we explained (you will learn about it in the chapters to come). With her physician's and her parents' consent, we decided that this plan might best help Jennifer begin to see results within a matter of days.

The Jump-Start Plan, we added, was for older children and teens; it was more stringent than our Step-By-Step Plan but it brought about a quick change in insulin and blood sugar balance. It would help eliminate cravings and hasten weight reduction, we continued, but the first phase of the plan could only be followed for a limited time, depending on her physician's recommendations.

"A jump start is just what she needs," her mother agreed, and the next day, after a quickly arranged doctor's visit, Jennifer began our Jump-Start Plan designed specifically for older children and teens.

At our following meeting two weeks later, Jennifer was all smiles and so was her mother. "It's incredible," Jennifer began.

"It's amazing," her mother cut in enthusiastically. "She's like a different kid." Then, smiling at her daughter, she encouraged her to continue.

"Within a day, two at the most, really, I just wasn't hungry anymore. It was like it wasn't me! I couldn't believe it. I didn't want to eat anything . . . I mean I was hungry but I wasn't starving, you know."

"It was like nothing I've ever seen in her," her mother continued. "After school, she would get lost in her room and forget to come out for dinner. I mean, I used to have to push past her to try and get dinner ready and I'd be yelling at her all the time for picking at the food while I was still trying to get it on the table and now . . . Tell them about Julie's phone call," her mother encouraged.

"Okay," Jennifer began. "Well, yesterday my friend Julie called just as I was walking in the door after school. I went to my room and we talked for a long time. The next thing I knew, my mother was calling me for dinner. I had forgotten about my snack, I mean I completely forgot about it. That has never, ever happened," she added.

"And one more thing, I'm not as tired after school. I used to come home, eat, and a lot of times watch some TV and fall asleep until dinner. Twice this week I finished my homework before dinner. That's never happened before, either."

We were pleased and so were Jennifer and her mother. But the best was yet to come. Jennifer had lost over six pounds in two weeks. We explained that her weight loss was a bit too fast and we wanted the pounds to come off slowly and steadily, without effort.

"But it was, you know, no effort," Jennifer protested. "I wasn't even trying to take off the weight that fast. I'm just not hungry. It's not me, it's just that I Jump-Started really well," she added triumphantly.

We could not help but share in her enthusiasm, but we explained that we didn't want her to stay on The Jump-Start Plan for a prolonged period of time. Though the weight loss might slow, we wanted her to shape a program that she could live with for the rest of her life.

And, in the weeks and months that followed, we helped Jennifer move into the second phase of her plan, slowly increasing the number of meals that contained carbohydrate-rich foods. Though she preferred the quick changes and impressive weight loss of the first phase of The Jump-Start Plan, Jennifer adapted to the less demanding lifestyle changes that came with the second phase of the Plan, and her weight loss continued, a bit more slowly but steadily.

At her six-month check-in, Jennifer arrived dressed casually in jeans and a peasant blouse, tucked in at the waist! Though she was no taller, her slim appearance made her look long and lean. Happily she told us of her successes: in the program, at school, and, of course, in her social life.

"I've got two boyfriends," she confided, "but they aren't both really *boyfriend* boyfriends, one is still like a friend—right now. He used to tease me before but he says it was 'cause he really liked me. I'm not sure but Mom says it's okay." She shrugged. Our eyes met her mother's and we smiled.

"Dr. Martin[2] says I'm at a perfect weight. He says I'm just right. When he asked me if it was hard, I almost laughed. I told him what was hard was trying to deal with those little tiny diet meals or drinking that stuff or taking those pills. This is easy."

Jennifer looked at us solemnly and added, "It really is. I'm not hungry or anything. I can't believe it."

But we could. And we have seen the same success in youngster after youngster. When you give them a livable pro-

---

[2]In all cases, names and identifying details have been changed.

gram that corrects the cause of their cravings, you give them the "fighting chance" they need.

Last week we received a photo and an unsigned note in the mail. Jennifer, now two and a half years older and pretty as ever, was pictured next to a tall, wide-shouldered young man. Jennifer's white dress offset her beautiful dark hair, and her smile was sweet and genuine. She stood straight and proud and slim and looked truly happy; the prettiest girl at the prom, we were sure.

We read the note that accompanied her photo. It bore a few sentences in Jennifer's distinctive hand. "This is Tom; he's the one who used to tease me. Guess what else, the guy who used to go with Ann Marie just asked me out, too. He doesn't go out with Ann Marie anymore but I'm still not sure if I should go out with him anyway."

This, we agreed, would take some careful deliberation and consideration. After all, not every contingency is covered by The Carbohydrate Addict's Program for Children and Teens.

A Final Note

Parents of carbohydrate-addicted youngsters who struggle with their weight often vacillate between concern and frustration, guilt and hopelessness. We want you to know that if you are the parent of a youngster who is overweight or simply struggling to keep his or her weight "in check," this book was written with both you and your youngster in mind.

In addition to the practical help each chapter provides, you will also discover support in understanding and dealing with the feelings that go along with being a concerned parent, in dealing with well-meaning friends and family, and in coping with any other youngsters in the household who may not be carbohydrate-addicted. You will learn that much can be done to help resolve your youngster's weight problem. By changing the frequency, the quality, and the balance of carbos in your youngster's diet, you can normalize your youngster's insulin levels. Normal insulin levels can reduce or eliminate your youngster's cravings and stop the surplus storage of fat—without any need for artificial limitation or regulation.

The Carbohydrate Addict's Program for Children and Teens can help your youngster reach and maintain ideal insulin levels, without deprivation or sacrifice. With this balance established and maintained, you can help your youngster keep cravings low and weight right on target.

Take time to read all the chapters in this book; do not simply skim the pages or jump to the Program guidelines. The help that your child may need the most might well be on the pages that you have skipped. Do not help your child begin the Program until you have completed the entire book. You will find answers to questions and strategies to help ensure success all along the way.

But do take your time. After all, you both deserve it.

six

The Many Faces of Carbohydrate Addiction,

Part 2: Focusing In on Moods, Motivation, Learning, and Attention

Each day at least two million of America's children struggle to overcome a wide variety of emotional and learning problems that include, among others, hyperactivity, impulsivity, inattention, mood swings, inability to concentrate, and lack of motivation.[1] The prevalence of these problems may go far beyond the two million mark depending on who is speaking for or about the youngster, where the youngster lives, and his or her age and gender.

In one epidemiological study in England, for instance, only two children out of 2,199 were diagnosed as hyperactive (less that one-tenth of one percent). A study in Israel, on the other

---

[1]There are many causes for eating, weight, behavioral, learning, and emotional problems in youngsters, as in adults. It is essential to rule out any other cause for your youngster's difficulties before embarking on this program.

hand, found that 28 percent of children were rated as hyperactive by their teachers. In the United States, an earlier study reported that teachers rated almost 50 percent of boys as restless and over 40 percent as having a "short attention span" or being "inattentive to what others say." Some of these youngsters have been diagnosed as having attention deficit disorder (ADD). Others have not.

There is no single definition of this widespread and apparently growing set of problems or a single determination of its cause, most likely because we are looking at a group of disorders that have many different causes and manifest themselves in many different ways. In some cases, a congenital cause—one that was present at birth—lies at the root of a youngster's behavior, learning, or mood problems. In other cases, no such precise origin or reason can be attributed.

As in so many things, each child is different. And whether or not youngsters have been given an "official" diagnosis of ADD, whether carbohydrate addiction is the central cause of a youngster's problems or acts in combination with other problems, we have found that many children and teens show dramatic improvement in behavior, learning, mood, and interpersonal interaction when they follow this program.

While you must certainly pursue all appropriate avenues to determine and treat other possible causes of your youngster's difficulties, if your youngster is carbohydrate-addicted, you will most likely find that this program will be of great benefit.

Normal-weight and overweight carbohydrate-addicted kids alike often experience one or more difficulties that fall into three main categories: *hyperactivity* (including excessive running and climbing, inability or unwillingness to stay in one's classroom seat, fidgeting), *impulsivity* (including difficulties in waiting to be called on or in waiting turns, and repeatedly interrupting others), and *inattention* (including lack of organizational skills, lack of interest, forgetfulness, losing things). In addition, many parents also report difficulties involving mood and motivation.

> **Many carbohydrate-addicted kids have a
> "propensity for problems" that include
> a range of behavior, mood, and learning difficulties.
> Some have been diagnosed as having ADD or ADHD.**

Some, but not all, carbohydrate-addicted youngsters seem to have what has been termed a "propensity for problems": difficulties at home or at school, problems in relating to peers (sometimes with the exception of one or two special friends), low self-esteem, or an unwillingness or inability to abide by rules or to keep promises. Their difficulties seem to be cyclical: spiraling downward in a whirlpool of problems at home or at school, followed by a short reprieve during which parents and child alike may think they have made some headway, followed by a reemergence of the same problems or new challenges.

Some carbohydrate-addicted youngsters have been diagnosed with learning disabilities, some have been described as "destructive," some may show signs of depression or anxiety or both. Some youngsters are "clingy," some are unwilling to give or accept affection, some alternate between being physically aggressive and demanding of affection to being almost pathologically aloof. Still others become unusually attached to special objects or pieces of clothing, collections of objects, or a special pet.

It is not uncommon for some carbohydrate-addicted youngsters to be described as being hyperkinetic or having hyperactive child syndrome, attention deficit disorder, attention deficit hyperactivity disorder (ADHD), or minimal brain dysfunction and dyslexic-like syndrome.

Though the numbers suffering from carbohydrate-related emotional, behavioral, and mood-related problems is staggering, the good news is that in recent years there have been great advances in mapping and understanding the physical drives that govern food cravings, new insights into the ways in which our bodies use and store food energy, and important breakthroughs in the relationship between diet and behavior.

The Lowdown on Low Blood Sugar

As discussed in Chapter 3, in carbohydrate-addicted kids excess insulin levels may throw off vital blood sugar balance; cells may be inundated with an unneeded excess of blood sugar or left starving for their critical share of food energy; or, more likely, first one, then the other. Blood sugar swings can bring on adrenaline releases that result in extremes in increased activity as well as mood swings and a youngster's inability to concentrate or to control impulses.

Within one to two hours after eating carbohydrate-rich foods, a great proportion of young carbohydrate addicts find themselves unable to concentrate, unable to think clearly, or vulnerable to major changes in mood or alterations in awareness—all the result of dramatic blood sugar swings (sometimes made worse by sharp rises in adrenaline).

Although we touched on the topic of low blood sugar in Chapter 3, some additional information may help you fully appreciate the many ways in which blood sugar levels may be shaping your youngster's behavior, ability to learn, mood-reactiveness, and motivation. If, in the future, you want others to understand the link between your youngster's addiction to carbohydrates and behavioral, learning, motivation, and mood problems; if you want your spouse, family, or friends, and your youngster's teacher, counselor, or physician to understand the importance of this connection, we want you to be prepared with the facts. So let's start with the basics.

First, a clarification: There are several causes of low blood sugar, that is, *hypoglycemia.* The first type is found less often in the carbohydrate-addicted youngster. This is called *fasting hypoglycemia,* and it occurs when blood sugar levels drop slowly because of prolonged lack of food intake. If a youngster suffers from fasting hypoglycemia because he or she is unwilling or unable to eat, a cause and correction must be sought. This program was *not* developed with fasting hypoglycemia in mind. Rather, this program was designed to help correct a second type of low blood sugar, called *reactive hypoglycemia,* which occurs when blood sugar levels fall quickly (often due to the body's inability to appropriately distribute food energy because of high levels of insulin in the blood).[2]

> **In the midst of an overload of calorie-laden foods,
> the vulnerable bodies of young carbohydrate addicts
> of any weight may be starving for nourishment.**

Carbohydrate-addicted youngsters (whether normal-weight, underweight, or overweight) suffer repeated and often undiagnosed episodes of reactive hypoglycemia (low blood sugar). In the midst of an overload of calorie-laden foods, their vulnerable bodies may be starving for nourishment. Like the spendthrift who uses up all his or her money and is left with too little money on which to live, the *underweight* hypoglycemic quickly burns up both excess blood sugar and the minimal amount of essential blood sugar as well. Like the far-too-thrifty person who puts all the money into the bank and doesn't leave enough money to live on, the *overweight* hypoglycemic youngster channels too much blood sugar out of the bloodstream into waiting fat cells. Like a person who has money but is unable or unwilling to spend it on life's necessities, the *normal-weight* hypoglycemic youngster may appear to maintain an ideal weight level but, at the same time, his or her muscles, nervous system, and organs may not be receiving their desperately needed nourishment.

> **Sugar highs and sugar lows may be
> literally running your youngster's life.**

In all these cases, though carbo-addicted youngsters may overload on what appears to be excess sources of quick food energy, they are almost bound to find that, in time, not enough blood

---

[2]For a more detailed discussion of insulin and blood sugar levels in carbohydrate-addicted youngsters, see page 63.

sugar remains in their bloodstream to keep them going. They may burn it up in hyperactive responses or store it too readily in ever-waiting fat cells, but in either case, sugar highs and sugar lows may be literally running and ruining your youngster's life.

REACTIVE HYPOGLYCEMIA: SIGNS AND SIGNALS

An "official" diagnosis of reactive hypoglycemia (low blood sugar) calls for a five-hour laboratory sampling of blood, and even then results may be inconclusive, but here are some simple signs to help you determine if your Carbo Collector or Carbo Burner may have this blood sugar imbalance.

Within a short time after eating carbohydrate-rich foods, particularly simple sugars, Carbo Burners and Carbo Collectors[3] alike may become hypoglycemic.

Do you find that, within an hour or two after eating, your youngster:

- Shows extremes in energy levels—becoming *either* hyperactive or sluggish, tired, and drowsy—or vacillating between one and the other?
- Becomes unmotivated or experiences mood changes?
- Appears confused or uncoordinated?
- Starts to perspire without reason?
- Becomes irritable, distant, or isolated?
- Has difficulty focusing or simply sits and stares (or falls asleep)?
- Gets a headache, feels faint or shaky?
- Intensely craves more carbohydrate-rich foods?

If your youngster has one or more of these signs after eating carbohydrate-rich foods, he or she may be experiencing reactive hypoglycemia, and frequent and unbalanced carbos may be the culprit.

---

[3]For a more detailed description of Carbo Burners and Carbo Collectors see discussion beginning on page 63.

Hypoglycemia:
The Disappearing Diagnosis

When we were young, the signs of hypoglycemia[4] were recognized by the physician as well as by the average person. If it happened once in a while you were told to eat a bit of protein, and that would make you feel better. If it happened more frequently, your physician gave you a diet that was high in protein and low in sugars that would keep your blood sugar levels balanced throughout the day.

> **Today many health professionals seem
> quite reluctant to give a diagnosis of hypoglycemia.**

Today there is an odd and unexplainable trend in medicine. Just when hypoglycemia appears to be far more widespread than ever before, the medical establishment appears to be almost intent on disproving that reactive hypoglycemia exists.

Statistics on hypoglycemia are getting more difficult to obtain and will be almost impossible to produce in the future. The Endocrine Society and the American Diabetes Association have issued a joint statement declaring essentially that hypoglycemia appears to be greatly overdiagnosed and some reports question that such a condition as hypoglycemia even exists.

These dramatic shifts in attitude about a disorder from which so many suffer appear to stem from several studies that found that about one in four apparently healthy people report no hypoglycemic symptoms at the same time that they exhibit low blood sugar levels. Questioning the existence of a disorder because a small portion of people who have the problem don't have the same symptoms as others makes absolutely no sense to us, and it is unlike the way the medical establishment deals with almost any other disorder.

---

[4] Unless otherwise indicated, the term "hypoglycemia" will be used to indicate the medical condition reactive hypoglycemia only.

To get a real perspective, take another disorder, high blood pressure for instance, and look at how that medical problem is viewed. As you know, some people who have high blood pressure may not have any symptoms; they may not even realize they have a problem until they are told by their doctors. Other people with high blood pressure, on the other hand, may feel lightheaded, get headaches, or experience warm flushes. The fact that some people with high blood pressure do not have noticeable symptoms, however, does not negate the symptoms of others with high blood pressure, nor does it indicate that there is no such disorder as high blood pressure; that kind of thinking just doesn't make sense in relation to high blood pressure, anymore than it does in relation to hypoglycemia.

Yet today, to be given an "official" diagnosis of hypoglycemia, one has to undergo a lengthy laboratory test in which a liquid sugar drink (glucose) is consumed and blood is sampled, periodically, for the next five hours. The test is difficult as well as expensive for adults, and virtually overwhelmingly challenging for kids. And an official diagnosis of hypoglycemia will be made only when laboratory technicians note blood sugar levels of about half normal fasting levels at *exactly the same time* as the typical sweating, weakness, tremors, and other signs of hypoglycemia are experienced. Even then, there is the question of what are "normal" blood sugar levels among nonadults under such artificial circumstances.

To make matters worse, the assumption that sugar in the blood means that blood sugar is available for use by the cells that need it most is questionable. We now know that many people, especially those with long-term high blood insulin levels, are prone to be "insulin resistant" and that their muscles and organs may not take in the very energy that lies only a membrane-width away from the cells that need it. Insulin resistant youngsters may at times show high levels of blood sugar, but they may at the same time be "starving" for the very energy the blood sugar could provide if the cells could only take it in. As their young bodies compensate, their blood sugar levels can drop and drop fast from one moment to another. For these youngsters, blood sugar levels may reveal little, if any, useful information for a diagnosis of hypoglycemia.

> **It is no wonder that so few people know how to
> spot signs of low blood sugar or what to do about it.**

Given the almost impossible requirements for a diagnosis of hypoglycemia, it is no wonder that so few adults, much less children and adolescents, can get confirmation of this problem or help in getting rid of it.

The reasoning behind the current, almost bizarre attitude toward hypoglycemia escapes us. Scientists continue to document hypoglycemia's powerful influence as well as its connection to excess levels of insulin in the blood. Dr. J. T. Devlin and Dr. E. S. Horton in their medical textbook *Modern Nutrition in Health and Disease* noted that "insulin's hypoglycemic effect is potent, and when present in sufficient quantity, insulin can cause hypoglycemia despite the actions of all known counter-regulatory factors."

Yet in the face of this and so many other studies, the trend is to deny that reactive hypoglycemia is the widespread problem that has been documented by scientists and experienced by so many patients. We are truly at a loss to explain why so many in the medical establishment seem to want to act as if this problem does not exist. Whatever the reason, this problem will not be denied, nor will it go away by itself. As we see our youngsters falter and fall under its powerful influence, we must not be talked out of trusting our own perceptions of our youngsters' very real reactions.

*The Great Disrupter:
How Sweet It Isn't*

You may have been told that scientists have disproved any link between sugar consumption and hyperactivity, or sugar consumption and mood swings. We have found that nothing could be further from the truth.

It is true, indeed, that several researchers have compared sugar-laden drinks with a "control" drink (one that contained no sugar) and found no significant differences in behavior, activity, or mood in youngsters who had one type of drink or the other. That is not to say that these youngsters showed no signs of hyperactivity, inability to concentrate, mood swings, or the like. These scientists simply observed that there were no *differences* in the intensity or incidence of behavioral, learning, or mood problems in youngsters who had consumed either of the drinks. These same researchers then went on to conclude, wrongly, that since no differences were observed in behavior or learning or mood after subjects consumed what researchers assumed to be two different drinks, sugar (contrary to what so many parents have observed) did *not* provoke these problems.

The grand error that these researchers made, however, was that the drink to which the sugar-sweetened beverage was compared was sweetened with a sugar substitute. Since youngsters' bodies may perceive and react to artificially sweetened beverages much in the same way as they do to sugar-sweetened beverages, it is not surprising that these scientists found no differences after consumption of *either* drink. Following the consumption of either of the two sweet-tasting drinks, insulin is bound to pour into the bloodstream, and so the nervous systems of these youngsters would be expected to pulsate with excitement and energy. Hyperactivity or mood swings, especially in the carbohydrate-sensitive youngster, would be a predictable outcome after either sweet-tasting drink is consumed.

> **It many cases, sweet drinks that contain "real" sugar or sugar substitute can lead to behavior problems.**

The crucial point these researchers missed is that it is not what is *in* the drink that matters (whether it contains "real" sugar or sugar substitute), but rather how a youngster's body *responds* to the drink. In this case, all sweet-tasting drinks seem to bring about the same reaction in kids who are predisposed to hyperactivity, or mood changes, or the like. It makes no difference to many of these youngsters' bodies whether the sweet drink contains "real" sugar or sugar substitute.

Comparing behavior after the consumption of two sweet drinks makes as little sense as comparing behavior after the consumption of two different brands of cola—there may be a different label on the front of each but the body is generally going to react to both drinks in pretty much the same way. We may perceive subtle but important differences in taste, but in the general scheme of things, our bodies consider them, and will react to them, in similar ways.

If these researchers had wanted to determine if, indeed, sugar was the behavior disrupter that so many parents have witnessed, it would have made far more sense to compare a sugar-sweetened drink with plain water and then observed differences in youngsters' behavior. We believe that they would have witnessed the great differences that we ourselves have seen.

Health professionals, teachers, and counselors may wrongly advise parents that sugar-related hyperactivity and mood swings are nothing but a myth.

It is of great concern to us that, when it comes to what science has to say about what goes into your youngster's mouth, powerful financial and political influences are in play. Great vested interests have supported so many "scientific studies" that have made their way into medical journals and onto the evening news that it is hard to keep count. Indeed, many well-respected medical and scientific journals have published "supplements," collections of scientific reports that are supposed to investigate one particular issue, such as sugar consumption, for instance, but that, at the same time, may be funded entirely or in part by the very industry that produces the same foods these researchers are supposed to be investigating. One must assume that this may be a clear case of conflict of interest. These scientists' "findings" may be nothing more that "biased science." Yet these same "findings" may have a powerful influence in determining what you hear on the latest news report about the impact of a food or drink on your youngster's behavior, attitude, mood, ability to learn, and health.

When it comes to the reports that say they have "disproved" the sugar-hyperactivity connection, some of these scientists may have done real and permanent harm. For now, thinking they are backed by "valid" scientific research, physicians throughout the country may wrongly advise parents that sugar-related hyperactivity and mood swings are nothing more than a myth. To determine the truth, we want you to have a clear understanding of the deficiencies and the vested interests that may be influencing the research in this area, and we want to urge you to trust your own perceptions. Rather than convincing us that sugar is not harmful, we strongly believe these researchers may have simply proven that artificial sweetener can be just as bad as the "real thing."

Scientists in the Department of Pediatrics and Psychiatry at the University of Pittsburgh School of Medicine took a different approach, though they have confined their work, so far, to youngsters with juvenile diabetes. Not surprisingly, these scientists found that even mild low blood sugar levels caused temporary decreased functioning in the performance of youngsters' thinking tasks. Rather than attempting some artificial and complicated comparison between sugar-sweetened and sugar-substitute-sweetened drinks as so many other researchers have, these scientists simply did what parents do; they observed how well youngsters were able to handle mental challenges when their blood sugar levels were low. And, of course, they found that low blood sugar did indeed decrease a youngster's ability to think well.

Other researchers as well as parents have reported dramatic improvement in concentration, reduction in hyperactivity, and mood swings when additives were removed from their youngsters' diets. The premise was that many youngsters were allergic to colorings, preservatives, and the like that are added to the foods and that the undesired behaviors youngsters manifested were, in whole or in part, physical manifestations of their reactions to these allergens.

Allergen-free diets may be "accidentally" correcting your youngster's blood sugar fluctuations but they may call for unnecessary sacrifice and deprivation.

While many youngsters may be allergic to these substances, we found that many of them did even better on our program. At first we were at a loss to explain the relationship, but when we examined the allergen-free diets, we discovered the connection. The allergen-free diets that had called for the removal of all foods containing additives and preservatives and colorings had resulted in the removal, as well, of all heavily processed and highly sugared foods. For many of these youngsters, it was the removal of the simple sugar overload, rather than the allergens, that was helping to regulate their insulin and blood sugar levels and that led to the improvements in behavior, learning, and mood. Those youngsters with sensitivities to additives continued their allergen-free diets, of course, but many who thought they were sensitive to these substances found that, on this program, they achieved far more positive results, without sacrifice or deprivation.

Beyond the Great Sugar Debate

Taking a completely different approach to looking at sugar's influence on our youngsters, Dr. T. W. Jones and colleagues, reporting in the *Journal of Pediatrics* in 1995, examined the "mechanisms underlying the adverse effects of sugar ingestion in healthy children." These scientists examined the physical responses of youngsters between the ages of eight and sixteen as well as those of adults. All the youngsters and adults they studied had no history of diabetes or carbohydrate intolerance; none was taking medications or had any behavioral or psychological problems. After consuming a high-sugar (glucose) drink, blood samples were taken at regular intervals.

In this distinctive study, researchers found that, in response to their sugar drink, youngsters showed a markedly higher concentration of epinephrine (adrenaline) in the blood than did adults. The authors report that "Epinephrine [adrenaline] responses were exaggerated in children, even though a glucose load larger than the standard 75 to 100 gm was given to adults . . ." and add that "responses in the children were associated with an increase in symptoms such as feeling shaky and sweating, that are commonly attributed to stimulation of the sympathetic nervous system," which helps modulate and balances the body's internal system.

Dr. Jones's research team succeeded in doing what other researchers had failed to do: They documented that youngsters show an exaggerated adrenaline response to the consumption of sugar compared to adults because their young nervous systems are much more sensitive to reductions in blood sugar levels. Most important to parents is this report's conclusion that for healthy, symptom-free youngsters, the consumption of the amount of sugar roughly equal to that found in two twelve-ounce cans of cola or, we would add, in a sports drink, along with some cake or cookies or candy, is followed by enough of a fall in blood sugar to bring on both hormonal and neurological symptoms.

The consumption of sugar equal to that in two twelve-ounce cans of cola resulted in enough of a blood sugar drop to bring on both hormonal and neurological symptoms.

In looking over this research, it is even more remarkable to keep in mind that Dr. Jones and colleagues were studying the effects of sugar consumption on youngsters with no behavioral problems, who were taking no medications, and had no history of carbohydrate intolerance. One can only wonder how much more powerful their findings would have been had they observed the changes that come with sugar consumption when youngsters do indeed struggle with attentional, learning, mood, or behavior problems; when they are taking medications; or when they are known to be addicted to carbohydrates.

While there is still some debate about the exact physical mechanism that causes youngsters to experience hormonal mayhem and neurological agitation after they consume high-sugar drinks, parents can perhaps finally feel confirmed that the changes in behavior they have witnessed after their youngsters consume sugar-laden foods and drinks are not a figment of their imagination but, more likely, examples of their astute and discerning observations.

EXPERTS VERIFY WHAT PARENTS HAVE LONG SUSPECTED: THE POWERFUL DIET-BEHAVIOR CONNECTION

Let the Facts Speak for Themselves

"When I was a child," writes Dr. Thomas Armstrong in his book on attention deficit disorder, "Sunday morning breakfast usually consisted of some devilishly delicious sweet rolls my mother had gotten up early to bake. Sunday afternoons were spent sleeping them off (sometimes in church) or just feeling vaguely restless or irritable.

"It turns out," he continues, "that the effects of a sugar-laden high-carbohydrate breakfast of sweet rolls, or syrupy pancakes, or waffles dripping with jam, or even toast and butter, are particularly fierce on some biologically sensitive kids with attention and/or behavior problems."

Dr. Armstrong goes on to point out that, among other studies that have explored the diet-ADD link, "researchers at the George Washington University School of Medicine in Washington, D.C., gave high-carbohydrate breakfasts (two slices of toasted and buttered white bread) and high-protein breakfasts (two eggs scrambled in butter) to groups of 'hyperactive and non-hyperactive children' between the ages of eight and thirteen. Children in each group were given, on alternate days, a non-nutritive orange drink sweetened with either aspartame or sucrose. Blood samples were taken just before and up to four hours after the meals. Also, subjects took a brief test involving attention span at one-half hour, two hours, and four hours after breakfast."

Their results indicated that the "hyperactive kid" who consumed the carbohydrate breakfast and sugar drink did more poorly on the attention span test than any other kids in the study. On the other hand, when "hyperactive kids" ate a meal that was rich with protein, even though they had a sugary drink, they actually did better at the attention task than even the non-hyperactive groups. Dr. Armstrong goes on to report that the researchers proposed that "hyperactive children" may be more sensitive to changes in the brain chemical serotonin, which was brought about by the consumption of sugar and, we would add, other carbohydrates as well.

"Serotonin," explains Dr. Armstrong, "is the brain chemical that causes us to feel sleepy after a big meal (especially a meal that has a lot of carbohydrates in it). However, during the day it can also result in our feeling restless, irritable, or inattentive. Sudden surges of serotonin can also throw off levels of other neurotransmitters such as dopamine and norepinephrine. Protein, however, increases the level of amino acids, and these serve to block many of the effects of serotonin."

The upshot of the research, Dr. Armstrong concludes, as he brings his diet-ADD discussion to a conclusion, is that parents must provide their "hyperactive and inattentive kids" with breakfasts that are "balanced." (You will learn more about finding the Optimal Carbohydrate Balance for your youngster in the chapters to come.)

When two-time Nobel Prize-winning scientist Linus Pauling was told that certain hyperactive children's problems cleared up after removal of "sensitive" foods, he remarked, "It is from individual experiences of this sort that a great deal of progress has been made, rather than through double-blind controlled trials."

We believe that both individual experience and scientific experimentation are important means by which we can explore the diet-behavior connection.

Let's look at what the experts have to say regarding the carbohydrate–insulin–blood sugar–behavior link.

The very definition of the medical condition hypoglycemia (low blood sugar) indicates its powerful effect on the ability to think and function:

> Hypoglycemia—a deficiency in glucose in the bloodstream, causing muscular weakness and incoordination, mental confusion, and sweating.
> —*Bantam Medical Dictionary*, 1982

> Hypoglycemia is characterized by acute fatigue, restlessness, malaise [discomfort, uneasiness], marked irritability and weakness.
> —*Taber's Cyclopedic Medical Dictionary*, 1997

"Spontaneous reactive hypoglycemia is a poorly defined entity," conclude Drs. P. J. Lefebvre and A. J. Scheen, in their medical textbook chapter on hypoglycemia. These scientists go on to note that the symptoms occur when adrenaline is released in response to falling blood sugar levels or when nerve cells do not get enough blood sugar to function normally. These symptoms of hypoglycemia "are variable from one subject to another," and they include hunger, sweating, fast heartbeat, shakiness, and headache in addition to fatigue, drowsiness, feelings of growing faint or altered awareness, mind confusion, thirst, intense anxiety, irritability, and lack of motivation. And, these scientists add, "The symptoms may be episodic, sometimes aggravated by carbohydrate-rich meals. In addition, these researchers connect "abnormal insulin secretory patterns" to certain patients who suffer from this form of reactive hypoglycemia.

Other researchers have concern about the long-term effects of hypoglycemia:

Hyperinsulinemia, a common cause of persistent hypoglycemia in infants and children, can result in permanent damage to the central nervous system.
—R. L. Telander, et al., *Mayo Clin Proceedings*, 1986

(An important reason to correct the cause of the problem now!)

Hypoglycemia may contribute to or, in some, form the very basis of many allergic symptoms in youngsters. Dr. Doris Rapp, in her national best-selling book on discovering and treating allergies in youngsters, notes that many children who show allergic reactions to foods will, at the same time, show dramatic drops in blood sugar levels. These youngsters' symptoms, she concludes, include fatigue, irritability, mood swings, weakness, extreme hunger, wiggly legs, anxiety, and problems concentrating. If the blood sugar level should drop too far (below 60 mg/cc), she notes, "it can cause the brain to act sluggish or confused so that it becomes difficult to think, learn, remember, or act appropriately. Some children," she adds, "have this problem and learn poorly every day. They can't remember, get tired, become irritable, or misbehave, usually late in the morning and again late in the afternoon."

Dr. Rapp's research has revealed a rather large number of children who appear to act hypoglycemic every day and, at the same time, have blood sugar tests that are perfectly normal. "We give them a snack," she notes, "and in a few moments they, too, act normal." She adds that some of these youngsters "may have hypoglycemialike symptoms because they are addicted to a certain food . . . if they need their 'fix' they may have withdrawal symptoms." Dr. Rapp acknowledges, "As in much of medicine, what you've just read is not unanimously agreed upon among doctors."

But while physicians and researchers continue to explore the dynamics of the problem, hypoglycemia has been tied to behaviors so extreme as to be termed "delinquent." Publications by Alexander Schauss and Stephen Schoenthaler and books by Barbara Reed and Alexander Schauss indicate that delinquent behavior can, indeed, be related to diet. In support of the power of diet on "unacceptable behavior," one need only look to a final report of a one-year study of nineteen juvenile delinquents by one probation department in California that concluded that 80 percent of juvenile delinquents appeared to be hypoglycemic.

In an article published in the *Journal of Clinical Psychiatry*, Dr. Bonnie Spring and colleagues detail the sugar-insulin-hypoglycemia connection, noting that sugary foods can trigger hypoglycemia and its associated symptoms much the way that an injection of insulin might, that is, by means of low levels of blood sugar that can affect brain blood sugar levels and cause a release of adrenaline. "A reactive blood glucose fall to a hypo-glycemic level allegedly causes the behavioral effects of carbohydrate foods," they conclude.

And other researchers confirm and expand their findings. Drs. J. T. Devlin and E. S. Horton in their textbook *Modern Nutrition in Health and Disease* conclude, "Ingestion of carbohydrate produces a prompt increase in plasma insulin and a decrease in glucagon (the counter hormone to insulin) concentrations." They add, "When a carbohydrate-free protein meal[5] is ingested,

---

[5]These dietary alternatives constitute portions of both The Step-By-Step Plan and The Jump-Start Plan of The Carbohydrate Addict's Program for Children and Teens.

insulin concentrations increase [only] slightly and promote protein synthesis in skeletal muscle, with a parallel rise in glucagon, which prevents hypoglycemia."

It is not surprising, then, that after reviewing the research, Drs. Lefebvre and Scheen conclude, "Diet is the first treatment of alimentary and reactive hypoglycemia. Simple sugars should be omitted and replaced by complex carbohydrates," and "a high-protein, low-carbohydrate diet should be tried."[6]

The research results and conclusions above are a small sampling of the many findings and opinions of experts who have witnessed and reported on the diet-behavior connection. What they have to say may verify what you already know or suspect: that in many ways, your youngster's behaviors depend on what your youngster eats.

If your youngster is carbo-addicted, feelings, abilities, attitudes, behaviors, even his or her very personality, may be influenced by the foods and beverages consumed and the insulin and blood sugar swings that result.

---

[6]These dietary alternatives constitute portions of both The Step-By-Step Plan and The Jump-Start Plan of The Carbohydrate Addict's Program for Children and Teens.

Balanced Body, Balanced Mind

Whether your youngster is a Carbo Collector or a Carbo Burner; whether carbohydrates make your child or teen hyperactive, or lethargic, or first one then the other; whether or not your youngster would benefit by losing weight—if your youngster is drawn to carbohydrate-rich foods with recurring or intense cravings, this program can help correct the underlying imbalance that lies at the core of the problem.

Within a matter of days on the Program that follows, your youngster's excess levels of insulin should begin to normalize, and with it, insulin-related carbo cravings as well as weight, behavior, mood, learning, and motivation problems can resolve—naturally. As one parent so aptly put it, "I feel like I have my child back again. I almost forgot how wonderful that could be."

Alex in Charge:
A Very Special Story, Part 2

We talked to Alex directly and explained in simple terms what the Program might do for him and what he in turn would have to do. He agreed to try it, somewhat unsure of what was involved, then added, "I just want to get rid of this itchy feeling; I hate it and then, all of a sudden, everyone's yelling at me. It's not my fault," he said, revealing what we knew was Alex's personal truth.

After Alex's pediatrician was consulted, Alex began the Program using The Step-By-Step Plan in which he would gradually add one thing at a time to one meal each day. With his parents' help, Alex's only job was to make sure that he balanced his carbohydrate-rich lunches (which often included pizza, chips, juice, fruit, and cookies) with a good portion of leftover chicken or roast beef, a burger, or an all-meat hot dog or two. "Not just a slice of lunch meat," we cautioned, "a nice-sized portion." We added that if he wanted to get an extra jump on his program, he could do the same for his after-school snack.

We explained that the protein-rich food he would be adding to his carbo-rich lunch and snacks was meant to help keep his blood sugar levels more constant and reduce the cravings that drove him to seek additional carbos, which, in turn, started the low blood sugar–carbo-craving cycle all over again.

We kept in touch by phone, and at our next monthly meeting Alex was all smiles, and so was his mother. "It's incredible. All he did was make some simple changes and he's like a different kid. After school," she continued, "he used to slam through the front door and head straight for the refrigerator and grab some soda and cookies, and he was literally nonstop until he collapsed at night. He barely stopped for dinner, just grabbed something and kept going. Now he can do homework, and yesterday he sat down and told me what he did at school. His teacher wrote a note home, and I don't want to jinx it, but it's almost too good to be true."

Alex, unexpectedly open, had a report of his own success to add. "My teacher used to hate me. I know it. She used to scream at me all the time but the worst thing was when she had to go on an errand. She'd put one of the kids in charge of the whole class and they would all stay there except me. She used to make me go with her."

We waited in anticipation.

"Well, yesterday, when she left the room, she called me to the front and I figured she was going to make me go with her. I used to hate that. All the kids would make fun of me and call me 'baby' but this time, she put me in charge. She said, 'Alex, while I'm away, you're in charge and everyone has to listen to you' and they all did. She said I did a great job and that's when she sent the note home."

He looked up with what seemed like the proudest smile we had ever seen.

"Well done," we thought, and we smiled, too, knowing that from now on it would no longer be unusual to find Alex in charge.

seven

Carbohydrate-Addicted Kids: Classic Categories,

Can You Spot Your Youngster?

Make no mistake: carbohydrate-addicted kids come in all shapes, sizes, and varieties. There is no one profile. They show different signs of their addictions, in different ways, at different ages.

Here are some of the classic types of carbo-addicted kids we have encountered. Some youngsters fit into more than one category; others seem to be in a class by themselves.

The descriptions that follow may help you spot carbohydrate addiction in your own child as well as in others.

Locusts

These kids eat anything and everything, and they appear to be hungry all the time. They are voracious consumers of food although, depending on how well their young bodies burn up the onslaught of calories, they may be slim, normal-weight, or overweight. Overweight young Locusts are often blamed for their weight problems based on the assumption that they are fat basically because they eat too much. Not true! Slim Locusts often eat just as much as those who are overweight, and while activity is an important variable, a great deal depends on how the body itself handles the rush of calories.

Slim or overweight, the young Locust is driven by recurring hunger and cravings that signal an almost ever-present insulin imbalance that can take its toll on the youngster's emotional, psychological, intellectual and physical health. Do not be fooled! Still-slim Locusts can be as much at risk for insulin and low blood sugar–related problems as are overweight kids; perhaps even more, for the slim Locust's voracious hunger and cravings are more likely to be mistakenly attributed to an appetite that is "normal" in a growing youngster.

The good news is that the Carbohydrate Addict's Program for Children and Teens puts no limits on the amount of food the young Locust is allowed to eat. At the same time, the Program corrects the cause of the youngster's cravings and hunger so that a normal appetite emerges, one that peaks with hunger but that is, in time, satisfied with healthy, normal-sized portions of a variety of foods. For the Locust on this program, satisfaction is no longer fleeting, and the youngster's mind and body have time to recover.

Rabbits

Carbohydrate-addicted Rabbits seem to be always on the go. Like the furry variety, these Rabbits prefer nibbling rather than consuming large meals. If they had their choice, Rabbits would live on snack foods, junk food, sandwiches, and sweets. Unlike the animals from which they get their name, Rabbits do *not* favor salad vegetables as a mainstay of their daily diet, but rather, if allowed to, would live on chips, cookies, sodas, and other snacks and sweets.

Rabbits are often active kids, eating on the run, and parents are often at a loss to get them to eat anything that even remotely resembles a "real meal." Occasionally Rabbits may struggle with excess weight but often they are normal-weight (sometimes even underweight). Rabbits are vulnerable to the same health, psychological, learning, and emotional problems as any other carbohydrate-addicted kids.

The Carbohydrate Addict's Program for Children and Teens is a wonderful alternative for Rabbits, giving them the freedom to choose foods they enjoy while cutting the carbo cravings that often limit their willingness to eat "real food."

Bears

Bears are often renowned for the amounts of food they can consume, and like their furry counterparts, Bears get sluggish or tired after eating. Many Bears gain weight as winter approaches, and though their eating may not change from season to season, they often "naturally" lose weight during the summer months. Parents may be tempted into thinking that summer-slimming indicates the carbo addiction will resolve itself, but the pounds usually return with the onset of winter.

If not given appropriate help, Bears will continue to gain and lose weight with each major change in season, and the degree of weight change will often increase with each passing decade. As youngsters, Bears often suffer from low blood sugar swings that lead to depression or loss of motivation as winter approaches. Some parents may attribute these changes to a type of school phobia but the problem may be much more of a seasonal affective disorder-like problem. The frequent intake of carbos that Bears so love may be literally feeding the problem.

As Bears reach adulthood, seasonal-related weight changes often increase, and health-related problems can gain a firm foothold. The Carbohydrate Addict's Program for Children and Teens can help put your Bear back on the right track. On this program, your youngster will discover a wide variety of easy-to-follow alternatives that will help smooth summer-winter weight and energy fluctuations and help focus, motivate, and keep slim the Bear in your family.

Sponges

As their name implies, Sponges will soak up almost any type of liquid. From soda to fruit juice, sports drinks to chocolate milk, if it's fluid it disappears in the presence of a Sponge. Eternally thirsty, these lovers of liquid, drink as if they had been touring the Sahara. While all Sponges consume great quantities of liquid in either short spurts or consistently over time, they vary greatly in the amount of food they eat.

Sponges who, in addition to drinking a great deal, also eat great amounts of snack foods, junk food, and sweets are more easily identified as carbohydrate addicts by their parents and other relatives. Sponges who eat relatively small portions or a wide variety of foods, however, may not be recognized as having an addiction to carbos, and the carbo connection to their mood swings, learning or motivational difficulties, or weight problems may be missed.

Although Sponges may appear to be indulging in so-called healthy drinks, youngsters who experience recurring cravings for fruit juices, low-fat chocolate milk, sports drinks, and regular or diet sodas are simply exhibiting signs of a carbohydrate addiction. Repeated onslaughts of these drinks can shock the body with insulin insults and trigger rebounding low blood sugar cycles, creating a strong potential for weight and health problems, now and in the future. Even plain low-fat milk can spike your youngster's insulin levels if he or she has an genetic tendency to carbohydrate addiction.

If water is not your Sponge's beverage of choice, and if a never-ending parade of drinks finds its way into your youngster's grip, the Program that follows will help your Sponge get off the liquid sugar merry-go-round that may be running and ruining both of your lives.

Fruit Bats

Fruit Bats can usually be found in near proximity to the food that gives them their name. From grapes to melons, from fresh fruit to dried, one hand of the Fruit Bat is usually wrapped around something that's sweet and seemingly "healthy." Cherries, oranges, apples, peaches; what could be wrong? The answer: lots!

Fruit *is not* a complex carbohydrate. It contains *simple sugars*, and if your youngster is prone to carbohydrate addiction, the steady intake of fruit can cause the same insulin and blood sugar imbalances that come from frequent consumption of any other type of sugar. While the fiber and vitamin benefits of fruit cannot be denied, for the carbohydrate-addicted youngster, the continual intake of simple sugars can cause far more damage than a parent would ever suspect.

If anyone has told you that fruit is not fattening, think again. In itself, *a* fruit may not be fattening, but, as always, it's not what's in the food but what the food does to *your* youngster's body. For youngsters prone to carbohydrate addiction, fruit—either fresh or dried—can trigger the carbo-insulin connection to emotional, psychological, learning, and weight-related problems.

Some Fruit Bats are also Sponges, consuming fruit juice by the gallon. Remember that the human body was never designed to eat fruit all year long, or to handle the high sugar onslaught of juice (which is far more concentrated than when it is in its natural state, combined with the fiber of the whole fruit). While fruit has a wonderful public image, for the carbohydrate addict it may not be as "innocent" as you think.

Parents often have a difficult time accepting the idea that fruit might be a problem for their kids. If you cannot help but see fruit as an excellent snack choice, consider the following scenario. Imagine for a moment that every time your youngster eats strawberries, he or she breaks out in hives. Regardless of the healthy image that strawberries engender, most likely you would not allow your youngster to eat strawberries. You would find another way to ensure that your child got the nutritional benefit of this food without risking an allergic reaction.

In the same way, consider that your youngster responds to the frequent intake of fruit with insulin and blood sugar changes that are harder to see than the easily visible hives we have described.

Mood swings, activity-level spikes and drops, learning and motivation problems, and repeated cravings for more fruit or other carbos are rarely attributed to the frequent intake of fruit that is indeed causing the underlying insulin imbalance. If Fruit Bats continue their fruit addiction, weight problems can emerge in childhood or adolescence, or, for some, in adulthood.

Do not be fooled into thinking that all-fruit sweetened jams, cookies, or fruit rolls are addiction-free. Remember, fructose (fruit sugar) is a *simple* sugar, even simpler than table sugar (sucrose), and can cause the same sugar responses that any sugar can cause. The Carbohydrate Addict's Program for Children and Teens will allow your Fruit Bat to enjoy the fruit he or she loves, every day, while cutting the cravings that drive the Fruit Bat repeatedly to come back for more.

Whatever your type of carbohydrate-addicted kid, remember that the behavior is not the child. More often, your youngster's behaviors indicate what is going on inside, and given a balanced body, your child can be given the greatest chance of doing his or her best.

CAN YOU SPOT YOUR CARBO-ADDICTED KID?

These descriptions make it easy to spot a carbohydrate addict right before your eyes!

LOCUST
Whether slim or overweight, the Locust seems to be ever-hungry and can consume great quantities of food. Parents may be unsure if they're observing a "healthy" appetite or an addiction to carbohydrates.

RABBIT
Often very active, this nibbler would prefer to eat on the run, surviving on only snack foods, junk food, sandwiches, and sweets. Rabbits come in all shapes and sizes, and the parent of a rabbit may not realize that mood swings, extremes in

activity levels, and difficulties in concentration may be linked to an underlying carbo addiction.

BEAR

A dedicated lover of starches, snack foods, junk food, and sweets, a Bear can consume these foods in great quantities, and often feels tired and sluggish after eating. These kids often have a tendency to put on pounds easily, and changing seasons can bring changes in their appetite, activity levels, and weight.

SPONGE

If it's liquid, it disappears in the presence of the Sponge. Eternally thirsty, these kids consume great quantities of regular or artificially sweetened soda, sports drinks, fruit juice and fruit-flavored drinks, iced tea, lemonade, and the like. All these quick-response fluids in addition to milk (regular, low-fat, or chocolate-flavored) can feed the Sponge's carbo addiction. The thirst that drives a Sponge is usually a recurring craving for liquid carbos, or artificially flavored carbo taste-alikes, rather than a physical call for fluid. Sponges can experience the same low blood sugar–related problems as do other carbo-addicted youngsters.

FRUIT BAT

Great and frequent consumers of fruit of many kinds (fresh, canned, or dried), a Fruit Bat (of any weight) may appear to be eating "healthy" foods. Parents may miss the carbo connection that may be causing low blood sugar–related psychological, emotional, mood, learning, or weight problems.

For more detailed descriptions, see pages 136–141.

The Carbohydrate Addict's Program for Children and Teens

eight

Getting Ready: Strategies for Success Before You Begin

You and your youngster are about to embark on an exciting and promising journey—a journey that, with your help, could lead your youngster to a far healthier and happier life. Others may decide to come along as well, in their own time, and they may join you along the way. On this journey, you and your youngster will see and learn things you have never experienced before, pleasant surprises and unanticipated discoveries.

Although at times you both may encounter unexpected obstacles and challenges, we will try our best to offer the guidance and support you need every step of the way, so that you, too, can experience the triumph of success and the deep satisfaction of a victory worth striving for.

Most importantly, you and your youngster will change and grow together.

As you continue on this journey, you will have the gratification of witnessing firsthand the many ways in which your decisions, choices, and actions have helped—in real and measurable ways—to make your youngster healthier in mind, body, and spirit. As with any trip, planning is the key to making it a positive experience, so that it may best meet your needs and get you where you want to go. So, with the road ahead and waiting, let's prepare to get started.

Three Rights Can't Go Wrong

The ideal situation in life has been described as having three facets: the person with whom you want to be, all the time you desire, and all the resources you need to enjoy them both. Similarly, we have found that, when making any change, it is best if possible to bring together three elements: the right people and the right plan at the right time. We would add that the change should be made for the right reasons as well.

The Right People

As you prepare to help your youngster get started on the Program, the first question to ask is, "Who can help *me* to help my youngster be successful?" Ironically, when they are faced with almost any new endeavor, this is often one of the last questions many people consider. This question is usually posed when things do not go as anticipated, in desperation, and when all else has failed. But asking this question first, not last, can help you get the support and help you need to ensure success from the start.

Some parents challenge the importance of support. "I'd rather do it myself," they say. "It's easier, and when you deal with someone else, it's just not worth the hassle." Some of them are absolutely right. That decision, however, depends on knowing yourself and your youngster. If you and your youngster can communicate well, even when your child is not getting what he or she wants at the moment; if you are not likely to become the scapegoat for your youngster's feelings of frustration; if your youngster is able to understand and keep in mind—beyond the passion of the moment—that your intentions are only those of a loving parent, with his or her best interests in mind, then it is quite possible that you can "go it alone."

If, on the other hand, on the journey ahead you could use a few other hands, hearts, minds, and souls to help keep you sane and focused and to offer ideas and perspective when you need them most, then by all means consider enlisting some help before you begin.

Some parents with whom we have worked are quick to assume that not asking for help is best because, deep down, they did not think they could count on anyone else. Do not make that assumption. First, read the pages that follow. You may find valuable support in the most unexpected places, and you may discover some delightful surprises along the way.

Before securing support from the "right people" in your youngster's life, we strongly suggest that you finish reading this book, taking notes along the way if you wish, so that you have a complete understanding of what is involved and why it is being suggested before you attempt to explain the Program to someone else. After you've read the book, we recommend that you discuss the Program with the following people in the following order.

Primary Relationships Getting real-life support from your spouse, ex-spouse, mate, and/or the other parent of your child is a bit of a complex proposition. Securing full and genuine help can make your endeavor easier and, in some cases, more rewarding.

If, on the other hand, you cannot count on their support or have concern that they may not act in what you consider the best interests of your youngster, if past experiences tell you that these persons cannot be counted on to help *in the ways your youngster needs to be helped,* then it may be best to consider other support-related options.

A spouse who helps you in the way *he or she* thinks is best to get the job done, an ex-spouse who has other issues with which to cope, a mate who has agreed to help you in the past but has failed to do so, should not be counted on for help. You may certainly want to tell them about the Program and try to enlist their cooperation (or at least their noninterference) later on, and you might certainly respect their thoughts, desires, and opinions, but do not make the mistake of inventing in your mind a supportive partner where one does not exist. It will leave you angry and frustrated and your youngster's success could ultimately be jeopardized. In Chapter 11 we will give you strategies for coping with people who become obstacles and would-be saboteurs of your child's progress, but for now let's stay focused on making the best people-choices possible as you begin the Program.

As in many things, consider actions, not words.

When deciding whether to enlist the help of a primary relationship (or any other relationship), consider actions, not words. Have they been there when you needed them? Have they helped in the ways *you* needed help? Did they help you discover what you wanted to do, or did they tell you what should be done? Did they remain supportive or did they fade? Did they expect something in return? Was their support worth the price you had to pay? The answers to these questions will help you choose and refuse potential members of your support "team."

Physician Before starting this Program, you should consult your youngster's physician. Use the recommendations in the "Talking It Through" section that follows to help ensure that your doctor understands what the Program entails and why you think your youngster can benefit from it.

Immediate Family For ease of communication, we define immediate family not by bloodlines but rather as those with whom a child lives (siblings qualify as immediate family, but we have included them in a separate section that follows). In the case of divorce, the immediate family may entail family members from two households. In addition, if your child spends time with grandparents or other relatives, or caretakers or sitters regularly on a full-time or part-time basis, or during vacation periods, consider them part of the immediate family as well.

Getting any individual immediate family member to agree wholeheartedly to work actively with you on making changes in your youngster's life is wonderful; getting a child's entire immediate family to agree to work together is not something one should expect to happen (not within our short lifetimes anyway). We are not being cynical. We are simply sharing our experience that, given the wide diversity of opinions, expectations, and unfinished emotionally charged issues that exist in most families, one cannot reasonably expect cooperation, much less support, from all those involved.

It is best to face this reality from the start. It will save you disappointment and outrage later on, and most importantly, it will help you plan for alternative avenues of support and help. Occasionally a youngster's immediate family is able to agree (1) that a problem exists, (2) how they would like to handle it, and (3) who will take responsibility for making changes. This situation is rare, and if you find yourself in such a supportive environment, count yourself very fortunate.

If, on the other hand, a supportive and helpful immediate family is not in your cards, if you are alone by design or by fate, or if family members are unwilling or unable to agree, it is best to be forewarned. Many parents with whom we have worked counted on family members to be there for them and for their children, only to be disappointed when they needed support most.

So if family members are not going to support you, it is better to know now than later. This program does not require the help of other family members, though their support can make it a bit easier and a lot more satisfying. With or without their help, however, you can still offer your youngster all the help he or she needs. Interestingly, we have found that immediate family members who at first were unwilling or unable to offer support—who in many cases were quite negative—became involved and caring contributors to a youngster's success once they saw the changes that the Program brought.

In addition, along with family help comes the risk that personal issues such as power, control, jealousy, and unresolved anger may inappropriately be brought into play. In the chapters to come we will help you deal with family members' intentional or unintentional sabotage of the Program should that occur, but for now, in the getting-ready stage, consider whether you can count on the support of your youngster's immediate family, and if that is a realistic possibility, consider incorporating the suggestions we offer in the "Talking It Through" section that follows.

> **An important note:** Even if you are certain that you can count on support from your child's immediate family, enlist additional support from others. It can prove an important backup at times when you may find it most welcome.

Teachers Your youngster's teachers can be very helpful in promoting your child's success on the Program. We have found that many teachers can provide invaluable assistance in supporting and facilitating your youngster's success. In addition, the active involvement of your youngster's teachers can bring a great deal of pleasure and ease to the Program, and teachers can offer you important information on your youngster's progress in the learning environment. If, however, after following the suggestions we offer in the "Talking It Through" section that follows, you find that you are unable to enlist help from your youngster's teachers, or that you encounter obstacles at school, do not be concerned; as long as your youngster wants to succeed, he or she needs virtually no one else's commitment and support but yours. Even if your youngster's commitment rises and falls at times, his or her chances for success need not suffer.

In addition, as we have found with immediate family members, teachers who at first were unwilling or unable to offer support may later become staunch advocates of the Program once they see for themselves its many benefits and the positive changes they may have previously doubted or refused to support.

So try to enlist the assistance of your youngster's teachers, but if support is not forthcoming, keep communication lines open if possible, and continue to prepare to get your youngster started.

Your Child You may have wondered why we did not put your youngster at the top of the list of people to talk to about the Program. We have found that with this program, as with many things, it is best to sort out your ideas, get feedback from others, and rethink your approach before you discuss the matter with the person who is most involved.

Practice thrice, then say it twice.

A communication adage we teach our second-year medical students says, "Practice thrice, then say it twice." If you want a new idea to be understood and accepted, before you present it in two different ways to your "target" person, present it to three other people first.

Talking about the Program to others before you discuss your thoughts with your youngster will often help you discover the best way to tell your youngster why you think he or she needs the Program, as well as what the Program will entail. It is important to try out your thoughts on others first; in addition, some may surprise you with interesting and useful suggestions. Of greatest importance is that, in talking it over with others, confidentiality must be maintained. You most certainly do not want your youngster to hear that you have been discussing his or her problems or the Program itself with others before you have had a chance to discuss it directly with the child.

So if possible, first talk the matter over with others (assuming you can count on their discretion), and then using the suggestions you will find in the "Talking It Through" section that follows, sit down and talk it over with your youngster. Remember that everything you are saying is new to your youngster, so explain it as many times as necessary to ensure that your kid fully understands the benefits the Program can provide and what changes it will entail.

Siblings The sisters and brothers of our carbohydrate-addicted kids are like snowflakes in that each one is unique and unpredictably different. Each relationship is different as well. In communicating information about the Program to your youngster's siblings, you should consider two things: your experience as to the best way in which to present the information, and your evaluation, in real terms, of what you want from this sibling.

If, for instance, you believe that an older brother or sister is interested in helping your youngster, and if you are going to need to enlist the older sibling's cooperation (in the preparation of after-school snacks, for instance), it would be best to take the time and make the effort to communicate much of what you have learned from this book.

If, on the other hand, you do not think the sibling is willing or able to help *on a consistent basis*, or if you do not really think that it is necessary for a young sibling, for example, to get more than a few simple cursory statements regarding what changes can be expected, then by all means offer only the information that is necessary.

You will find suggestions on how best to enlist sibling support for the Program in the "Talking It Through" section that follows.

With siblings, however, another issue must be addressed. While each family is unique and the rules by which members abide may vary, in regard to the Program, your carbohydrate-addicted youngster must be protected from the "teasing" or insensitive remarks of siblings. Cruel words, thoughtless statements, even innocent but insensitive remarks can undo a great deal of hard and important work. So enlist the understanding and help of your youngster's siblings if you can but, in any case, make certain that your carbohydrate-addicted youngster is given the best possible chance for success.

Friends and Co-Workers You will certainly need to choose for yourself, but we generally recommend that to keep things simple, friends, acquaintances, and co-workers should be given information on your youngster's program strictly on a need-to-know basis.

Good friends, who might be counted on for support and suggestions, would naturally be given more information; other friends, who might be joining you and your family for dinner, for instance, need to know little if anything about the Program, for unless you wish to share your thoughts, feelings, or enthusiasm, no one will be able to ascertain that your youngster's dinners are different from any other kid's, unless perhaps they happen to note that the meal seems a bit healthier than might be expected.

> **You are going to have to be strong
> and you are going to have to stay strong.
> But you can do it and we will help.**

The Whole Wide World There is a great big world of people out there; some waiting to help you and your child, some waiting to sabotage, most not really caring one way or the other. It will be your job, in part, to work within this system to get your youngster what he or she needs. You may have to ask an unreceptive wait-ress to take back your youngster's meal because it was not what your child ordered; you may have to ask the counter person at the deli to go back into the freezer and check the label for hidden sugars; you may have to deal with other parents who don't quite understand why your youngster has to have a salad or protein with every snack or meal when the child stays over at a friend's house. You are going to have to be strong and you are going to have to stay strong. And you can do it.

Use the recommendations in the "Talking It Through" sec-tion that follows to help increase the probability that you will get the support and cooperation you need, but in any case, stand tall; this is your youngster's life and you may, at times, literally find yourself fighting for it.

TALKING IT THROUGH
Whether you are talking with your youngster's physician or teacher, a grandparent who keeps an eye on your youngster after school, your spouse, a friend, a stranger, a sibling, or your carbo-hydrate-addicted youngster, here a few suggestions that have proven quite successful in getting yourself heard and getting the cooperation you would like.

1: Choose your time and place.

Choose the right time and the right way to say what you want others to hear, based on when they can best hear you, and when they are best able to consider what you have to say. When speaking with your youngster's physician, for instance, do not squeeze your concerns and request for assistance into the tail end of a quick appointment. Instead, call ahead, explaining that you want to discuss a new program and that you need a specific amount of time in which to do it. If you are calling for an appointment, don't go into too much detail over the phone. You want a chance to explain your concerns and the details of the

Program and to listen to the physician's feedback in person.

If you want to discuss the matter with your spouse, wait until he or she has had some time to relax, or ask when the two of you might talk. Explain that what you want to discuss is not something negative, or an issue between the two of you, but rather that you want to get your spouse's opinion. People will tend to press you to tell them everything at that moment, so be prepared to talk about it on the spot, but try to explain that you want to discuss it in some detail; at the same time, hold out for the best time to be heard and understood.

When you are ready to discuss the Program with your youngster, be considerate of the timing as well. If your child has a test the next day or is waiting for a phone call, hold off for a few hours or for a day or two. Even though you are aware that the Program is far more important than a phone call from a friend, you may need to wait until your youngster can give you undivided, or at least less-divided, attention.

It just may be that no time is a good time. Your youngster or your spouse may always be tied up with other thoughts and other demands. If this is the case, let your child or spouse choose the timing of the first discussion but be sure to decide together how he or she intends to accommodate any future communications in so busy a schedule.

2: Do not make assumptions.

Do not assume that someone will or will not understand your concerns, will or will not support or help you, or will or will not value what you have to say. Say your piece, ask for what you want, and listen to the response. Sometimes you will find that those on whom you thought you could count are not willing to offer any assistance or support. Sometimes you will discover that those you thought would be critical and unsupportive are more than willing to help.

Your carbohydrate-addicted youngster's response to your first suggestions regarding the Program may surprise you. We have had many parents tell us that they never thought they could broach certain topics like weight or learning problems without upsetting or distressing their youngsters, but found their kids open and anxious to discuss a solution. Others tell us that they thought this would be an easy topic to approach, that they felt as if their youngsters had been waiting for them to bring it up, but found their kids hesitant, defensive, or resistant. Expectations may be confirmed or disproved. You can't make assumptions because, in Gilda Radner's words, "You just never know." So gently broach the topic and hope for the best.

Chances are, your youngster will be eager to discuss the matter, but if this is not the case, do not push. A refusal to talk, even a furious response, can reverse within a short time—if your youngster is given the time and opportunity to work through the feelings in his or her own way.

We recommend that parents communicate in "I" statements that deal with the goal (getting the youngster on the Program) rather than starting the conversation off with a review of the problem (undesirable eating habits, excess weight, behavioral problems, and so on). For instance, a statement that starts with "We have been aware that your weight (or difficulty in concentrating) is causing you problems . . ." is almost certain to make your youngster feel embarrassed, ashamed, or defensive. On the other hand, a statement like, "I was reading this book and it says that in many cases weight problems (or difficulties with concentrating) in kids can come from . . ." is best because it puts the focus on the solution right from the start.

3: Communicate both feelings and facts, but when possible, keep them separate.

Whether you are requesting help, support, cooperation, understanding, or involvement, it is often helpful to communicate the facts about your youngster's addiction to carbohydrates and its impact as well as your feelings and concerns. After explaining to relatives, for instance, in very simple terms, that your youngster is sensitive to carbohydrate-rich foods and that you would like them to stop giving your youngster candy, you might add that it is difficult to watch the effect that the candy has on your child's behavior. This approach gives validity to your feelings and allows the listeners to empathize with your concerns, at the same time.

If they challenge your perception, for example, that giving your youngster candy is causing the problem, or that there is in fact any problem at all, we have found that it is best not to argue fact. Remain, instead, in the area of feeling—feelings cannot very well be disputed. No one (well, hardly anyone) can argue with the statement, "I know you don't see it as a problem, and perhaps that's not the issue, but *I* really have concerns and I would rather you didn't offer the candy."

On the other hand, when you speak to your carbohydrate-addicted youngster, keep statements about your feelings at a minimum. While you may share your concerns and hopes with others, it may be a bit too much to expect your youngster to deal with your feelings and his or her feelings at the same time.

4: Describe the problem and the solution in positive terms.

Use constructive images. When talking with your youngster you might say, "This program will help you get and stay slim without depriving you of the food you love" rather than, "If you do this you won't be so heavy." To a teacher you might say, "Eating in this way may help stabilize my child's blood sugar levels, reduce the adrenaline that may be coming from blood sugar swings, and help my child stay focused" rather than say, "If you would just stop giving sugar, my child would not be so difficult to deal with."

5: Gloss over the details of biology unless asked.

Some parents make the mistake of trying to explain too much. It would take hours and hours to read aloud what you have read so far. Add to that time all you will read in the pages to come. Most people don't want or don't need to know all the details. Let them guide you. You might tell others that your youngster "has a physical imbalance" that leads to carbohydrate cravings, weight gain, hyperactivity, learning difficulties, and mood swings.

If asked, you can add that the imbalance is related to blood sugar swings. Only if asked for more detail or when speaking with your youngster's physician, your primary relationship, your child's teacher, or others in similar situations does it make sense to bring in details of the biological-behavioral imbalance or to ask them to look over the book.

Depending on your youngster's age, level of maturity, and desire to know, and in as simple terms as possible, describe to your youngster the physical imbalance that is causing the carbohydrate addiction. Explain in just enough detail that there is a physical reason for the cravings and problems.

6: In real-life terms, explain what you are requesting of others and what you anticipate. Whenever possible, make it clear and easy.

When visiting your youngster's physician, rather than simply handing the doctor this book, explain that you want the doctor's opinion of the Program, recommendations, and monitoring. Take the time to write out an example of three days' typical food intake and activity choices, so that the proposed program can be quickly reviewed. Leave the book as well, so that the physician can leaf through it or read it in detail if desired. If the doctor requires more information, provide it as requested.

Whether you want cooperation from a spouse, approval from your youngster's physician, or cooperation from a teacher, clearly indicate exactly what you are requesting. You might ask a teacher to "make sure that you keep me informed of any changes in behavior," or you might ask your spouse to "make certain you serve the food I will leave in the fridge" or to "include one of these foods in snacks," rather than asking for some vague promise of "help" or "cooperation."

Some parents may read this book along with their carbo-addicted youngsters; some simply may make the book available for their kids to read as desired, without any demands or pressure. Ages, attitudes, and needs differ in each kid. We recommend that, if possible, you ask your youngster to decide how he or she would like to learn about the Program—that is, by reading the book alone, by reading it with you, or by having you encapsulate the essential points.

7: Fix the problem, not the blame.

Do not get caught in communications that attempt to place blame on you, on others, or on your child. Keep focused on what needs to be done and the best ways to do it. If things get difficult, allow some time and space and try again, listening for others' fears or feelings of failure.

8: If you hit resistance, suggest a trial period.

When dealing with a carbohydrate-addicted youngster, a primary relationship, or an immediate family member who is not particularly enthusiastic about the Program for whatever reasons (rational or irrational), suggest a trial period during which they will offer their full cooperation and support. "Let's try the Program for two weeks" (or three or four if they can handle it), you might offer. "Then we can reevaluate it at that time."

Some family members may argue theory, most kids will just resist, but few people can rationalize refusing to agree to a trial period. Depending on the plan and your youngster's response, even a short time may be enough to bring about big differences. A limited trial period and a time for reconsideration gives everyone a chance to see that not much is required and that the results may be more than worth the effort.

Physicians, as well, often prefer giving a new program a short trial period, after which they can more realistically evaluate your youngster's progress.

The Right Plan

To ensure that any health-promoting program is right for your youngster, and to choose one that is most likely to be successful, look for a program that corrects the cause of any problems with which your youngster is coping. In this case, by definition, The Carbohydrate Addict's Program for Children and Teens has been designed to correct the insulin imbalance that lies at the core of your youngster's cravings and blood sugar swings, as well as the many weight, behavioral, mood, and learning problems that may result.

Although all carbohydrate-addicted youngsters share a common physical imbalance, they have a wide variety of preferences and priorities. As no parent needs to be reminded, each youngster is a unique combination of needs and desires and must be treated as such.

No successful program can offer a one-size-fits-all approach. Our program offers two different plans: The Step-By-Step Plan and The Jump-Start Plan— with lots of choices in each.

Different ages, levels of maturity and independence, peer-pressure influences, personal preferences, and social demands make it essential to select a program that has been designed to fit the needs of your youngster. No successful program can offer a one-size-fits-all approach to any group of people—much less to kids.

The Carbohydrate Addict's Program for Children and Teens is made up of two plans, The Step-By-Step Plan and The Jump-Start Plan. With your physician's input, you and your youngster will choose the plan that is more appropriate to your needs, preferences, lifestyle, and goals. Both plans will guide your youngster in reducing or eliminating cravings and balancing insulin and blood sugar levels, but, as you will see, each plan moves at a different pace, is appropriate for different age groups, and requires a different level of involvement and commitment.

In the chapters that follow, you will learn a great deal more about the plans that will guide you through the Program. For now, keep in mind that for a program to be "right" it must correct the *cause* of your youngster's cravings, and at the same time greatly enhance your child's probability of long-term success.

The Right Time

Some people will say that there is no wrong time to get started on the road to success. We disagree. We believe that choosing a good time to get started can help you and your youngster not only get on the road to success but stay there. The basis for what constitutes the "right" time, however, may surprise you.

When we first began to do research with parents and children, we worked with many parents who, against our initial recommendations and for reasons of their own, started their youngsters on the Program at less-than-perfect times: when kids and parents were under powerful and transient stresses, during the holidays, or right before vacation. Many of these families surprised us with their easy and long-lasting successes—although we should add that by the choosing to start when they did, they faced some unnecessary and most likely avoidable obstacles.

In the years that have followed, we have learned one simple truth: No time is the "right" time if you don't want to do something, and almost any time is the right time if you do.

No time is the "right" time if you don't want to do something and almost any time is the right time if you do.

If you and your youngster are ready to begin the Program, if you are both excited about breaking the addiction cycle for good, or if the promise of losing weight and resolving behavioral and learning problems inspires you both, then now may very well be the right time to start.

If, on the other hand, either you or your youngster feels that this is not the right time to begin "just yet," if either of you think that at some time in the future, either on a specific date or at a time that remains to be agreed upon, it would be better to start, then certainly consider waiting to begin.

In the interim, use the time available to examine the reasons for delay and be certain that these reasons are valid and reflect the real concerns of child or parent. A youngster who wants some time to think over the Program is presenting a valid point. A couple of days or a week might be appropriate. Needing more time than that, however, indicates to us that the youngster may have additional concerns that should be explored, examined, and, if possible, resolved.

Parents and youngsters can disagree on when to begin.

A point of potential conflict arises when one person is ready to begin the Program and the other is not. There is no easy answer to this dilemma, although we have found that communication often reveals that timing is of less importance than are other hidden or unspoken concerns. If you and your youngster are at odds over the right time to begin the Program, talk it over, and then talk it over again. You may be surprised at the potential problems you can circumvent before you ever begin if you learn to listen to what is meant when the words "not ready" begin to surface.

Some parents ask us our advice about whether to begin the Program when vacations or holidays are approaching, whether to wait until after an upcoming family affair or birthday, or whether the beginning or ending of the school year is the best time to start.

We will not say that outside events do not matter. We have indeed found that vacations away from home, holidays, birthdays, and family affairs can, for some, provide additional challenges to success when they take place *when a youngster is first starting* the Program. When beginning the Program, some parents and children alike prefer to have a little more time to read over labels, be able to shop at familiar stores where the stock is predictable, and eat at restaurants where the menu is known. These parents and youngsters find that the comfort of time and the certainty of knowing what is available have allowed them to get into the swing of the Program without having to cope with added surprises. Once they feel comfortable with the Program, of course, vacations away from home, holidays, family affairs, and similar situations present no problems.

For some, when they are learning anything new, it is always preferable to have the luxury of concentrating on acquiring that skill without the pressure of competing demands or time.

A program for all seasons.

For others, upcoming vacations, holidays, and family affairs offer added incentives for beginning the Program. While events such as these should never constitute a reason for losing weight or getting behavioral problems under control, they can offer foreseeable moments of anticipated success. Many parents and youngsters find that summer vacations provide a wonderful chance to concentrate on beginning the Program. The warm months stretch out and offer more time to concentrate on change and a greater number of activity options as well. For others, camp activities or summer jobs present unnecessary challenges to the starting of a new program.

Some parents and youngsters find that the beginning of the school year is an ideal time to start the Program; for those who want to lose weight, beginning the Program in the fall will allow them to maintain weight loss they may have attempted or achieved during the summer months. In addition, for those anticipating the stresses and challenges of the coming school year, starting the Program in the fall can provide real hope and real help in handling many of the upcoming school-related demands.

So seize the moment or wait for the right time, depending on which is appropriate to your situation, but in all cases, as you plan it out, as you think it out, be certain to talk it through with your youngster.

The Right Reasons

As you know, The Carbohydrate Addict's Program for Children and Teens has been designed to correct a physical imbalance; the fact that it can help resolve many insulin and blood sugar–related problems is a wonderful added benefit, but these bonuses should not become overpowering reasons for following the Program.

If, for instance, weight-loss expectations too strongly fuel a teen's motivation, it becomes harder to make sure that he or she will eat all the foods necessary to provide a well-balanced, nutritious eating program. If a parent encourages a child to begin the Program but at the same time places unrealistic demands for behavior "control" on the youngster, the child may be more likely to rebel and sabotage the very program that would normally bring about these changes naturally. So while you may keep in mind the weight, behavioral, mood, and learning changes you want for your youngster, balance these goals with your desire for a healthy and happy child or teen who feels free to reach for success without unnecessary pressure or fear of failure.

Katie Can Do:
A Story of Success Without Limits

Katie was only ten years old, but this pretty little girl already saw herself as a failure. Overweight and out of control—that was how her stepmother, Blair, presented the situation.

"She simply has no limits," Blair began, speaking as if Katie were not there listening, quietly witnessing the litany of her own failures. Before we could intercede, Blair continued. "She can't stop eating, she can't stop talking, she's loud and demanding, and she just can't keep her hands off things that aren't hers."

We were speechless. We had never witnessed so negative a presentation of a child's problems. We jumped to bring about damage control and halt the conversation before new and hurtful accusations could be flung at Katie.

We stopped the interview and suggested that we wait until Katie's father could join us. Blair's inventory of faults shifted to the reasons that her husband would not be able to come to see us but we held our ground, and in the end we were successful in meeting with Blair and her husband, this time without Katie present.

At the meeting we learned that Katie's eating and weight had become problematic during the last two years, within six months of her parents' divorce and her father's quick remarriage. Katie had apparently taken to stealing food and money (presumably for food) from her parents and her classmates as well. She had been suspended from school for stealing and for disorderly classroom behavior. We were told that at times she seemed to do "whatever she wanted" and that she appeared to have "no limits." Though Katie's father, Tom, was certain that his daughter's behavior was a reaction to the divorce, Blair was not as sure.

"I thought at first that it was just her way of showing anger," Blair explained, "but over the summer, I saw something that makes me wonder." Blair went on to describe a repeating pattern of behavior in which Katie would awaken feeling somewhat calm though sleepy. Her appetite was strong, that is, she was clearly hungry, but the normal breakfast she ate seemed to satisfy her.

As the day progressed, however, Katie's hunger and behavior became more extreme. "She is already asking for lunch by eleven A.M. If I give her a snack, it's never enough. She's constantly demanding attention and sometimes it seems like she just won't stop talking or grabbing at me, or else she's ignoring me completely while making a mess somewhere in the house. Sometimes I can't tell if she's just out of control or just doesn't care, or intentionally trying to be destructive.

"I know how I sound," Blair went on, "but you need to understand that I knew that Katie was going to live with us from the start, and I know it doesn't sound like it now, but I wanted to be a mother to her." Blair explained that Katie's mother had a problem with alcohol and was not able to be with Katie on a regular basis. Katie had had virtually no contact with her mother for months.

"It's all mixed up," Blair went on. "I feel responsible, Tom feels responsible, too, and we try to make it up to her, but nothing we do seems to make any difference. She's just out of control and her weight is just part of it, and to tell you the truth, we're at our wits' end."

For a moment we saw the situation from Blair's point of view, and though we did not agree with the way she had acted in front of Katie, we could empathize with her frustration and Tom's unresolved guilt that his marrying Blair had led to Katie's changes in behavior.

We recommended that Katie should be evaluated by a psychologist. We agreed that after the initial psychological work-up, we would all meet with the psychologist to work together on treatment recommendations that could complement the changes the Program would bring. In the interim, Blair and Tom took the Carbohydrate Addict's Quiz for Parents of Children and Teens. Tom's evaluation placed Katie right on the borderline between mild and moderate addiction, but Blair's evaluation placed Katie high in the strong addiction range.

"I'm with her all the time," Blair explained, "and Tom still sees her as she used to be." Tom agreed but seemed to want to tell us something else.

"It's just that we're under pressure to get this worked out," he explained. "We can't just let this go on." It was then we learned that Blair was pregnant and that both she and Tom were very concerned for the well-being of a newborn in the house.

"I know I should be worried about my daughter," he confessed, "but it's really hard. She can just push you to the limit, you know?" he asked rhetorically, and while we did, we also knew, only too well, how alone and desperate this young girl must be.

Rachael had been a difficult kid herself; too loud, too strong, too demanding, too hungry. She was too much for too many people. She pushed everyone's limits and she stopped only when she had pushed them too far.

Now Katie was under a deadline that she did not know existed; she had to shape up soon or, as her father indicated, the only thing left was to "send her away to school." We thought nothing could be worse for this young child who had, essentially, already lost her mother.

We tried to explain that deadlines do not make for good healing—the mind, body, and soul do not understand time-related demands; they work at their own pace with or without our consent. We cautioned Blair and Tom that, first and foremost, the reason for Katie to start the Program had to be as a way of helping Katie find balance in her body and, as a natural consequence, attain a balance in her feelings and behavior as well.

They said they understood but we knew they had barely heard us. They wanted Katie to lose weight and get control of her behavior, and they hoped that this program would give them what they wanted rather than offering Katie what she so desperately needed: balance in thought and feelings and actions. They wanted change and they wanted it now, and while many parents get the changes they hope for on the Program, quickly and without struggle, others may find that some changes take more time.

After a few weeks on The Jump-Start Plan (you'll read more about it starting on page 209), Katie's hunger had normalized, her weight had begun to drop, and her behavior was dramatically improved. We were surprised, then, when we received another call from Blair and Tom requesting an appointment to discuss additional therapeutic interventions.

Katie, it seemed, was changing but not fast enough for her father and Blair, and while we were unable to get them to clarify what problems remained unresolved, we got the distinct feeling that virtually nothing Katie was able to accomplish was ever going to be good enough. We wondered if perhaps they secretly hoped that Katie would just disappear so they might be free to start their own family anew.

Well, fate is funny and, in this case, very kind. Within a day or two of our meeting with Blair and Tom we received an unexpected phone call. It was from Katie's mother. It seemed she had been in rehabilitation but had hesitated contacting Katie until she was certain that she was in control of her drinking problem. Now, under continuing supervision, she was hoping to reestablish her relationship with Katie under much more positive terms. Having spoken with Tom and Blair, she had contacted us so that she might learn about the Program and help her daughter with it.

The weeks passed quickly. We met with Tom and Blair and Katie's mother on several occasions. Katie's school psychologist and a social worker joined us as well. Almost without discussion, everyone, including Katie, agreed that Katie would go to live with her mother with regular monitoring by social worker and psychologist.

When we met again three months later, Tom and Blair seemed thrilled with their life away from Katie, and while that bothered us a bit, we focused on the fact that Katie was blossoming; her grades were excellent, she received only praise from her teacher, her mother adored having her back, and with the loss of weight and the calmness that seemed to surround her, she appeared almost graceful, not a term one would ever have used to describe the Katie of the past.

We received a postcard from Katie not too long ago. She had been to NASA's exhibit at the Kennedy Space Center. The postcard had on it a picture of an astronaut walking in space with the earth's surface far below. Katie's note was short but to the point. "I want to be an astronaut," she wrote. "Can do!" she added, confirming the success that was finally hers, now and in the years to come. A success that, it seemed to us, was without limits.

nine

Getting Started:
The Step-By-Step Plan

The Carbohydrate Addict's Program for Children and Teens offers two different plans: The Step-By-Step Plan and The Jump-Start Plan. Though each plan moves at a different pace, they are both designed to accomplish the same goal: to restore balance to your youngster's body.

The Step-By-Step Plan of the Program includes a wide array of small-step options (called Choices) that have been designed to fit easily into the special world of the child and teen. As its name indicates, The Step-By-Step Plan takes your youngster through a series of small steps, designed to slowly and steadily correct the insulin imbalance that drives your youngster's intense carbo cravings and blood sugar swings, and their associated difficulties. Each small change builds on others and, almost without realizing it, your youngster has made important lifestyle changes.

On The Step-By-Step Plan, youngsters move directly toward their Optimal Carbo Balance, that is, the right combination of foods and activity to restore their insulin and blood sugar balances and to reduce or eliminate the problems imbalances can bring (details to follow on page 199).

With the approval of your youngster's physician, and while maintaining enough carbohydrates in the diet for your youngster's optimal health, The Step-By-Step Plan can be followed for an indefinite period of time by both children and teens.

In contrast, The Jump-Start Plan is a special accelerated program that is aimed only at older children and teens who are in need of quick change.

The Jump-Start Plan is divided into two phases. Phase One is a time-limited,[1] rapid-result plan for the older child or teen who, with the physician's approval and monitoring, is in need of quick change. The Jump-Start Plan is not meant to be followed for long periods of time, nor is it meant to be followed by younger children.

Phase One of The Jump-Start Plan involves rapid change and should be followed:

1. Only by the older child or teen.
2. Only for a limited time.[2]
3. Only with your youngster's physician's approval and monitoring and in accord with the physician's recommendations.

Within a matter of days on Phase One of The Jump-Start Plan, youngsters usually experience a significant reduction in cravings and blood sugar–related problems and an increase in control of their eating and behavior. It is important to note that while this phase of The Jump-Start Plan brings remarkable results rapidly, it asks for greater change in a shorter time than does The Step-By-Step Plan.

During Phase Two of The Jump-Start Plan, youngsters gradually add Carbohydrate-Rich Foods, activities, and other options so that, by achieving their Optimal Carbo Balance, the Program can be maintained—without losing its benefits and without deprivation or sacrifice—for life.

[1,2]Appropriateness and duration of phase and program should incorporate recommendations by your youngster's physician, who should approve your youngster's participation and monitor progress, as should be done with all programs that call for changes in the child's eating and activity regimen.

First Things First

Okay. Let's get started. When beginning The Carbohydrate Addict's Program for Children and Teens, the first choice you will make with and for your child will be whether to start on The Step-By-Step Plan or The Jump-Start Plan.

No problem! Since changing plans is always an option, the first choice is only where to *begin*. In the pages to come, you will be given guidance for switching plans at any time. As always, consult with your youngster's physician; bring this book (and an inventory of several days' sample meals and activities if you like). If you have not looked it over already, make certain you read Chapter 8. It's filled with many helpful suggestions for communicating with your youngster's physician and with teachers, family members, and many others.

IMPORTANT: Before selecting which plan is best for your child or teen, it is essential that you read this chapter and Chapter 10, detailing The Jump-Start Plan, through to the end, so that you have a complete understanding of both plans.

Remember, when choosing which plan to start with, the decision is not carved in stone. If your youngster begins one plan and decides to switch to the other, that can be done at any point. (You'll find some helpful suggestions for changing plans on page 204.) We recommend, however, that you do not keep switching back and forth from one plan to the other.

In choosing a plan, consider the following: If your youngster is more likely to prefer gradual changes, that is, those that will not ask a great deal all at once but that, over time, will come together to make slow but steady progress, begin with The Step-By-Step Plan. If, on the other hand, your older child or teen is in need of quicker change and is motivated to take on greater challenges in exchange for more immediate results, begin with The Jump-Start Plan. As always, keep your youngster's age, physical requirements, preferences, and motivation in mind.

QUICK COMPARISON OF PLANS* IN THE CARBOHYDRATE ADDICT'S PROGRAM FOR CHILDREN AND TEENS

	THE STEP-BY-STEP PLAN	THE JUMP-START PLAN
Who is it for?	Carbo-addicted youngsters who prefer a series of small steps, designed to bring about slow and steady beneficial lifestyle changes.	Older children and teens who are carbo-addicted and in need of quick results. Phase One should be followed for a limited time only.* Phase Two will help bring about beneficial lifestyle changes.
What will my youngster do?	**STEP #1:** Add-On an Insulin-Balancing Food to one daily meal or snack. **STEP #2:** Add-On a once-a-week Activity.	**PHASE ONE: Guideline #1:** At all meals and snacks, other than during one rewarding Combo Meal each day, choose only Insulin-Balancing Foods.
	STEP #3: During one meal or snack each day, eat *only* Insulin-Balancing Proteins or Vegetables (Hold-On and until the next meal or snack to enjoy carbo-rich foods).	**Guideline #2:** At one rewarding Combo Meal each day, enjoy a *balanced* combination of both Insulin-Balancing Foods and Carbohydrate-Rich Foods.
	STEP #4: A *one* daily Swap Meal (or Snack), replace all Quick Trigger Foods with any Slow Trigger Foods.	**Guideline #3:** Complete all meals and snacks within sixty minutes.
What should my youngster do in the weeks that follow?	Continue to select one new Add-On Food, Add-On Activity, Hold-On, or Swap Choice each week until an Optimal Carbo Balance is reached.	Move to Phase Two of The Jump-Start Plan: Once each week add Carbohydrate-Rich Food to an Insulin-Balancing Meal (or Snack) along with a weekly activity and, if desired, a weekly Swap.
		Continue Phase Two until cravings, or weight, motivation, learning, mood, attentional, or other difficulties first begin to reemerge. Then remove *last* added Carbohydrate-Rich addition to reach an Optimal Carbo Balance.

*A full understanding of your youngster's Plan is needed to help insure your youngster's success. Do not use this summary in place of the chapter(s) which fully describe the options and guidelines of your youngster's Plan. Appropriateness and duration of phase and program should incorporate recommendations by your youngster's physician who, as with all programs that call for changes in your youngster's eating and activity regimen, should approve your youngster's participation and monitor his/her progress.

Additional information on determining your youngster's Optimal Carbohydrate Balance may be found on pages 199 and 221.

For slower, steady change for all youngsters, choose The
Step-By-Step Plan. For quicker change for older children
and teens, choose The Jump-Start Plan.[3]

The Step-By-Step Plan

Remember, The Step-By-Step Plan is made up of Choices:
gradual, easy changes in either diet or activity.

Each week, with your guidance and approval, your youngster
will make one selection from four different types of Choices:
Food Add-Ons, Activity Add-Ons, Hold-Ons, or Swaps. We will
guide you with a preferred order of selection, but you and your
youngster will be free to make Choices that fit both your needs.
Each Choice on The Step-By-Step Plan will involve a very small
change, a change that is neither difficult nor demanding.

As each Choice is selected, it is added to your youngster's
daily routine and to any previous week's Choices that have been
selected in the past. It's as simple as that! In any one week, no
more than one Choice should be added. After a week of having
incorporated a new Choice, if your youngster is ready, he or she
can select the next Choice (preferably in sequence). As the
weeks go by and the Choices add up, the small changes that each
Choice requires add up as well. Since each Choice is added to
the others that have been selected in previous weeks, the combined impact of the Choices join and work together to correct
the physical cause of your youngster's carbohydrate cravings and
to break the body's physical imbalance that lies at the very base
of the blood sugar and insulin swings. Though each Choice is in
itself small, as the weeks go by, the transformations you see will
surprise and delight you.

Depending on the age and maturity of your youngster, you
will probably want to guide him or her in selecting each weekly

---

[3]Appropriateness and duration of phase and program should incorporate recommendations by your youngster's physician, who should approve your youngster's participation and monitor progress, as should be done with all programs
that call for changes in the child's eating and activity regimen.

Choice; some children and teens can be relied on to pick appropriate and sensible choices for themselves, though most need
guidance. Listen not only to what your youngster says but also to
what he or she is not saying. Is there enthusiasm in making a
Choice? If so, make plans about how best to incorporate the
newest Choice. If not, try to uncover the concerns and conflicts
that your youngster may not know how to express.

Most parents find they and their youngsters gain understanding from the process of Choice selection. They discover a
great deal more about each other than they thought possible—
when, and if, they listen to each other's words, tones, hesitations,
and signals.

If your youngster is in conflict about a Choice, give him or
her the time needed to work it out by talking it out. Once you
understand the concerns, give your youngster first crack at
solving the problem or planning the strategies that are needed.
Don't offer your help until your kid has had a chance to work it
out alone. It's difficult for parents not to supply the answers, but
it's important for kids to learn to solve these problems for themselves—with your experience and guidance but not with your
answers. Encourage but don't push; most of all, try to help your
child or teen focus on any fears, concerns, or reluctance and
then discover his or her own way out.

We recommend a single rule of thumb: It is better to have a
youngster willingly continue past Choices and select no new
Choice than to have a youngster so resent a new Choice that all
the previous progress is jeopardized. As most parents have discovered, patience is not only a virtue, it is a clear necessity.

So if, at the end of any week, your youngster is *not* ready to
select an additional Choice, or if you think selecting an additional Choice is not appropriate at that time, encourage your
youngster to stop making new selections and, as appropriate,
simply continue with the Choices already selected. As always,
encourage your youngster to move at a pace that's right for him
or her.

The Order of Things

We recommend that, on The Step-By-Step Plan, Choices should be selected in the standard order that follows, that is, first a Food Add-On, then an Activity Add-On, a Hold-On, a Swap, then a repeat of the sequence. This standard sequence that we suggest is not essential, however, and though it has proven an easy, logical sequence that helps build momentum and moves toward progressive success, you and your youngster may prefer an alternative sequence of Choices.

Step #1: Incorporate a Food Add-On

Overview

Incorporating a Food Add-On simply entails adding one Insulin-Balancing Food to one of your youngster's daily meals or snacks. Most Insulin-Balancing Foods are high in protein or fiber and low in carbohydrates. The addition of protein-rich or high-fiber foods to the high-carbohydrate meals or snacks that your youngster usually enjoys (which contain breads, pasta, or other starches; snack foods; or sweets), creates a new balance that can help stabilize your youngster's insulin levels. As insulin levels normalize, blood sugar is no longer swept from the bloodstream to waiting fat cells and can freely enter and nourish the brain and other organs and muscles. Youngsters are free of the ravages of unwarranted weight gain and the mood swings, behavioral problems, and hyperactivity that hypoglycemia can bring. As insulin and blood sugar levels stabilize, recurrent and intense cravings for carbohydrates as well as problems in motivation and concentration can literally disappear. This balance in diet can bring with it a balance of mood, mind, and being.

If you use the standard sequence of Choice selection that we recommend, your child's first step in The Step-By-Step Plan will be to Add-On a high-protein or fiber-rich food (Insulin-Balancing Food) to the same meal or snack each day, so that the insulin-raising effects of Carbohydrate-Rich Foods may be better balanced by the Insulin-Balancing Foods. We call these meals Combo Meals, because they combine Insulin-Balancing and Carbohydrate-Rich Foods.

Insulin-Balancing protein-rich foods include meat, fish, poultry, eggs, cheese, and tofu.[4] Most children and teens have no problem finding one or more Insulin-Balancing Foods that they are willing to Add-On to their usual high-carbo foods, changing an unbalanced carbohydrate-laden meal or snack into a more balanced Combo Meal or Snack.

In addition to protein-rich foods, Insulin-Balancing Foods also include fiber-rich vegetables: nonstarchy vegetables that can be prepared in a variety of ways (stir-fried or sautéed, for instance) or eaten raw in salads (which your youngster can top with an especially good dressing or dip). Adding high-fiber foods to your youngster's usual carbo-laden meals or snacks will, again, turn it into a more balanced Combo Meal or Snack. You will find a complete list of Insulin-Balancing Foods starting on page 183 and details on how best to incorporate Step #1 into your youngster's typical eating pattern in the pages that follow.

**We will provide you with help for
dealing with the vegetable-phobic youngster.**

"Veggie" Important Note: Don't be concerned if your child typically refuses to eat anything that even remotely resembles a vegetable. For the vegetable-phobic child, Insulin-Balancing Vegetables may be bypassed for the time being; you may choose protein-rich Insulin-Balancing Foods for now, and later you will find veggie-promoting recipes and hints for making vegetables appealing.

---

[4]Pressed soybean curd preferred by non-meat-eaters and available in larger supermarkets and health food stores.

CHOICE SELECTION:
YOUR CHOICE OF SEQUENCE

The order in which Choices are incorporated into your youngster's Step-By-Step Plan is not crucial to his/her success. Individual needs, likes and dislikes, time and financial considerations may make a different order more desirable or may make one kind of Choice preferable over another.

While the standard sequence of Choice selection that follows has proven an easy and logical sequence and has helped many of our youngsters, others have succeeded as well by picking and choosing their own order and combinations of Choices.

If you and your youngster have no strong preference regarding the sequence of Choice selection, we recommend that you follow the standard sequence of Choice selection that follows. If you or your youngster prefer a different sequence of Choice selection, feel free to adapt the order and combination to meet those needs.

EXAMPLE OF A STANDARD SEQUENCE OF CHOICE SELECTION

(Food Add-On, Activity Add-On, Hold-On, Swap):

Week #1:	Food Add-On	Add some chicken, meat or fish and/or some Insulin-Balancing vegetables or salad to usual lunch each day
Week #2:	Food Add-On Activity Add-On	While continuing previous Choice: Add dancing, walking or aerobics for ½ hour on Saturdays
Week #3:	Food Add-On, Activity Add-On, Hold-On	While continuing all previous Choices: Hold-On and have no carbohydrate-rich and foods each day, during evening snacks
Week #4	Food Add-On, Activity Add-On, Hold-On, and Swap	While continuing all previous Choices: Swap Slow Trigger Foods for typical Quick Trigger Foods at afterschool snacks (for example have pretzels, baked chips and dip, and/or fruit instead of usual candy, cookies, and juice)
Week #5	Food Add-On, Activity Add-On, Hold-On, Swap and new Food Add-On	While continuing all previous Choices: Add some chicken, meat or fish and/or some Insulin-Balancing vegetables or salad to dinner each night.

And so on . . .

TWO (OF MANY POSSIBLE) *ALTERNATIVE* SEQUENCES OF CHOICE SELECTIONS:

SAMPLE ALTERNATIVE #1:
Mary McC.* was twelve years old. She loved to run and dance and move but she hated vegetables. Here's a sample of her alternative order of selection of Choices:

Week #1:	Activity Add-On	Add Dancing, Walking or Aerobics for $1/2$ hour once each week
Week #2:	Activity Add-On, and new Activity Add-On	While continuing previous Choice: Add another $1/2$ hour of Dancing, Walking or Aerobics (new total time for workout: 1 hour per week)
Week #3:	Activity Add-On, Activity Add-On, and new Swap	While continuing all previous Choices: Swap Slow Trigger Foods for typical Quick Trigger Foods at evening snacks (have pretzels, baked chips and dip, and/or fruit instead of usual candy, cookies, and juice)

And so on . . .

SAMPLE ALTERNATIVE #2:
Joshua D.* was fourteen years old. He enjoyed salads and would eat *some* vegetables and he liked meat and chicken. On the other hand, he strongly preferred to work at his computer rather than exercise or participate in sports. Here's a sample of his alternative order of selection of Choices:

Week #1:	Food Add-On	Add some chicken, meat and/or some Insulin-Balancing vegetables or salad to usual dinner each day
Week #2:	Food Add-On and new Food Add-On	While continuing previous Choice: Add some chicken, meat and/or some Insulin-Balancing vegetables or salad to usual afterschool snack each day
Week #3:	Food Add-On, Food Add-On, and new Food Add-On	While continuing all previous Choices: Add some chicken, meat and/or some Insulin-Balancing vegetables or salad to usual breakfast each day
Week #4	Food Add-On, Food Add-On, Food Add-On, and Activity Add-On	While continuing all previous Choices: Add walking (around mall) for $1/2$ hour once each week (giving him an opportunity to check out all the new gadgets in his favorite stores).

And so on . . .

* In all cases, names and identifying details have been changed.

How to Incorporate a Food Add-On

1. Look over the list of Insulin-Balancing Add-On Foods that begins on page 183. This list contains a wide variety of high-protein and fiber-rich foods that your youngster can Add-On to any one meal or snack.
2. Keeping your youngster's preferences and needs in mind, help your child select one daily meal or snack each day to which an Insulin-Balancing Protein or Vegetable will be added.

The type of food your youngster adds can vary from day to day as long as it is an Insulin-Balancing Add-On Food and it is added to the same meal each day.

The type of food your youngster adds can vary from day to day as long as (1) it is any one of the protein-rich or high-fiber foods that is included on the Insulin-Balancing Foods List, and (2) it is added to the same meal or snack each day.

For some kids, snacks may vary from day to day; incorporate an Add-On to a snack only if that snack is a regular part of your youngster's daily eating routine.

If your youngster is making an Insulin-Balancing Add-On Food Choice for the first time, have him or her choose a meal or snack that would normally *not* include protein-rich or high-fiber foods, in other words, one that consists almost totally of high-carbohydrate foods (starches, snack foods, junk food, and sweets (including fruit). That after-school snack that used to contain only fruit, for instance, might be a perfect choice to which to Add-On some Insulin-Balancing Protein, like mini-cheese squares or sliced chicken one day, or some celery stuffed with regular or low-fat cream cheese the next. If this is *not* your youngster's first Food Add-On Choice, see the "In the Weeks to Come" section that follows for help in adding new foods to meals that already include Insulin-Balancing Foods.

So for this first week, your youngster will add at least one Insulin-Balancing Food to the same meal or snack each day. Each Add-On portion should be equal to an "average portion," given your youngster's age. When adding a new food, it is sometimes a good idea to reduce the total amount of other foods to make room for this new addition, but if your youngster can and wants to eat all of the regular meal or snack in addition to the Add-On food, that's quite all right, too. If your youngster cannot or does not want to finish all the food at that meal or snack, remove or reduce any foods *other* than those that are Added-On.

**The goal is *not* to force kids to reduce their food intake
or to limit or prohibit foods, but rather
to correct the *cause* of the hunger and cravings.**

The goal is *not* to reduce food intake by prohibiting or limiting foods, but rather to add Insulin-Balancing Proteins or Vegetables to those carbohydrate-rich foods your youngster routinely eats in order to balance these meals. As your youngster's intake of carbos is balanced by protein-rich or fiber-rich foods, insulin levels should naturally drop and with them, intense and recurring carbo cravings and blood sugar swings.

Remember, the particular Insulin-Balancing Food that your youngster selects can change from day to day (a variety of choices is a good idea), and the food choice may be an Insulin-Balancing Protein, a high-fiber Insulin-Balancing Vegetable, or a food that incorporates both (chicken salad made from chicken and celery, for instance), as long as all new additions can be found in the Insulin-Balancing Foods List that follows and as long as the food is added to the same meal or snack each day.

It is important to be certain that during the week you have on hand a wide variety of Insulin-Balancing Add-On

Foods. You will find wonderful new recipes, and quick and easy suggestions beginning on page 291.

Remember also that Insulin-Balancing Foods that are added to meals and snacks are meant to balance and complement other foods—particularly Carbohydrate-Rich Foods—that your youngster may prefer and crave, not to replace them totally. Carbohydrate-Rich Foods such as bread, pasta, rice, and other complex carbohydrates are needed for both enjoyment and health. For the carbohydrate-addicted youngster, Carbohydrate-Rich Foods can—and should—be part of each day's eating, but as time goes on a greater number of carbo-loaded meals and snacks will, with the addition of Insulin-Balancing Proteins and Vegetables, become well-balanced Combo Meals and Snacks. A common mistake that parents make is to demand that a youngster give up a food that he or she enjoys and cherishes. Don't even try to do it. You will be faced with rebellion, and the success of any program will be jeopardized.

Food Add-Ons, on the other hand, are less likely to put you in conflict with your youngster. Since Food Add-Ons are meant to be just that—food to be added on to your youngster's usual meals and snacks—and because they take away nothing your child enjoys, you can usually avoid the defiance and resistance that "diets" often generate. Some youngsters may resist the thought of adding something new (we'll give you some help as we go on), others will be willing to accommodate, but, in either case, Add-On Choices are not likely to put you and your youngster into a "no win" situation.

Food Add-Ons may not put you and your youngster into an emotional battle but they can help win the war; Food Add-Ons can do wonders. As Insulin-Balancing Foods are slowly added to your child's previously unbalanced high-carbohydrate meals, you will find that your youngster's blood sugar swings may disappear, naturally.[5] Mood and

---

[5] If, as additional Choices are added on The Step-By-Step Plan, your youngster does not experience dramatic reductions in blood sugar–related problems, as appropriate, consider switching to The Jump-Start Plan. See page 204 for complete details on switching plans.

impulse control problems often resolve easily as your
youngsters reflect a new balance within their bodies.
Energy levels stabilize and can be maintained without periodic and sometimes unpredictable swings.

**When high-carbohydrate meals are
balanced by the addition of Insulin-Balancing Foods,
blood sugar levels can stabilize—naturally.**

In the chapters that follow, you will find recipes and hints
on how best to make Add-On Insulin-Balancing Foods most
appealing to a youngster's particular tastes, as well as strategies for dealing with the most finicky eater (yes, even yours!).

If there is no Insulin-Balancing Food Choice that you
feel is appropriate for your youngster or that he or she is
willing to add, feel free to move to the Step #2's Choice List
and make a selection from that list instead. If and when
appropriate, come back to the Food Add-On Choice List at
some future time. But for now, continue to Step #2.

3. After your youngster has incorporated a Food Add-On for
   at least one week and is ready to move on, read the
   "Step #2" section that follows.

Step #2: Incorporate an Activity Add-On

Overview

Incorporating an Activity Add-On simply entails adding easy,
time-limited, and enjoyable movements, exercises, and activities
to your youngster's regular routine. While most people will agree
that activity, in general, is essential to the health and well-being
of most youngsters, we include activity as part of the Program not
only because it is generally good common sense to do so but
because, in addition, activity has been shown to reduce and stabilize insulin levels.

INSULIN-BALANCING FOODS*

Insulin-Balancing Foods contain fewer carbohydrates than Carbohydrate-Rich Foods and your youngster's body will release less insulin after eating Insulin-Balancing Foods than the flood of insulin that usually follows the consumption of Carbohydrate-Rich Foods.

The following Insulin-Balancing Foods can generally be eaten (as part of the Program) without concern for hunger-rebound, that is, the cravings cycle that brings your youngster back for more and more carbohydrate-rich foods.

Important: Choose low-fat varieties, as appropriate, based upon recommendations of your youngster's physician. (see page 417 for low-fat choice guidance).

Remember, if a food is not listed in the Insulin-Balancing Foods list that follows, it should automatically be considered to be a Carbohydrate-Rich Food.

On The Step-By-Step Plan*:
Add-On Choices: Add–On any Insulin-Balancing food to your youngster's formerly high-carbo meals or snacks. These meals, now containing both Insulin-Reducing and Carbo-Rich Foods, have become Combo Meals. The addition of high-fiber or protein-rich foods can help reduce your youngster's addictive response to carbohydrates. Choices are based on adding any of these foods to the same daily meal or snack. Each Insulin-Balancing Add-On should be equal to an "average portion" for a child or teen your youngster's age. In time, quantities of Carbohydrate-Rich Foods will naturally reduce as Add-Ons add up.

Hold-On Choices: At one daily meal or snack, help your youngster "Hold-On" by refraining from all Carbohydrate-Rich Foods (including starches, snack foods, junk food, and sweets). When a Hold-On is chosen that meal contains only insulin-balancing proteins and/or vegetables and other foods on the Insulin-Balancing food list. Youngsters "hold-on" and wait to have any Carbo-hydrate-Rich Foods (pages 184–185) for the next regular meal or snack that would typically contain them. You will find fun and easy insulin-balancing meal recipes starting on page 308.

On The Jump-Start Plan*:
Combo Meals: Combine Insulin-Balancing proteins and/or vegetables from this Insulin-Balancing Foods list with carbohydrate-rich foods (especially breads, grains, fruits, and carbo-rich vegetables, see pages 184–185) to make a *balanced* Combo Meal. During Phase One, for a timelimited period, one Combo Meal will be eaten each day and all other meals and snacks will be Insulin-Balancing Meals containing Insulin-Balancing Foods only. During Phase Two, an additional Combo Meal will replace an Insulin-Balancing Meal, once each week. See page 214 for balancing guidelines.

Insulin-Balancing Meals: Combine proteins and vegetables from this Insulin-Balancing Foods list to make delicious meals and salads. Insulin-Balancing Meals should contain Insulin-Balancing Foods only.

INSULIN-BALANCING PROTEINS

Insulin-Balancing proteins should be baked, pan-fried with very little fat, roasted, broiled, boiled, sauteed, steamed, stir-fried, but not breaded.

MEATS*:

All regular and lean meats that contain no added filler or sugars, including:
Bacon
Beef
Corned beef
Ham
Hot dogs (all meat, no filler)
Lamb
Pastrami
Pork
Sausages (no sugar added)
Veal

FOWL

Chicken
Cornish hen
Duck
Goose
Turkey

FISH AND SHELLFISH

All varieties, canned or fresh

INSULIN-BALANCING DAIRY* AND MEAT ALTERNATIVES:

Regular or low-fat varieties of ONLY :
Eggs and egg substitutes
Cheese
Cream cheese
Cottage cheese
Sour cream
Tofu (soybean curd)
Vegetarian meat alternatives (that contain 4 grams of carbohydrates or less per serving)

Note: *Always make selections as in keeping with physician recommendations. For low-fat suggestion see "Incorporating Health Recommendations Into Your Youngster's Eating Program," page 417. Appropriateness and duration of phase and program should incorporate recommendations by your youngster's physician who, as with all programs that call for changes in your youngster's eating and activity regimen, should approve your youngster's participation and monitor his/her progress.
**For simple, fun ideas, see our kids-friendly recipe section starting on page 289.

INSULIN-BALANCING VEGETABLES

Many fiber-rich vegetables are tasty raw; they make wonderful finger foods when eaten plain or topped with one of our sensational dips,** when steamed, stir-fried, or sauteed.

VEGETABLES:

IMPORTANT: *Not* all vegetables are low in carbohydrates (that is, not all are Insulin-Balancing Foods).Vegetables that are *not* listed below as Insulin-Balancing vegetables, are Carbo-Rich vegetables and should be treated as any Carbohydrate-Rich Foods (see page 185 for a list of Carbohydrate-Rich vegetables).

Alfalfa sprouts
Arugula
Asparagus
Bamboo Shoots
Beans (green, snap, or wax)
Bean Sprouts
Cabbage (all varieties)
Cauliflower
Celery
Cucumbers
Dill pickles
Greens (all varieties)
Kale
Kohlrabi
Lettuce
Mushrooms
Okra
Onions (up to two tablespoons)
Parsley
Peppers (green only)
Radishes
Scallions
Spinach

ADDITIONAL LOW-CARBOHYDRATE FOODS:

NOTE: THESE FOODS MAY BE INCLUDED IN INSULIN-BALANCING AND COMBO MEALS BUT SHOULD NOT BE USED AS ADD-ONS
Herbs and spices Soy flour (used sparingly as incidental in recipe)
Oils and fats:*
Butter, margarine, mayonnaise (regular), olives.

CARBOHYDRATE-RICH FOODS

This chart includes examples of *some* of the many Carbohydrate-Rich Foods typically found in youngsters' diets. Carbohydrate-Rich Foods, particularly starches, fruits and high-carbo vegetables, are essential to good health and well-being and some must be included each day as a part of your youngster's well-rounded diet. Quantities depend on your youngster's individual needs. Unless your physician advises otherwise, choose "average-size" portions appropriate for your youngster's age. There is no need to measure or weigh food and your youngster can come back for more, as long as Carbohydrate-Rich Foods are consumed only at appropriate meals and are balanced with Insulin-Balancing Foods. See page 214 for balance guidelines.

On The Step-By-Step Plan*:
    Add-On Choices and Combo Meals: Carbohydrate-Rich Food portions should be decreased slowly and be supplemented and replaced by increasing portions of Insulin-Balancing Foods that have been "added-on" (see page 174).

    Hold-On Meals and Insulin-Balancing Meals: as a Hold-On choice, these Carbohydrate-Rich Foods should be removed from a meal or snack and saved for the next meal or snack that would typically contain them. The Carbohydrate-Rich Foods that would normally be eaten during this meal should be replaced entirely by Insulin-Balancing Foods. (see page 190).

On The Jump-Start Plan*:
    Combo Meals: Be sure to include a variety of healthful Carbohydrate-Rich Foods (particularly starches, fruits, and high-carbo vegetables) in your youngster's Combo Meals and balance them with portions of salad and Insulin-Balancing vegetables and protein (see page 214).

    Insulin-Balancing Meals: Do not include any of the Carbohydrate-Rich Foods in this chart in your youngster's Insulin-Balancing Meals (see page 212).

CARBOHYDRATE-RICH FOODS

Breads, grains and cereals
All varieties including regular or low-fat:

Bagels	Grits
Biscuits	Pancakes
Bread	Tabuli
Cereal (hot or cold)	Tahini
Corn meal	Tempura coating
Couscous	Stuffing
Croissants	Waffles, etc.

CARBOHYDRATE-RICH FOODS (*continued*)

Vegetables

Carbohydrate-Rich vegetables are usually starchy or root vegetables and include all of the following vegetables.

These vegetables should *not* be included in Insulin-Balancing Meals but can be part of all balanced Carbohydrate-Rich Meals:

Beets
Broccoli
Brussels Sprouts
Carrots
Corn
Eggplant
Onions (when more than small amount)
Peas
Peppers (red)
Potatoes
Squash and Zucchini
Turnips
Tomatoes (when more than 1/4 tomato per meal)

Fruits and Fruit Juices

All varieties including fresh, dried or cooked:

Apples
Bananas
Blackberries
Blueberries
Cantaloupe
Cherries
Coconut
Dates and Figs
Grapes
Grapefruit
Honeydew
Kiwi fruit
Lemons and Limes
Mangoes
Nectarines
Oranges
Papaya
Peaches
Pears
Pineapple
Plums
Raisins
Strawberries
Tangerines
Watermelon

Dairy** and Meat Alternatives

Regular, frozen and low-fat varieties of:
Cream
Milk
Yogurt
Ice cream
Ice milk
Vegetarian meat alternatives (which contain 5 grams of carbohydrates or more per serving)

Legumes, Seeds, and Nuts

All varieties of beans, seeds and nuts including:
Beans (black, kidney, lima, etc.)
Cashews
Chestnuts
Garbanzos (chick peas)
Peanuts
Pistachios
Pumpkin seeds
Soy "nuts"

Snack Foods**:

All varieties

Luncheon Meats with Filler**:

All varieties

Sweets, Sugars, Desserts, Cakes, Candies**:

All varieties; any food containing sugar or honey

Beverages

All fruit juices and juice drinks
All sweetened drinks

Carbohydrate Act-Alikes**:

All foods, drinks, gums and mints that contain sugar-substitutes or artificial sweeteners of any kind.

Note: * Appropriateness and duration of phase and program should incorporate recommendations by your youngster's physician who, as with all programs that call for changes in your youngster's eating and activity regimen, should approve your youngster's participation and monitor his/her progress.

** These foods have been included for the sake of completeness of categorical listings. Appropriateness of the inclusion and/or appropriate amounts of these foods in your youngster's diet should be determined by a conference with his/her physician.

Sports-loving and physically active children and teens (Carbo Burners) may not need help in this area, but some carbohydrate-addicted youngsters, especially those who are Carbo Collectors, need motivational support and real-life, kid-friendly suggestions to help them fight their body's physical tendency to conserve energy and remain inactive.

**The not-so-active carbohydrate-addicted kid
is probably *not* lazy.**

Contrary to what most parents have been told, not-so-active carbohydrate-addicted kids are usually not lazy; their bodies may simply not process food energy well and, in doing so, signal their bodies to conserve energy. Though these youngsters may seem at times to eat a great deal and do little, their muscles may literally not be getting the energy they need. For the carbohydrate-addicted youngster, food energy may be channeled to fat cells rather than to muscles. Though many of the food-related Choices you will select may help correct this imbalance, it is also helpful to add some activity and movement to your youngster's program.

Through mechanisms that scientists are still uncovering, activity clearly lowers insulin levels. Some scientists say that with activity the body becomes less "insulin resistant"—able to use insulin and burn blood sugar more appropriately. Other researchers contend that activity signals the body to release more of the "spending hormone" glucagon, rather than the "saving hormone" insulin, and so insulin levels are kept low and blood sugar levels stable. In either case, no matter what the explanation, we have found that easy, fun, and youngster-friendly Activity Add-Ons not only motivate the not-so-active youngster but, in addition, help move his or her body toward an ideal insulin and blood sugar balance.

**Some activity and movement is important,
but vigorous exercise regimens are
not a requirement of the Program.**

It is important to understand that vigorous exercise is not necessary on The Carbohydrate Addict's Program for Children and Teens. Activities such as dancing, walking, in-line skating, bike riding, skateboarding, and basketball can be a fun part of the Program and can help normalize your youngster's insulin levels.

Keep in mind that if your youngster is not able to, or simply does not want to choose an Activity Add-On, there are other Choices. This is a step-by-step program, and as your youngster begins to look and feel better, activity and movement will hold greater appeal. Give your child or teen a free hand for the moment, move on to the next Choice for now, and in time, as the body comes into balance, the mind and spirit may follow— without struggle.

Although like weekly Food Add-Ons, Activity Add-On Choices are simple in themselves, in combination with the other Choices, these selections can make important and dramatic changes in your youngster's insulin balance and in the areas of weight, behavior, learning, and mood as well.

So encourage but don't demand, persuade but don't push. Your youngster's resistance is simply a sign of the physical imbalance that the Program itself will help remedy.

How to Incorporate an Activity Add-On Choice

1. Look over the Add-On Activity Choice List on page 188. It contains a wide variety of fun activities that your youngster can enjoy.
2. Keeping your youngster's needs and preferences in mind, help him or her pick one Activity Choice as a second step selection.

    Once during the week, your youngster will add this activity to his or her regular routine, *while continuing* the first week's Add-On Food Choice. As with all Choices, encourage and guide but, if at all possible, respect your youngster's strongest desires.

    If there is no Activity Add-On Choice that you feel is appropriate for your youngster or that your youngster is willing to add, feel free to move to Step #3's Choice List and make a selection from it instead. If appropriate, come back to the Activity Add-On Choice List at some future time. But for now, continue to Step #3.

3. After your youngster has incorporated an Activity Add-On for at least one week and is ready to move to the next step, read the "Step #3" section that follows. Remember that each Choice, in combination with other Choices, works toward lowering your youngster's addiction to carbohydrates and will make the incorporation of the following week's Choice that much easier.

ADD-ON ACTIVITY CHOICES

Though it is always a good idea to start with a light Add-On activity choice and work up to more challenging ones, activity choices can be selected from *any* of the categories listed below. Each activity choice is based on one half-hour workout, once each week. Have your youngster pick a day and time and encourage him or her to stick to it.

Note: There will be other opportunities to increase the frequency of these workouts, but we have found it best to add one workout period per week at a time.

LIGHT ACTIVITY

Biking (regular or stationary bike): easy, gliding, at even pace or on flat surface

Bowling

Dancing: moderate pace

Gymnastics: light play or tumbling

Pool play: easy paddling or swimming, beach ball throwing, or any light pool fun

In-line skating, roller skating, or ice skating: mostly coasting on flat surfaces

Skateboarding: at very easy pace

Sledding or tobogganing: easy play

Walking: briskly, at home, outside, or in mall

MODERATE ACTIVITY

Aerobics: light to moderate pace

Baseball, basketball, football, soccer, volleyball, tennis: light, easy pace

Biking (regular or stationary bike): moderate pace

Dancing: fast-paced, without interruption

Gymnastics: moderate activities or tumbling

Jogging: light, brisk running

Pool play: brisk, intense play or paddling, without interruption

Rope jumping: light to moderate pace

In-line skating, roller skating, or ice skating: light to moderate pace

Swimming: moderate, even-paced

Skateboarding: moderate pace

Skiing (cross country/downhill): light to moderate; count periods of skiing only

Sledding or tobogganing: moderate pace, with some rest

Walking: fast-paced, without interruption, at home, outside, or in mall

VIGOROUS ACTIVITY

Aerobics: intense, fast-paced

Baseball, basketball, football, soccer, volleyball, tennis: moderate to fast pace

Biking (stationary bike): strong, fast pace

Gymnastics: intense workouts or tumbling

Jogging: intense running

Rope jumping: fast-paced, consistent

Swimming: fast-paced

Select choices only if they do not conflict with recommendations of your youngster's physician.

Step #3: Incorporate a Hold-On Choice

Overview

Hold-On Choices involve delaying the consumption of all carbohydrate-rich foods (including starches, snack foods, junk food, and naturally sweetened or artificially sweetened goodies) that are usually eaten at a particular daily meal or snack, and "holding on," that is, waiting to have carbohydrate-rich foods until the next meal or snack that would normally include them. Hold-On Meals and Snacks, then, will not have any Carbohydrate-Rich Foods. Kids "hold on" and have the Carbohydrate-Rich Foods they desire at the next meal. While youngsters may not be thrilled to forego their special treats, this Choice is "do-able" because kids can count on having the food they love at their next meal or snack. By that time, their insulin is more likely in balance and their cravings and blood sugar swings are greatly reduced.

When Carbohydrate-Rich Foods are eliminated from a meal, the meal will now contain low-carbohydrate Insulin-Balancing Foods only. For that reason, meals in which all Carbohydrate-Rich Foods have been removed (meals in which youngsters "hold on" until later to eat Carbohydrate-Rich Foods) are referred to as Insulin-Balancing Meals. (Combo Meals, in contrast, balance and combine Insulin-Balancing Foods with Carbohydrate-Rich Foods in one meal.)

It is very important to know that our research has shown that the more *often* Carbohydrate-Rich Foods or artificially sweetened foods are eaten over the course of a day, the more they can trigger insulin imbalances that lead to recurring carbohydrate cravings and low blood sugar cycles. For this reason, we refer to Carbohydrate-Rich Foods as Trigger Foods.

**It is essential to give your youngster's body
the time it needs to recover from
carbohydrate-induced insulin insults.**

Reducing the number of *times* each day that your youngster eats Trigger Foods gives your youngster's body a greater opportunity to "reset," that is, to regain its optimal insulin balance through a longer recovery time between insulin insults.

A Simple Note About Complex Carbos: It is essential to remember that complex carbohydrates are necessary for good health and *must* be included in your youngster's diet every day. Sweet treats, though not necessary for good health, are often quite important to some youngsters, and in most cases cannot be eliminated. Hold-On Choices offer an easy and practical solution.

Hold-On Choices can help reduce or eliminate the negative insulin impact that Trigger Foods can have on your youngster's carbohydrate-sensitive body by decreasing the number of times each day your youngster consumes these Carbohydrate-Rich Foods. In this way, Hold-On Choices can help your youngster regain insulin and blood sugar balance without sacrificing either good nutrition or the enjoyment of their greatly cherished treats.

**When kids "hold on" and consume Carbohydrate-Rich
Foods less often, they still get the food they love
but their cravings diminish or disappear—naturally.
Even goodies lose their power.**

Though treats and goodies can remain in each day's fare, they can now become a portion of it, rather than its central focus. These foods will probably no longer hold as great a "power" over your youngster. And best of all, this balance will come naturally, easily, and without struggle.

With your guidance, your youngster will still be able to enjoy treats but simply eat them less often.

**Your youngster will learn quickly that the goodies
he or she enjoys so much will not be taken away.**

When youngsters know they can count on having treats at specifically agreed-upon meals, snacks, or occasions, they grow secure in the knowledge that their favorite foods will not be taken away, and as high-carbohydrate snacks become *less frequent* and insulin levels return to normal, youngsters experience a natural reduction in cravings for starches, junk food, snack foods, and sweets. This circle of restored health perpetuates itself just as the addiction did in the past.

> **The changes that come about naturally
> can be truly astounding.**

Freed of feelings of resentment, rebellion, deprivation, and the drive for carbohydrates, youngsters quickly gain confidence and control as well as a new ability to delay gratification.

During a Hold-On (Insulin-Balancing) Meal or Snack, your youngster is free to choose from any of the Insulin-Balancing Foods listed beginning on page 183, knowing that favorite goodies will still be forthcoming. To make things even easier and more pleasurable, you will find recipes for fun, easy, and satisfying Insulin-Balancing Meals and Snacks beginning on page 308.

> **Treats and goodies can remain in each day's fare,
> but they can now become a portion of it,
> rather than the central focus.**

How to Incorporate a Hold-On:

1. Look over the list of Insulin-Balancing Foods on page 183.
2. During one meal or snack each day, your youngster will "hold-on" and delay the consumption of all Carbohydrate-Rich Foods until the next meal or snack that would normally include these foods. During Hold-On Meals and Snacks, your youngster should eat *only* Insulin-Balancing

Proteins, Vegetables, and other Foods that are found in the
Insulin-Balancing Foods List (page 183). Because these
meals include only Insulin-Balancing Foods, they are
referred to as a Insulin-Balancing Meals or Snacks.

Keeping your youngster's preferences and needs in
mind, help your youngster select one daily meal or snack
during which he or she will refrain from eating all carbohydrate-rich foods, including all breads, cereals, and other
starches, as well as all snack foods, junk foods, and sweets,
and instead eat only foods found in the Insulin-Balancing
Foods List. Remind your youngster that Carbohydrate-Rich
Foods will be saved and enjoyed at all other meals or snacks
that would normally include them. As always, while
selecting a Hold-On Choice, continue all previous Choice
selections. (If your youngster's new Hold-On Meal contains
any other Choice, see the "Special Circumstances" section
that follows). No additional meals or snacks should be
added to compensate for the addition of Hold-On Choices.

3. You can help your youngster make Hold-On Meals or
Snacks even more fun and satisfying by using some of the
many Insulin-Balancing recipes you will find beginning on
page 308.

As Hold-Ons are incorporated, you will find that your
youngster's intense drive for junk food, snack foods, and
sweets diminishes naturally.[6] Other foods will become more
interesting to your child, not because of threats or
promises, but because the child's body—now itself in balance—will naturally desire a more balanced diet.

If there is no Hold-On Choice that you feel is appropriate for your youngster or that he or she is willing to add,
feel free to move to Step #4's Choice List and make a selection from that list instead. If and when appropriate, come
back to the Hold-On Choice List at some future time. But
for now, continue to Step #4.

---

[6]If, as additional Choices are added on The Step-By-Step Plan, your youngster
does not experience dramatic reductions in cravings, as appropriate, consider
switching to The Jump-Start Plan. See page 204 for complete details on
switching plans.

4. After your youngster has incorporated a Hold-On Choice for at least one week and is ready to move to the next step, read the "Step #4" section that follows.

Step #4: Incorporating a Swap

Overview

Incorporating a Swap Choice entails choosing one meal or snack each day and at that meal or snack, trading one type of Carbohydrate-Rich Food for another.

When making a Swap Choice, your youngster will replace a Quick Trigger Food, one that is likely to cause a strong physical reaction, with a Slow Trigger Food, one that is less likely to cause as quick or intense an insulin and blood sugar response.

Slow Trigger Foods are less likely to bring about intense insulin and blood sugar swings.

TRIGGER FOODS DEFINED

All starches, snack foods, junk food, sweets, and many of the foods that we call carbohydrate act-alikes (those that contain artificial sweeteners or sugar substitutes) can cause the carbohydrate addict's body to release excess levels of insulin that can bring on carbohydrate cravings and blood sugar swings. Since, for many, both Carbohydrate-Rich Foods and carbohydrate act-alikes "trigger" these changes, we refer to both Carbohydrate-Rich Foods and carbohydrate act-alike foods as Trigger Foods.

Not all Trigger Foods will have the same impact on your youngster.

But not all Trigger Foods will have the same impact on carbo-hydrate-addicted youngsters. We have found that recurring and/or intense cravings and blood sugar swings occur most often after the consumption of foods that contain the simpler sugars (sucrose, fructose, dextrose, lactose, galactose, glucose, corn syrup, and "high-fructose corn syrup"). Simple sugars are made up of single or double molecules of sugar that cross the stomach barrier quickly and raise blood sugar rapidly. In nature, simple sugars are usually found in the presence of fiber, which helps slow down digestion and blood sugar responses, but food manufacturers have removed nature's fiber balance.

> **The human body was *not* built to digest juice**
> **without the pulp or to consume artificial sweeteners**
> **or soda . . . or candy!**

So youngsters find themselves in a nutritional dilemma, craving the sweet taste of foods their bodies were never designed to handle. Table sugar, candy, cookies, and the like do not exist in nature. The human body was never meant to deal with artifi-cial sweeteners and low-fat substitutes or with refined or processed foods. These foods can throw a youngster's entire blood sugar regulating system out of kilter.

Even the way we consume so-called healthy foods such as fruits are not in keeping with the natural order of things. The human body was meant to digest fruit only a few weeks out of the year, when it was ripe; the body was never meant to digest the bombardment of sugars found in fruit juice, where the balancing fiber or pulp has been removed. These foods, which so quickly impact on insulin and blood sugar levels, we call Quick Trigger Foods.

While complex carbohydrates such as those found in whole grain cereals, pasta, rice, potatoes, and other starchy foods stimu-late insulin responses, cravings, and blood sugar changes, partic-ularly in carbo-addicted kids, the physical response is usually not as intense or immediate. These foods are made of long strings of sugars that come apart more slowly in the digestive process. Most youngsters find that these foods do not bring about insulin and blood sugar swings as quickly or as intensely as do simple sugars. For this reason we refer to starchy foods and whole fresh fruits (containing all the natural fibrous pulp) as Slow Trigger Foods.

At a Swap Meal or Snack, your youngster will replace Quick Trigger Foods (such as candy, cake, or cookies) with Slow Trigger Foods (such as popcorn, chips, rice cakes, and pretzels).

Your involvement, your cooperation in making sure that a variety of Slow Trigger Foods is available for your youngster's "treat times," and your encouragement will play an important role in your youngster's learning how to successfully "Swap" Quick Trigger Foods for Slow Triggers. You will find a simple Swap List on page 197 and sample snack recipes on page 298.

How to Incorporate a Swap

1. Look over the Simple Sample Swap List on page 197. Notice the difference between Quick Trigger Foods and Slow Trigger Foods.
2. Help your youngster select *one* daily meal or snack, designated as the Swap Meal or Swap Snack. Using the Simple Sample Swap List that follows, remove all Quick Trigger Foods that are usually eaten at that particular meal or snack and replace them with any of the Slow Trigger Foods listed.

   If there is no Swap Choice that you feel is appropriate for your youngster or that he or she is willing to add, feel free to move to the "In the Weeks to Come" section that follows. If and when appropriate, come back to the Swap Choice List at some future time.
3. After your youngster has incorporated a Swap Choice for at least one week and is ready to move to the next step, read the "In the Weeks to Come" section that follows.

SIMPLE SAMPLE SWAPS

Quick Trigger Foods are intensely sweet and often bring on strong insulin and blood sugar reactions. They may be sweetened with table sugar, fruit sugar, or any other sweetener, real or artificial. While *Slow* Trigger Foods also raise insulin levels, they may be more slowly metabolized and provide a better choice when carbohydrate-rich treats are unavoidable.

SWAPS: At the same meal or snack each day, remove all Quick Trigger Foods that are usually consumed at that meal or snack, and replace with Slow Trigger Foods instead.

Remove all of these Quick Trigger Foods	And replace with any of these Slow Trigger Foods instead
Fruit juice,* dried fruits, fruit rolls, fruit leathers	Whole fresh fruits and vegetables of any kind along with their natural fibrous pulp
Candy, cake, cookies	Chips, dips,** pretzels, popcorn
Ice cream, ice pops, fruit pops	Non-frozen yogurt, either plain or containing real fresh fruit (no preserves, sugar or artificial sweetener)
Donuts, snack bars, cookies, cake	Rice cakes (without sugar), chips and popcorn, pretzels (low-fat, if appropriate)
Sugar-sweetened cereals	No-sugar cereals
Soda (sweetened with sugar or sugar substitute), fruit juice,* "sports drinks," fruit-flavored drinks	Water, milk (regular, low-fat, or skim; not flavored), decaffeinated iced tea (no sweetener—neither sugar nor sugar substitute), plain seltzer

* Fruit juice can be swapped for either fresh fruit or a drink substitute as indicated in chart above.
**See our great recipe section for slow trigger suggestions, including dips, that kids enjoy. As appropriate, choose low-fat varieties.

In the Weeks to Come

After your youngster has added to his or her regular routine one of each of the four Choices in The Step-By-Step Plan (that is, an Add-On Insulin-Balancing Food Choice, an Add-On Activity Choice, a Hold-On Choice, and a Swap Choice), your youngster is then free to go back and select any of these same types of Choices, in any order, for additional meals or activities.

For new Food Add-Ons, have your youngster once again look over the foods in the Insulin-Balancing Foods List on page 183 and choose another meal or snack to which these foods can be regularly added. Your youngster may choose to add another Insulin-Balancing Protein or Vegetable to the same meal to which he or she previously added such a protein or vegetable, for instance, or your child might prefer to add an Insulin-Balancing Add-On Food to another meal or snack altogether. Just be sure to have your youngster add Insulin-Balancing Foods to no more than one *new* daily meal or snack at a time, continuing it for a full week before making any other selections. With each new Choice, at the same time, your youngster should continue the previous Choices.

To Add-On new activities, continue to choose any selections that look interesting and fun, adding no more than one new Choice per week while continuing all previous Choices.

When it comes to Add-On Activity Choices, you may find that instead of adding a new Activity Choice to previous Activity Choices, it makes more sense to increase the length of time your youngster participates in an activity, the number of times each week he or she participates, or the level of activity (from light to moderate, for instance).

Your youngster can opt to increase the length of time of any activity—by half-hour increments[7]—or to increase the level or the frequency of any previous Activity Choice. In all these cases, consider the increase in time, frequency, or level as a new Choice selection. If, on the other hand, your youngster prefers to add a whole new Activity Choice to the weekly schedule, that, too, is perfectly acceptable. This is, after all, a program of Choice.

---

[7]With approval from your youngster's physician.

When your youngster wants to make a new selection other than a Food or Activity Add-On, be sure to remember that a new Hold-On Choice or Swap Choice can also be selected, one at a time, no more than once each week, while continuing all previous selections. (If your youngster's new Hold-On Meal contains any other Choice, see the "Special Circumstances" section that follows). Continue adding Choices until an Optimal Carbo Balance is reached (see details below).

The Step-By-Step Plan: Achieving an Optimal Carbo Balance

The Step-By-Step Plan leads and encourages your youngster to reach Optimal Carbo Balance directly, by incorporating Choices that balance Carbohydrate-Rich Foods with protein-rich or high-fiber foods (Food Add-Ons), increasing physical activity (Activity Add-Ons), slowly reducing the number of times each day Carbohydrate-Rich Foods are consumed (Hold-Ons), and replacing simple sugars with complex carbos (Swaps).

Each of these changes has been shown to lower insulin levels. As insulin levels decrease, blood sugar levels balance, and cravings, weight, and other related problems will usually begin to disappear. As problems begin to disappear and continue to disappear, this is the body's way of signaling that an ideal balance of carbohydrates and other foods in combination with activity has been reached.

Pinpointing Your Youngster's Optimal Carbo Balance

Unless otherwise indicated, your youngster should continue incorporating Choices until he or she reaches an Optimal Carbo Balance, that is, the ideal combination of food and activity that balances insulin and blood sugar levels and reduces or eliminates cravings, weight, behavioral, mood, and other related problems.

To pinpoint your youngster's Optimal Carbo Balance on The Step-By-Step Plan:

1. Continue incorporating weekly Choices according to The Step-By-Step Plan while you remain aware of your youngster's progress until one or more of the following changes occurs (as appropriate to your youngster):

   Carbohydrate cravings become far less *frequent* or have disappeared, or
   Carbohydrate cravings become far less *intense* or have been eliminated, or
   Weight problems start to resolve themselves[8] (that is, your youngster is losing weight or has stopped gaining weight as appropriate to your youngster), or
   Behavioral, mood, learning, or motivation problems are greatly reduced, have become far less frequent, or have disappeared.[9]

2. When one or more of the changes found in number one and appropriate changes in your youngster's carbohydrate addiction have occurred, stop *adding* new Choices.
   Continue all past selections. As long as your youngster's cravings, weight, and other insulin and blood-sugar-related problems continue to diminish or remain resolved, no new Choices need to be added. This combination of Choices can be said to have brought your youngster to Optimal Carbohydrate Balance; affording your child or teen Carbohydrate-Rich Foods while eliminating or keeping to a minimum the negative responses often related to insulin and blood sugar swings.

[8,9]For purposes of pinpointing Optimal Carbo Balance, you need not wait until all excess weight has been lost or until all behavioral, learning, motivation, or mood problems have been totally resolved. When your youngster has achieved *continued movement* in the direction of resolving difficulties in any of these areas, the first step in pinpointing an Optimal Carbo Balance should be considered to have been achieved (that is, the program has put your youngster *on the road* to success in this area).

3. If, after you have stopped adding Choices, the problems begin to reemerge, return to adding Choices until the problems once again are decreased or eliminated, that is, until the child has reached an Optimal Carbo Balance.

Important Note: Your youngster should always, unless clearly instructed by a physician, include an appropriate portion of Carbohydrate-Rich Foods in at least one balanced Combo Meal *every day*.

The Step-By-Step Plan: Special Circumstances

Suppose my youngster was doing that already?

Chances are, you will find that your youngster was incorporating one or more of the steps as part of everyday routine before ever coming to the Program. For instance, your youngster may regularly consume an Insulin-Balancing Protein as part of each night's dinner or your child may already be involved in an activity or sport. Your teen may regularly prefer Slow Trigger Foods for snacks.

These "natural" steps toward insulin balance are exciting and important but they do not take the place of the Food Add-Ons, Activity Add-Ons, Hold-Ons, and Swaps of the Program. You should build on your youngster's healthy tendencies with the intentional changes of the Program. So if your youngster is already eating meat, chicken, fish, or (dare we say it?) salad or vegetables, and is doing so of his or her own accord, that's terrific! Take your youngster's normal eating routine as the starting point and begin adding Add-Ons, Hold-Ons, and Swaps from there.

What do I do when a Choice disappears?

While it may be hard to imagine, you may find that as cravings drop, your youngster may voluntarily give up a once-routine afternoon snack; a kid may "forget" to eat a meal, or your once-voracious eater may not "feel" like eating. We understand that you may find this occurrence hard to picture but you may indeed find it happening, and you may not know what to do when the meal at which your youngster is supposed to incorporate a food-related Choice suddenly disappears.

If your youngster skips a meal or snack because cravings are so diminished that he or she has no desire to eat, then certainly count this as in keeping with an incorporation of a food-related Choice in question. While one could argue that your youngster is not strictly adhering to the letter of the law regarding a Food Add-On, Hold-On, or Swap, your child is indeed eliminating the rise in insulin levels that each Choice is designed to achieve. Do *not* encourage your youngster to skip meals for the sake of weight loss or other goals, check with your physician to rule out any other cause, and certainly make sure that your child is getting the nutrition necessary for good health and well-being, but, with all that said, if snacks or some meals are skipped because of a lack of "hunger," understand that, indeed, the Program is working.

In a similar way, when Hold-Ons are selected they can appear to eliminate Food-Add Ons and Swaps that have already been incorporated into that meal or snack. If your youngster's new Hold-On Meal contains past Choices, consider that these Choices are still being incorporated into the new Hold-On Meal.

The Step-By-Step Plan: Making a Change

Changing a Choice

There may come a time when your youngster wants to exchange one Choice for another. He or she may not have fully understood what was involved in a particular Choice selection.

There comes a time when we all need a change.

Changes in scheduling or the school year may present different challenges, and sometimes we all just want some variety. Exchanging Choices is never a problem.

When possible, try to make an exchange using the same list by changing meal or snacktime selections. If a change in meal selection is not suitable, feel free to look at other Choice Lists for an appropriate exchange. Try not to change more than one Choice at a time.

The Carbohydrate Addict's Program for Children and Teens was designed to decrease the hunger and cravings that drive our youngsters to eat unbalanced diets. Each new Choice brings new opportunities for improving your youngster's physical balance and well-being. For a program to be livable, however, it is important to recognize that children are, after all, only human.

Time Off

Time crunches, social and school demands, an unexpected cold or the flu, unforeseen situations, holidays, vacations, and more, all may slow or halt the addition of a new Choice each week. In some cases, your youngster may just want to lie back and temporarily "glide" on previous good behavior. Or the child may just not feel like adding anything new to the routine. No excuse is needed.

Once in a while, everybody needs some time off.

This is your youngster's program. If your child or teen would like to stop adding Choices at any place along the way, that is perfectly acceptable. For that week, or for several weeks to come, select no additional Choices. Try not to let too long a time go by without again beginning to add new Choices, but remember that almost all of us need a breather now and then.

And most important, during this "time out," your youngster should continue to follow the Choices that have already been selected. Don't backslide. If your youngster stops following the previously selected Choices, even for a short time, it will be that much harder to begin again.

Encourage your youngster to hold the ground he or she has gained. Remind your youngster of how good he or she felt and looked, each step of the way. If your child is overweight, make sure your youngster continues to wear new smaller-sized clothes that may now fit, and continue weighings every day and the charting of your child's weight. If your youngster has made progress in over-coming school or behavioral problems or has resolved some mood swings, be supportive and remind your child of the changes the Program has brought. Speak out, describe the changes and the pride your youngster has felt, and, without blame, keep the memory of recent victories alive. If you are concerned that your youngster may lose ground, consider moving to The Jump-Start Plan for a quick charge of change and motivation.

Before choosing to "take a week off" from new Choices, make it clear that even if no additional Choices are selected, the ones that have already been chosen should be continued.

Changing to The Jump-Start Plan

At any point on The Step-By-Step Plan you will find that it is easy to move into The Jump-Start Plan. Previously selected Add-On Activity Choices should be continued, but all Add-On Food Choices, Hold-Ons, and Swap Choices that your youngster made in The Step-By-Step Plan will temporarily be left behind when switching to The Jump-Start Plan. Using the guidelines in The Jump-Start Plan "Getting Started" section that follows on page 209, have your youngster maintain all previously selected Add-On Activity Choices and begin Phase One of The Jump-Start Plan. If your youngster needs a boost in motivation or a faster change than The Step-By-Step Plan provides, The Jump-Start Plan switch may be right on target. As always, consult your youngster's physician.

The Jump-Start Plan: An Overview

The Jump-Start Plan is a quick-start program for older children and teens. The Jump-Start Plan accelerates changes in insulin, blood sugar, and cravings, and in turn can bring about more immediate progress in the resolution of behavioral, emotional, mood, and weight problems. Phase One of The Jump-Start Plan is time-limited;[10] youngsters choose foods from the Insulin-Balancing Foods List (beginning on page 183) for all their meals and snacks other than one balanced daily Combo Meal (which many parents and youngsters refer to as the Reward Meal). During the other Insulin-Balancing Meals, only those foods found on the Insulin-Balancing Foods List should be consumed; during your youngster's daily Combo Meal, however, your youngster will enjoy a balance of high-fiber and protein-rich Insulin-Balancing Foods along with Carbohydrate-Rich Foods, including pasta, rice, potatoes, bread, fruit, even desserts.

On The Jump-Start Plan your youngster will experience remarkable changes—quickly.

By confining all Carbohydrate-Rich Foods (including not only starches, snack foods, and junk food, but also naturally or artificially sweetened goodies) to one balanced Combo Meal each day, carbo-addicted kids usually experience remarkable improvement quickly. With this new experience under their belts, with the knowledge that the Program can correct the cause of their cravings, blood sugar, behavioral, learning, mood, and weight problems, with an often first-time understanding that they are not to blame but that they do hold change in their own hands, carbo-addicted youngsters are often more powerfully motivated than they could ever be with words or promises.

During Phase Two of The Jump-Start Plan your youngster achieves Optimal Carbo Balance, and ideal insulin, blood sugar, and weight levels can be maintained—for life. By adding additional Carbohydrate-Rich Foods to their eating plan on a regular basis, along with activity and other options, youngsters can maintain the success they have so quickly achieved during Phase One

---

[10]Appropriateness and duration of phase and program should incorporate recommendations by your youngster's physician, who should approve your youngster's participation and monitor progress, as should be done with all programs that call for changes in the child's eating and activity regimen.

of the plan, which has come to mean so much to them and to their parents.

Important: Before your youngster begins The Jump-Start Plan, carefully read Chapters 8 and 10. These chapters contain essential information you will need as well as guidelines and helpful suggestions.

A LIQUID NECESSITY

Whether beginning with The Step-By-Step Plan or The Jump-Start Plan, youngsters must drink enough liquids (preferably water) to keep them well hydrated and healthy. As cravings drop, some youngsters need to be reminded to consume enough water to meet their physical needs. Without the cravings and hunger they have experienced for so long, youngsters may literally forget to drink or find that they have a lessened desired for liquids. Remind younger children to drink; for older children and teens, we recommend a special carry-along water bottle (some have attractive shoulder strap holders). Fill the bottle with water and urge your youngster to drink often. Make sure that whatever goes in the bottle and in your youngster (again, preferably water) meets the guidelines of your youngster's plan.

Charting Your Youngster's Progress

Progress Points

Each week you will be able to keep track of your youngster's progress and visualize the many ways in which the Program's Choices and guidelines are helping your child or teen grow lean, fit, healthier, and happier. Keeping track of your youngster's progress is completely optional, though many parents and kids find it important and very motivating.

> **You will be able to chart your youngster's success.**

In Chapter 11, "Strategies for Success," you will learn how to chart your youngster's progress so that you, your physician, and, most of all, your youngster can best keep track of breakthroughs as they occur.

On the Other Hand

The Carbohydrate Addict's Program for Children and Teens would not be complete without contingency guidance for times when your youngster may be unmotivated, resistant, or downright impossible. We more than understand. In Chapter 11, "Strategies for Success," and in Chapter 13, "Straight Talk: Questions, Answers, and Real-Life Help," you will find some real-life guidance for real-life problems—practical help in choosing the best action—or no action—to take, and when each is appropriate. In addition, you will find advice on how best to secure support from those who might be set on sabotaging all your hard work as well as how to handle peer pressure and family interference.

Alone No More: A Special Note

Until now, the parent of the carbohydrate-addicted youngster has been alone; alone in not understanding the silent influence that low blood sugar can have on a youngster's behavior, mood, and attitude; alone in an impossible struggle to control a youngster's eating, weight, or both; alone and concerned for a youngster's health, happiness, and well-being; and alone in a world often filled with frustration, worry, and self-doubt.

We wrote *Carbohydrate-Addicted Kids* for two reasons. Certainly, primarily it was written to help carbohydrate-addicted youngsters, to spare them the shame and pain and problems in life that are neither their burden nor their fate, but without doubt, this book was also written for the parent who all too often suffers alone for two.

ALEX'S STEP-BY-STEP PLAN*

Before The Step-By-Step Plan:
One Day's Sample Menu before beginning the Program:

Breakfast	*Snack*	*Lunch*	*Snack*	*Dinner*	*Snack*
sugared	bubble	pizza	cookies	macaroni &	cookies
cereal,	gum	potato	juice	cheese	juice
fruit	candy	chips		garlic	
milk		fruit juice		bread	
juice		cookies		ice cream	
				soda	

On The Step-By-Step Plan:

Week One:
Food Add-On: Added burger without bun or other protein-rich Insulin-Balancing Food to lunch each day.

Week Two:
Alex was already very active. Instead of an Activity Add-On, he and his parents chose a Hold-On as a second week Choice. At breakfast, Alex "held-on" and during the week had Insulin-Reducing varieties of muffins, pancakes, hash, and french toast – all made without any carbohydrate-rich ingredients (see page 308 for Insulin-Reducing breakfast treats).

Week Three:
Alex agreed to Swap his Quick Trigger cookies and ice cream evening snack for pretzels and a fruit.

Week Four:
Alex agree to swap crackers for cookies at his afterschool cookies and juice snack.

Week Five:
Alex chose another Food Add-On and added cheese to his afterschool crackers and juice snack.

Week Five:
Alex's Swap: Fruit in place of juice at his afterschool snack. A snack that was once cookies and juice (and almost sure to trigger blood sugar swings) had gradually changed to cheese, crackers, and a whole fruit – far less likely to trigger radical blood sugar changes.

In the Weeks That Followed:
Although Alex's cravings and behavioral problems started to disappear within a short time, he continued adding Choices as per his parents' and physician's recommendations. He was willing to do so and reached his Optimal Carbo Balance quickly and easily. His hyperactivity, mood swings and inability to control his impulses continued to resolve. By maintaining his program, Alex maintained his progress at home and his success at school.

*Sample eating plans are meant to illustrate the ways in which some of the Guidelines and Choices within each respective Plan may be incorporated and are not meant to substitute for specific eating and activity programs designed to meet youngster's individual needs.

Getting Started:
The Jump-Start Plan

The Jump-Start Plan is a quick-start program for older children and teens that accelerates changes in insulin, blood sugar, and cravings, and in turn can bring about more immediate progress in the resolution of behavioral, emotional, mood, and weight problems. The dietary needs of younger children may not be met by The Jump-Start Plan, and as with all nutritional programs for all youngsters, your youngster's physician's advice should be sought and followed.

The Jump-Start Plan is made up of two phases. Phase One of The Jump-Start Plan is intended as a time-limited program for older children and teens;[1] to help them experience immediately a freedom from addiction, cravings, blood sugar swings, and problems that result from insulin imbalances. Phase One of The Jump-Start Plan calls for greater changes in your youngster's eating than do the Choices that make up The Step-By-Step Plan. In exchange for the greater effort, carbo-addicted youngsters usually reap more immediate and dramatic benefits. Cravings are typically eliminated or greatly reduced in a matter of days; weight loss is usually quick and easy, and balanced blood sugar levels usually rapidly bring about a resolution or significant bettering of psychological, emotional, learning, mood, and motivation-related problems.

---

[1]Appropriateness and duration of phase and program should incorporate recommendations by your youngster's physician, who should approve your youngster's participation and monitor progress, as should be done with all programs that call for changes in the child's eating and activity regimen.

A short time on The Jump-Start Plan is often enough to motivate youngsters who, on first coming to the program, are in need of immediate change. Some newcomers find themselves under pressure related to their appearance or behavior and need help quickly, others need "proof" that the program will indeed work; some need confirmation that their problems are not their "fault." Phase One gives them what they need. Though it calls for greater change, a short time on The Jump-Start Plan can provide the quick changes some youngsters require—and more.

In addition, The Jump-Start Plan can be used by youngsters who have been on The Step-By-Step Plan and find they want to make progress more rapidly or by those who need a boost in motivation.

The Step-By-Step Plan provides a lifetime of
addiction resolution in exchange for
small-step changes, added one at a time.

The Jump-Start Plan first gives a boost and quick help,
in exchange for making greater changes.
Once immediate change is accomplished,
the Plan then moves to lifelong maintenance.

While The Step-By-Step Plan provides a lifetime of addiction resolution in exchange for small-step changes (called Choices) that are added one at a time. Phase One of the Jump-Start Plan, on the other hand, can give your youngster the lift or help needed more quickly if your child is willing to make greater changes all at once. Phase Two of The Jump-Start Plan will help your youngster maintain success through a lifestyle change maintenance program. For a quick start or a needed boost, The Jump-Start Plan is often a good choice; for slower and easier change or for the younger child, The Step-By-Step Plan may be the answer.

Important: Before selecting which plan is best for your child or teen, it is essential that you read this chapter and the preceding Chapter 9, "Getting Started: The Step-By-

Step Plan," through to the end, so that you have a complete understanding of both plans.

Phase One: Three Essential Guidelines

Overview

In Phase One of The Jump-Start Plan, your youngster will eat two types of meals: Combo Meals and Insulin-Balancing Meals and Snacks. At Insulin-Balancing Meals and Snacks your youngster will eat Insulin-Balancing Foods only (mainly high-fiber and protein-rich foods). During these meals and snacks your youngster will "hold on" and refrain from all Carbohydrate-Rich Foods as well as any carbohydrate act-alikes.

**During Phase One, all daily meals and snacks
will be Insulin-Balancing except for one daily
well-rounded Combo (Reward) Meal.**

In addition, your youngster will enjoy a daily Combo Meal, a well-rounded meal of protein and vegetables, along with the Carbohydrate-Rich Foods he or she so enjoys (including pasta, rice, potatoes, bread, fruit, even desserts). We call this meal a Combo Meal because it combines both Carbohydrate-Rich Foods and Insulin-Balancing Foods, but most parents and kids alike have come to refer to it as the daily Reward Meal. (Specific guidelines on how to balance the Combo Meal and incorporate Phase One follow.)

By eating Insulin-Balancing Foods for most of the day and saving all Carbohydrate-Rich Foods (including starches, snack food, junk food, and naturally or artificially-sweetened goodies) for one balanced Combo Meal (or Reward Meal) each day, carbo-addicted kids usually experience remarkable improvement quickly. With this new experience under their belts, with the knowledge that the program can correct the cause of their crav-

ings, blood sugar, behavioral, learning, mood, and weight problems, with an often first-time understanding that they are not to
blame but that they do hold change in their own hands, carbo-
addicted youngsters are often more powerfully motivated than
words or promises could ever help them to be.

Important: Before your youngster begins The Jump-Start
Plan, carefully read Chapters 8 and 9. These chapters contain essential information you will need as well as guidelines and helpful suggestions.

How to Incorporate
Phase One's Guidelines[2]

Phase One, Guideline #1

At all meals and snacks, other than during the Combo Meal each
day, your youngster should eat only those foods found in the
Insulin-Balancing Foods List (page 183). Make sure that no
Carbohydrate-Rich Foods or carbohydrate act-alikes (pages 184–185)
find their way into Insulin-Balancing Meals. Carbohydrate-Rich
Foods will reverse the insulin-lowering power that an entirely
Insulin-Balancing Meal can produce. So, in all Insulin-Balancing
Meals, include *only* Insulin-Balancing Foods. For low-fat guid-
ance, see page 417.

At any meal, the amount of insulin that is released is based on
the body's expectation of how much Carbohydrate-Rich Food
will be consumed. It bases this expectation on the experience of
the meals that have been eaten in the recent past. If little Carbohydrate-Rich Food has been consumed in the recent past, the
body "assumes" that little Carbohydrate-Rich Food will be eaten
at the next meal and, appropriately, it releases less insulin. When
your child eats meals that are low in carbohydrates for most of

---

[2]Remember, the Jump-Start Plan is intended for a limited time only and should
be followed only by older children and teens with a physician's approval and
monitoring.

the day, the body releases less insulin, and less insulin translates into less hunger, fewer and much milder cravings (if any), and fewer blood sugar swings (if any) as well.

Within a matter of days of refraining from Carbohydrate-Rich Foods (and carbohydrate act-alikes) during all daily meals but one, your youngster will experience a freedom from cravings that he or she may never have known before. This release from cravings makes staying on The Jump-Start Plan easier than you or your youngster ever thought possible. Do not judge your child's ability to forego much-loved carbos for most of the day based on past evidence of addiction. The physical changes that the Program brings makes staying on the Program far easier than you might anticipate. Much like the addictive cycle, this cycle of balance continues to perpetuate itself.

> **Note:** All Insulin-Balancing Foods are low in carbohydrates. The greatest portion of Insulin-Balancing Foods is made up of protein-rich meats, fowl, fish, or dairy (and tofu), as well as high-fiber vegetables. Since high-fat foods like butter, margarine, and oils are also low in carbohydrates, for completeness they must be included in the Insulin-Balancing Foods List as well. So if your physician recommends a low-fat regimen for your youngster, see page 417 for some guidance in making low-fat selections from the Insulin-Balancing Foods List.

Phase One, Guideline #2

In addition to your youngster's Insulin-Balancing Meals, once each day your child should enjoy one Combo Meal, that is, a *balanced* combination of Insulin-Balancing Foods *along with* Carbohydrate-Rich Foods such as pasta, rice, potatoes, bread, fruits, and, if appropriate, a well-loved and deserved dessert or treat as well.

As your youngster begins to eat this meal, insulin is released. The good news is, however, that because this Combo Meal comes after your child has eaten several Insulin-Balancing Meals and Snacks, the amount of insulin that will be released will be close to, or the same as, that of a nonaddicted youngster. Based on past meals, your youngster's body will assume that it does not need to release excess levels of insulin, and it will naturally normalize the amount of insulin it releases. Without the pull of excess amounts of the "hunger hormone," your youngster is able to eat with pleasure but not gluttony. Without the insulin's powerful demand for Carbohydrate-Rich Foods, your youngster will find a wider variety of foods desirable and palatable. You will see a new youngster emerge, one who is free to enjoy many foods without the undeniable drive for carbos experienced in the past.

As in All Things, Balance

While you and your youngster may refer to the daily Combo Meal as a Reward Meal™ because it is so enjoyed and anticipated, the balance of your youngster's daily Combo Meal is essential. Too much carbo, eaten out of balance, even during a daily Combo Meal, can push your youngster to seek more and more carbos in an attempt to balance out the excess release of insulin. No need for concern, however; a bit of balance goes a long way.

With your doctor's approval, the Combo Meal should be divided into quarters of *approximately* equal amounts:

¼ salad (with dip or dressing of choice).
¼ vegetables (raw or cooked, preferably from the Insulin-Balancing Foods List whenever possible, with or without special, enjoyable toppings). Help for the vegetable-phobic youngster can be found on page 284.
¼ protein (meat, fish, fowl, dairy, or tofu).
¼ Carbohydrate-Rich Foods including primarily complex carbohydrates (that is, starches like bread, potatoes, rice, and pasta), as well as fruit and, if appropriate, snack foods and dessert.

The amount of food that makes up each of the quarters should look about equal; no need to measure or weigh—just estimate "by eye" that they are about equal portions, "average" portions for your youngster's age level.

> **It is essential to maintain a balance of all foods in your
> youngster's Combo Meals but don't worry, there is help
> for the vegetable-hater and the non-meat-eater as well.**

If your youngster wants a second helping, that is perfectly acceptable as long as he or she takes *and eats* additional portions of all foods on the plate and as long as they are equal portions. It is *not* acceptable for a youngster to go back for seconds (or thirds) of Carbohydrate-Rich Foods only. The meal will be unbalanced and your youngster's body, weight, and behavior will probably show it.

There is no need to worry if your youngster hates vegetables or won't eat meat. You'll find practical guidance and alternatives for the vegetable-phobic youngster on page 284 and special recipes for the vegetarian youngster starting on pages 354 (Insulin-Balancing) and 391 (Combo Meals).

Phase One, Guideline #3

All meals and snacks should be completed in no more than sixty minutes. A second stage of insulin release takes place while food is being consumed. It is the body's way of checking to see if enough insulin has been released in relation to the Carbohydrate-Rich Food that has been consumed. This second stage of insulin release peaks about sixty-five to seventy minutes after Carbohydrate-Rich Food is first consumed. To keep your youngster's insulin release low, he or she should stop eating before insulin reaches this peak release stage. So from first bite to last, meals and snacks should never last longer than one hour. It is not a good idea to nibble on food while it is being prepared, and we strongly recommend against it, but if your youngster starts nibbling, keep it balanced and remember that no more than sixty minutes should elapse from first nibble to the end of the meal.

In summary, during the time-limited Phase One of The Jump-Start Plan, your youngster will consume only those foods found on the Insulin-Balancing Foods List for most meals and snacks. In addition, each day your youngster will enjoy a special Combo Meal (or Reward Meal), which will consist of a balance of both Insulin-Balancing Foods (high-fiber and protein-rich foods) and Carbohydrate-Rich Foods (including pasta, rice, potatoes, bread, fruit, juice, and some desserts, if desired). All Insulin-Balancing Meals and Snacks, and Combo Meals and Snacks as well, should last no more than one hour.

A SPECIAL STRATEGY FOR THE BATTLE OF THE BULGE

For the youngster who needs to lose weight, it is a great idea, if possible, to begin each Combo Meal with a salad. Salad, rich with fiber, slows down the rate at which blood sugar levels rise when carbos are consumed later in the meal. A slower blood sugar rise often means that less insulin will be released and your youngster will experience greater satisfaction more quickly and more easily. Low insulin levels make it easier for your youngster's body to burn the energy stored in fat cells as well.

So starting the meal with a salad is a great way to get off the weight more easily and more quickly. Do try to have your youngster *finish* the salad before moving on to the rest of the meal. (Once a kid gets a taste of carbos, the salad has far less appeal.) Top the salad with a great dressing (low-fat, if your doctor recommends) or with regular or low-fat bacon bits or cheese—whatever will make the greens appealing. Many kids like finger salads—raw carrot and celery sticks, green peppers, mushrooms, cucumbers, all sliced and ready for dipping.

Just keep in mind that, for the youngster who wants to lose weight, finishing the salad before beginning the main portion of the Combo Meal can be very helpful (though it is not absolutely necessary). By the way, remind your youngster that the sixty-minute time limit begins with the first bite of salad.

See Chapter 5, beginning on page 91, for some important information and surprising new tactics in the "Battle of the Bulge."

> **To shape the accelerated results of Phase One into a lifetime program, your youngster will move into Phase Two.**

Phase One, Special Circumstances

Many times, on The Jump-Start Plan, youngsters will experience an immediate drop in cravings that is so powerful that they will skip their usual snacks or meals. We know that you cannot imagine that that might ever happen to your youngster, but indeed as insulin and blood sugar levels normalize, your youngster may "forget" to eat or may inform you that he or she does not "feel" like eating.

If your youngster skips a meal or snack because of lack of hunger, then consider that he or she is indeed still following the guidelines of the Program, for without the stimulus of any Carbohydrate-Rich Foods, no insulin rise will take place and the purpose of the guidelines is still being advanced. Do *not* encourage your youngster to skip meals for the sake of weight loss or other goals, however, and make certain to check with your physician to rule out any other cause. Also make sure that your child is getting the nutrition necessary for good health and well-being. Still, with all that in place, if snacks or some meals are skipped because of a lack of hunger or desire to eat, chances are you are seeing the success of the Program in action.

Phase Two: A Program for Life

Overview

When you are ready to shape the accelerated results of Phase One of The Jump-Start Plan into a lifetime program, your youngster should begin Phase Two; now your child will start to add carbohydrates *slowly* until Optimal Carbo Balance is reached (guidelines follow). During Phase Two your youngster will add activities and, if desired, once each week begin to replace some simple sugars with more complex carbohydrates (Swaps), so that insulin and blood sugar levels can stay in balance and the weight loss and other benefits that were so quickly achieved during Phase One can be maintained. As their Optimal Carbo Balances are reached (see page 221, youngsters can maintain, for life, the successes they have so quickly achieved during Phase One of the plan. Best of all, kids quickly learn that they can predict and control the progress that has come to mean so much to them and to their parents.

Phase Two guidelines will take your youngster from the quick changes of Phase One to an Optimal Carbo Balance and, in doing so, will help your youngster move into a program that can be maintained for life.

Phase Two, Guidelines

Using Phase One's guidelines as a basic plan, *once each week*, have your youngster add an average portion of Carbohydrate-Rich Foods to one Insulin-Balancing Meal or Snack. The addition of Carbohydrate-Rich Foods changes an Insulin-Balancing Meal into a Combo Meal.

The new Combo Meal or Snack should be planned beforehand. Ideally it should be added at the same time each week, as a Sunday morning breakfast, for instance. As an alternative, an added meal can be a "special" or "free" meal or snack that is used for a special occasion; replacing a typical Insulin-Balancing Meal anytime during a weekend or for a birthday party, for instance, or, for the teen, to be enjoyed during a date or at the mall with friends. Make certain that the new Combo Meal or Snack is planned in advance, not added on the spot, and, as always, it should be kept balanced.

Combo Meals may feel like rewards but they are not intended to be carbo feasts. Balance is absolutely essential.

It makes no difference whether you and your youngster add the Carbohydrate-Rich Food into a meal or snack, as long as it is added once each week and replaces what was formerly a Insulin-Balancing Meal or Snack.

Combo Meals must always maintain the same balance of one-quarter salad, one-quarter vegetables, one-quarter protein, and one-quarter high-carbohydrate foods as described on page 214 for all Combo Meals. Combo Snacks should maintain a similar balance but contain smaller portions. For Insulin-Balancing Foods see page 182, and for Carbohydrate-Rich Foods see pages 184 and 185.

Remember, as your youngster moves into Phase Two of The Jump-Start Plan, Carbohydrate-Rich Foods should be added to transform only one meal or snack each *week*.

What Else Changes in Phase Two?

During Phase Two of The Jump-Start Plan, along with each Carbohydrate-Rich Food that is added each week and *on the same day*, your youngster should also choose an Activity Add-On as well. See page 188 for a wide variety of Activity Add-Ons. Just as Carbohydrate-Rich Foods are added to one meal or snack at a time, each week, in the same way, activities should be added once each week. Your youngster may choose an activity from any level although we recommend that he or she starts with a level that will be easy and fun; it is better to move from a less-demanding level to a more-demanding level than to move in the opposite direction.

Don't forget: Add-On Activities should be completed on the same day that the Combo Meal or Snack is added.

For an extra boost in weight loss or for stabilizing blood sugar levels, your youngster may, in addition, select a Swap Choice once a week or as often as he or she chooses. Swap Choices ask your youngster to replace a high-carbohydrate Quick Trigger Food (which can cause strong insulin and blood sugar responses) with a Slow Trigger Food (which is less likely to cause such intense responses). A typical Swap might include exchanging sugar-laden cookies for less densely sweet treats like popcorn, pretzels, or chips. Another Swap might entail exchanging a glass of fruit juice (which may tend to trigger blood sugar swings) with a snack of whole fruit (which contains much-needed blood sugar–stabilizing fiber). See page 197 for some sample Swap Choices.

In the Weeks to Come

Phase Two of the Jump-Start Plan will continue to move your youngster, week by week, into a lifelong maintenance program that will help your youngster sustain an Optimal Carbo Balance for a lifetime.

Each week, you and your youngster should go back and, using Phase Two's guidelines, select another Insulin-Balancing Meal during the week to which Carbohydrate-Rich Foods will be added. Another activity should be added, on the same day, to help keep insulin and blood sugar levels in balance. In addition, encourage your youngster to replace simple sugars with complex carbos (Swaps) whenever possible until an Optimal Carbo Balance (described below) is reached.

Each week will build on the week before; during the first week of Phase Two your youngster will add Carbohydrate-Rich Foods to one meal or snack, and one weekly activity session and an optional Swap to the original guidelines of Phase One; during the second week, a second *weekly* portion of Carbohydrate-Rich Foods along with an activity session will be added, and so on. Do not add Carbohydrate-Rich Foods to more than one additional meal or snack per week unless directed by your youngster's physician, and always try to have your youngster add a weekly activity session and at least one Swap on the same day.

> **Special Activity Note:** As each week brings another Add-On Activity Choice, your youngster may find that, instead of adding a new activity to previous weeks' activity selections, it makes more sense either to increase the length of time of the activity, the number of times each week for the activity, or the level of activity (from light to moderate, for instance).

Your youngster can either increase the length of time of any activity—by half-hour increments—or increase the level of the activity or the frequency of any previously selected activity, and count the increase in length of time, level, or frequency as a "new" activity selection for the week. If, on the other hand, your youngster prefers to add a whole new activity, that, too, is perfectly acceptable.

Carbohydrate-Rich Foods should be added to a meal or snack once a week *only until an Optimal Carbo Balance is reached* (see the section that immediately follows). The selection of additional activities and the selection of Swaps are always encouraged, unless otherwise indicated.

Pinpointing Your Youngster's Optimal Carbo Balance on The Jump-Start Plan

During Phase One of The Jump-Start Plan, for a limited time, your youngster consumed Carbohydrate-Rich Foods only once each day in a meal that was balanced with Insulin-Balancing Foods. All your youngster's other meals and snacks contained Insulin-Balancing Foods only. During that time, you and your youngster probably noticed a quick and dramatic reduction in cravings as well as an almost immediate resolution of motivational, mood, and other insulin and blood sugar related problems. For the overweight carbohydrate-addicted youngster, weight loss will most likely seem almost effortless as compared with struggles of the past.

During Phase Two of The Jump Start Plan, you have learned that your youngster will add Carbohydrate-Rich Foods slowly, to one meal each week (along with activities and optional Swaps) until Optimal Carbo Balance is reached.

Remember, an Optimal Carbo Balance is that combination of foods and activity that will allow your youngster to consume the best and most carbohydrates possible while maintaining balanced insulin and blood sugar levels, and controlling or eliminating related problems. Just as youngsters' bodies vary, so Optimal Carbo Balances are different for every youngster. One youngster's Optimal Carbo Balance most likely will not be the same as that of another youngster.

Pinpointing your youngster's Optimal Carbo Balance on The Jump-Start Plan is approached from the opposite direction than for The Step-By-Step Plan. On The Jump-Start Plan, the maximum amount of dietary carbohydrates has been removed temporarily in Phase One. Elimination or reduction of carbo-associated problems occurs quickly. In Phase Two, Carbohydrate-Rich Foods are slowly *added* back (along with balancing activities and optional Swaps) until problems begin to reemerge. When problems begin to reemerge, this is the body's way of signaling that the ideal balance of carbohydrates has been overstepped, and accordingly the last carbo addition should be removed (so that problems once again resolve). When this last carbohydrate addition has been removed and problems once again begin to resolve, an Optimal Carbo Balance is considered to have been reached.

To pinpoint your youngster's Optimal Carbo Balance on the Jump-Start Plan:

1. Continue incorporating weekly additions of Combo Meals as described in Phase Two Guidelines and stay aware of your youngster's progress until one or more of the following changes occurs (as appropriate to your youngster), indicating an ideal carbo balance has been *overstepped*:

   Cravings return or become more intense or the desire to "cheat" on the program begins to emerge, or
   Emotional, behavioral, mood, attentional, and motivational problems begin to reemerge,[3] or
   Weight loss (in the overweight youngster) slows, stops, or reverses.[4]

2. At the first sign of *any one* of these changes, remove the last added weekly Combo Meal or Snack and replace it with an

---

[3] For purposes of pinpointing Optimal Carbo Balance, you need not wait until all excess weight has been regained or until all behavioral, learning, motivation and mood problems have reemerged. When your youngster has shown a *definite reversal* in the resolution of difficulties in any of these areas, the first step in pinpointing an Optimal Carbo Balance should be considered to have been achieved (that is, continued addition of Carbohydrate-Rich Foods will hinder the child's progress).

Insulin-Balancing Meal or Snack. When the problems once again resolve, you have found your youngster's Optimal Carbo Balance.

3. If the problems persist, continuing removing Combo Meals or Snacks until problems once again resolve. At that point, you have found your youngster's Optimal Carbo Balance.

Important Note: Remember that although your youngster, with a physician's approval, can always return to Phase One of the plan and, in doing so, enjoy an almost certain freedom from cravings and other insulin-related problems, finding your youngster's Optimal Carbo Balance will help you both to discover the maximum amount of Carbohydrate-Rich Foods your youngster can enjoy without negative repercussions. Your youngster should always, unless clearly instructed by a physician, include Carbohydrate-Rich Foods in at least one balanced Combo Meal *every day.*

Making a Change

Changing from Jump-Start to Step-By-Step

To move from The Jump-Start Plan to The Step-By-Step Plan, youngsters have to take a step sideways, and your youngster may experience what seems to be a plateau or even a temporary backstep for a while, but for some youngsters the more flexible Step-By-Step Plan may be well worth it. First be certain that a change in plans is not your youngster's way of getting back into an addictive pattern. There should be a good reason for changing plans; make certain that a desire to change to The Step-By-Step Plan is not simply an excuse to indulge in more carbos.

Once you are certain that your youngster is not looking for an excuse to go back to old addiction-driven habits but is truly in need of *slower progressive change,* you can begin to move into The Step-By-Step Plan. First, determine how many Combo Meals and Snacks as well as Insulin-Balancing Meals and Snacks will be your youngster's starting point on the new program. This should be a joint decision, made in consultation with your youngster, as to a new starting point from which your youngster will slowly move towards a more balanced eating plan of less frequent, less intense, and more balanced carbo-rich foods. This new starting point will most likely include a greater number of Combo Meals and Snacks than your youngster has been eating on The Jump-Start Plan, and at first, there may be an increase in insulin and blood sugar–related problems, including a plateau or a gain in weight and a possible increase in previously controlled emotional, psychological, behavioral, learning, and motivational problems.

In time, as new Choices on The Step-By-Step Plan are selected and followed and as a greater number of Insulin-Balancing Meals and Snacks replace more carbohydrate-rich Combo Meals and Snacks, however, these plateaus or reversals will again resolve. Using your newly determined number of Combo Meals and Snacks and Insulin-Balancing Meals and Snacks as your starting point, enter The Step-By-Step Plan and follow the guidelines beginning on page 172. Remember, progress on The Step-By-Step Plan will be slower than in The Jump-Start Plan, but the Choices will be far less demanding and, ultimately, your youngster will reach the same goal. So change plans if it seems appropriate but do not change your focus, your motivation, and your awareness of how important it is to get your youngster "back in balance."

Charting and Rewarding Your Youngster's Progress

Don't forget to read about charting and rewarding your youngster's progress as well as other effective strategies for success in Chapter 11.

JENNIFER'S JUMP-START PLAN*

Before The Jump-Start Plan:
One Day's Sample Menu before beginning Program:

Breakfast	Snack	Lunch	Snack	Dinner	Snack	Snack
donuts	potato	chicken	cookies	pizza	cookies	popcorn
juice	chips	nuggets	diet soda	french	diet soda	juice
	candy bar	french		fries		
	juice	fries		corn		
		juice		rolls &		
		ice cream		butter		
				juice		

Phase One:
The Jump-Start Plan: One Day's Sample Menu

Breakfast	Snack	Lunch	Snack	Dinner	Snack
cheese	celery	baked	crudités	salad with	tuna salad
& mush-	sticks	chicken	(finger	dressing	celery
room ome-	stuffed	fingers (no	salad with	pizza	sticks
lette,**	with	breading),	dip)	side order	
cucumber	cream	salad with		of meat-	
coins,	cheese**	dressing,		balls	
herbal iced		cheese		green	
tea		slices,**		beans	
		herbal iced		almondine	
		tea		sorbet and	
				cookies	
				herbal iced	
				tea	

Phase Two:
Carbohydrate-rich foods were added to one meal or snack each week along with a weekly Activity Add-On (dancing and mall walking) and a weekly Swap until Jennifer noticed an increase in her cravings. When cravings *first* began to reemerge, Jennifer's last weekly carbo-rich addition was removed and, having reached her Optimal Carbo Balance along with her physician's approval, she remained with her own personalized version of the Plan.

*Sample eating plans are meant to illustrate incorporating of some of the Guidelines and Choices within each respective Plan and are not meant to substitute for specific eating and activity programs designed to meet youngster's individual needs.
**Low-fat choices were chosen as appropriate.

PART III

The Sweet Taste of Success

eleven

Strategies for Success

"The only trouble with success," said Ben Franklin, "is that so few people know it when they see it."

If you think that, contrary to Franklin's contention, you know success when you see it, you may be in for a bit of a surprise. One of the greatest difficulties we encounter when helping parents of carbo-addicted youngsters is getting them to recognize and appreciate the progress and success that is taking place right before their eyes.

> **Most of us are tend to focus on the "misses" in life rather than on the "hits."**

Most of us are conditioned to see the "misses" in life rather than on the "hits"; we are taught to pay attention to those actions that miss the mark and take for granted those actions that are right on target. It's hard; the misses seem to stand out so much more than the hits, and one miss seems to wipe out all the hits that have come before. It seems almost second nature that what goes wrong seems to have a greater effect on us than what goes right, and we react accordingly. While we might smile in surprise and satisfaction, for instance, on the rare occasion when youngsters hang up their clothes, we are apt to react much more strongly when we are greeted by yet another pile of dirty clothes strewn on the floor.

It is essential, then, to remember two important points when assessing your youngster's progress. First, remember that change often takes place in small increments. In fact, change is often what we refer to when we are describing the final result, the accumulation of many smaller changes that are viewed, in the end, in combination.

When a child learns to walk or talk or read, we are actually viewing the sum total of a multitude of smaller masteries and accomplishments. In the same way, changes in eating and lifestyle habits, changes in weight, behavior, mood stability, motivation, and the ability to concentrate are difficult to pinpoint from moment to moment; each must be viewed as a process, and success is the sum total of the many smaller successes that take place along the way.

The second important point to remember when assessing your youngster's progress is that almost none of us move in a straight line in trying to achieve our goals. We move three steps forward, one back, and often one to the side as well. Your youngster is not a machine; there will be moments of amazing breakthroughs but, likewise, there will be moments of doubt, concern, frustration, and even despair. Most likely, your youngster will experience similar feelings and you, as a parent, must help your child or teen maintain perspective and, with it, motivation.

Positive change comes not only as a result of many smaller successes but also by learning from some failures along the way. As long as the failures are fewer than the successes or as long as the failures provide lessons that will increase the probability of future success, progress is being made and positive change will be attained.

Maximizing Motivation: Tracking Success

You are on the trail of a wild animal. You are not far behind it but it is not yet clearly visible. You follow its tracks, noting changes in direction, and you feel the excitement build as you sense that you are almost upon it.

Your youngster's success may be just as close and just as elusive as a wild animal, but the excitement you will experience as you close in on it can barely be communicated in words.

It is essential, however, that you learn to recognize the "tracks" or signs of success, the small actions or achievements that will ultimately lead your youngster to the freedom, happiness, and health that is so desired.

Progress Points: Signs of Success

There are as many signs of success as there are kids, probably many more. What is success to one youngster may be less than success to another. Each youngster must be judged by past behavior and by what designates "progress" for that child alone. If your teen has no problem giving up candy in exchange for a pretzel snack, for instance, although this Swap will help him or her stabilize blood sugar swings, it is not as great a sign of success as it is for the youngster for whom this exchange is quite a challenge.

You and your youngster,[1] therefore, should determine together which changes most clearly mark progress, and together you can decide on the point value for each change. We refer to these points as Progress Points because they mark your youngster's movement toward long-term goals and they can help keep change in view and motivation high. In addition, Progress Points can be used to determine reward levels (more about that in a moment).

Progress Points can be awarded for important achievements as well as for smaller changes along the way.

Progress Points can be any number of points that you and your youngster assign to the changes and Choices that are required as your youngster moves through the guidelines and steps of the

---

[1]If your youngster is too young or otherwise unable or unwilling to participate in tracking progress, you can determine the point values to be assigned to accomplishments and keep score yourself. We recommend that you place the Progress Chart where your youngster can see it and note the changes that are taking place.

Program. A Swap, for instance, may be equal to 5 points, while a Hold-On, if it is more challenging for your youngster, may be worth 10. We recommend that point values fall between 5 and 30 points and that they be earned and evaluated weekly. In some cases younger children, or those needing more immediate gratification and motivation, do better with daily awards of Progress Points. Progress Points can also be awarded for the end result of smaller changes; for each pound lost,[2] for instance, or for getting a certain grade on a test. Use the chart on page 242 to help keep track of your youngster's progress and, for a real-life example, read "Its Own Reward: Lauren's Story" (page 236).

The Case of the
Disappearing Progress Points

The addition of Hold-On Choices (in The Step-By-Step Plan) and moving from Phase One to Phase Two of The Jump-Start Plan can eliminate the need for past Choices and the Progress Points a youngster would normally earn by following them. A past Swap at an evening snack, for instance, disappears when that entire snack is changed to a Hold-On (and all carbos are eliminated).

If changes in your youngster's plan eliminate the ability to earn Progress Points for previous Choices or for the following of prior guidelines, Progress Points awarded for the new change should be great enough to compensate for the lost opportunity to earn Progress Points.

On The Step-By-Step Plan, for instance, the addition of a Hold-On eliminates a youngster's ability to earn Progress Points that had been awarded for a Swap for that meal. In this case, let's say the Swap was worth 5 points. Rather than making the Hold-On worth 5 points as well, we recommend you make it worth 10 points to compensate for the lost opportunity to earn swap Points and to keep motivation high. On The Jump-Start Plan, moving from Phase One to Phase Two requires no additional effort in regard to food changes, and Progress Points earned

---

[2] Weight loss should be based on weekly averages as detailed on page 244.

should stay the same. The addition of a weekly Activity Add-On and an optional Swap Choice during Phase Two, however, should be rewarded with additional Progress Points, as appropriate.

Just Rewards

The question of whether youngsters should be rewarded for making the very changes that will ultimately make their lives better is a tough one that must ultimately be a personal decision. In general, we recommend that parents reward their youngsters' progress. In the same way that we earn grades on our way to the ultimate goal of graduation and just as we may be inspired therefore to work harder to earn good marks along the way, so carbo-addicted youngsters often do well when smaller achievements—those that move them toward greater goals—are rewarded.

Progress Points can be especially useful for youngsters whose achievements are not easily quantified, for those who have trouble with mood swings, or for those with difficulty concentrating, for example. Assigning point values to the changes that are not usually noted, praised, or rewarded can help youngsters gain self-esteem and value their own progress. Even though pounds and grades can be easily quantified and rewarded, here, too, Progress Points help youngsters celebrate their own success.

A word of caution: Some youngsters may appear reluctant to become involved in accumulating Progress Points. They may say that it's "baby stuff" or they may just shrug and indicate that they have no desire to participate. We have found that a lack of interest in accumulating Progress Points often indicates a hidden fear of failure. The best way to handle this situation? First, open up the subject without being pushy or demanding. See if you can get your youngster to help *you* understand why the point system holds little or no interest. If you hit resistance (and most likely you will), let it go for the time being. But only for the time being. As your youngster progresses on the Program, remind him or her that "you know, by now you would have earned this many Progress Points." From time to time, you might suggest that you begin counting at that point and award the points retroactively. As your youngster feels more and more confident in success, you may be surprised to find that what used to be "baby stuff" becomes far more appealing.

Progress Points can act as rewards themselves, and using the Progress Chart that follows, your youngster and you can see his or her movement toward success. Progress Points can also be used to determine when a reward of a more tangible nature has been earned.

**Rewards can both mark and celebrate
your youngster's success.**

By accumulating Progress Points, youngsters can earn an agreed-upon reward. Some rewards may include experiences, privileges, or items that the youngster wants but that have no connection to his or her long-term goal: a trip to the movies or a sleep-over with a friend, for instance. Whenever possible, however, we encourage parents to relate rewards to one of their youngsters' long-term goals; for a youngster whose goal is to lose weight, a new piece of smaller-sized clothing would be ideal, as would a previously disallowed privilege for a youngster whose long-term goal is to be better able to handle impulse control. In this way, as your youngster's participation in the Program earns Progress Points, the rewards that your youngster earns both mark and celebrate the signs of success.

When it comes to rewards, we have found that parents and kids can be amazingly creative. Discuss the idea of rewards with your youngster and you may find out a great deal of new information about what is important to your youngster as well as how hard he or she is willing to work for it.

Progress Points can be accumulated until a reward is earned.

Rewarding Goals

First, a short-term goal must be set. Short-term goals are the small changes that will mark your youngster's progress along the way to long-term goals. Some examples of typical short-term goals include the maintaining of a Swap Choice for a week on The Step-By-Step Plan, following Phase One of The Jump-Start Plan for a week, recording each pound lost (based on a weekly average), doing homework, or talking about feelings of frustration rather than acting them out. These small changes will help to bring about greater long-term changes such as losing weight, eating healthfully, getting a better grade in math, or maintaining control of one's temper. Once a short-term goal is agreed on, it should be assigned a number of Progress Points that will be awarded upon its attainment. In the same way, rewards should be agreed upon, specifically, and the number of Progress Points needed to earn a reward should be specified and written down.

For example, Ashley and her mother agree that for each pound Ashley loses, she will earn 5 Progress Points. They also agree that when she has earned 25 Progress Points she can buy a new pair of jeans. In this case, the loss of the weight will, happily, necessitate new clothing anyway.

Jordan, on the other hand, needs more immediate point accumulation to maintain his motivation. He has difficulty staying focused, and getting him to do his homework has always been an almost impossible challenge. For each day he is able to finish all his homework assignments, he earns Progress Points that can be immediately redeemed for special privileges. Progress Points can be awarded on a daily or weekly basis for the guidelines and Choices or for other accomplishments and can be changed immediately into rewards or left to accumulate until a larger reward can be earned.

Never, never choose a reward that takes your youngster off the Program. If your youngster were taking a certain medication, you would never consider rewarding him or her by allowing the skipping of a dose or two. In the same way, do not allow your youngster to celebrate success by negating the excellent progress that has been already accomplished. A reward should *never* be a day off the Program. As a reward you might want to add a food that is particularly desirable but too expensive or time-consuming to make every day. Just be certain that the food is eaten in keeping with your youngster's eating plan. In the same way, a much-enjoyed trip to a restaurant can be a well-sought-after reward, with the same stipula-tion—that it never negate your youngster's program.

The best rewards are those that are earned, at just the right pace, by the accumulation of Progress Points, that make your youngster feel proud of his or her accomplishments on the program, and that are reasonable given your own financial and time constraints. Being a good parent means encouraging your youngster, of course, but be considerate of your own needs as well. Celebrate with your young-ster; both of you have most certainly earned it.

Its Own Reward: Lauren's Story

Lauren W.[3] had been on the program for only two weeks, but already her motivation was lagging. Lauren's long-term goal was to lose fifteen pounds in time for the senior class trip a few months away; to accomplish this weight loss and, more importantly, to meet the long-term goal of keeping the weight off, Lauren's parents knew she had to gain control over her carbo addiction.

Although Lauren had already lost four pounds during Phase One of The Jump-Start Plan and although she had lost the weight without struggle or deprivation, Lauren's parents could tell that her commitment was growing less strong. She began complaining about not being able to have pizza at lunchtime and wanted money for "special treats" after school.

We asked Lauren if she had been experiencing cravings or hunger or if she felt deprived. She admitted that she was far less hungry on the Program than she had been before beginning it and that she felt more energetic and, in general, happier as well. Still, she admitted, she was feeling pressured to go off her program by her friends at school, who couldn't understand why she wouldn't eat the school lunch or join them in eating after-school snacks. We could see that the influence of her friends was beginning to take its toll.

[3]In all cases, names and identifying details have been changed.

It was clear that, for Lauren, her long-term goal of a weight loss of fifteen pounds was a little too distant to get her through the daily demands and challenges that lay immediately ahead. We asked her to tell us more about the senior class trip that had initiated her coming to see us about her weight. We hoped to rekindle her commitment as well as to learn what might be used as a meaningful reward for her.

Lauren's face lit up as she talked about the trip. It was a weekend away from her home in Jacksonville, Florida. The whole class was going to Disney World, she explained, then added that although there would be teachers and parents in attendance as chaperones, it was going to be a lot of fun. "We'll go to the parks on the first day and," she added, her face darkening with concern, "to Blizzard Beach, the water park there, on the second day—" Lauren abruptly stopped talking.

"Do you like to swim?" we asked.

Her face brightened again as she began to recount how fine a swimmer she was. She loved the water, she said, then admitted that when she went to the beach with her friends she always wore a big T-shirt and cutoff jeans. She was clearly ashamed of the way she thought she looked in a bathing suit and only went swimming in the presence of very close friends. Even then, she wore this makeshift outfit so as to bridge her desire to enjoy the water with her need to keep her body out of view.

We encouraged Lauren to talk more about what the weekend would hold if she had her way. After a bit of encouragement she revealed that, like all of us, she would want to be free to enjoy the sun and surf and wear a "real" bathing suit without concern for what her friends might say. In an especially intimate moment, she voiced the fantasy that she would even look "good" in a two-piece bathing suit, though she added self-consciously, "I know that's not really possible."

We explored, in detail, Lauren's feelings about herself and her weight and, in consultation with Lauren's parents, set up a reward schedule. With ten weeks to go before the trip, there was time for Lauren to lose the weight at an ideal rate and, with rewards to encourage her and keep her focused, we believed she might better be able to withstand the pressure from her peers.

Each pound lost based on a weekly average, we decided, would equal 10 Progress Points. Each Progress Point, in turn, was equal to $1 that could be applied to the purchase of new clothes for the class trip. For each pound lost, then, Lauren could count on $10 worth of new clothes. Lauren's parents had confided in us that Lauren needed some new clothes for the trip anyway but agreed to allow her a bit more toward the purchases in hopes that a schedule of rewards would help keep their daughter on track.

To start Lauren off with an extra boost, her parents agreed to retroactively credit their daughter with 40 Progress Points for the four pounds she had lost to date. We all agreed that one proviso had to be added: The money could not be used until one week before the trip (although she could put her desired purchases on layaway). If she gained any weight, any Progress Points and the money she earned would be deducted accordingly, based on the same rate.

Lauren's parents voiced concern about what would happen after the class trip. They hated to think of her gaining back all the weight she had lost and added that if a reward was needed to keep her motivated, they were troubled by the thought that when she reached her goal weight and no rewards were forthcoming, she would gain all the weight back. We explained that although each youngster was different, most kids felt so good after reaching their long-term goal and received so much positive reinforcement that maintaining their progress was less of a problem than parents anticipated.

The weeks flew by, and when we next saw Lauren she was fifteen pounds slimmer. The class trip was only three days away and Lauren brought in several items for us to see. She opened each bag, one by one, and finally with slow deliberation, as if to extend the moment, she brought forth a very pretty two-piece bathing suit. Not quite a bikini, it still allowed no place to hide any unwanted pounds.

Though, at the start, she had wanted to lose only a total of fifteen pounds, Lauren explained that after "falling in love" with this bathing suit (and the way she was beginning to feel about herself, we would have added), she had decided to lose twenty. Her physician thought that the extra weight loss was actually a good idea; her parents agreed, and Lauren had continued to lose at a steady rate. Now, only one pound short of her long-term goal, she stood before us proud and happy and, for the first time, confident.

We shared her excitement and before we could ask how she might reward herself in the future for maintaining her eating program and her weight loss while on the class trip, Lauren answered our not-yet-voiced concerns.

"I can't wait," she told us. "I have it all worked out." In great detail, she recounted how she had called Disney World and had discovered that she would have no problem getting the Insulin-Balancing salads and proteins she needed for some of her meals. They were available, she discovered, at almost any restaurant in the parks. For her Combo Meals, she explained, she could "play it by ear" and enjoy all the new experience of food and fun. Although most of that would probably be at Blizzard Beach, she added, thoroughly enjoying her own joke.

It was clear to us that in making plans to stay on her program while on her trip, even though rewards of money and clothes were no longer forthcoming, Lauren was confirming that her weight loss had brought with it its own rewards. Still, as they say, only time would tell.

And tell it did. We kept in touch by phone periodically, and the next time we saw Lauren was over a year later in a nearby mall. Once again she carried a new clothes purchase. This time, however, money for the clothes had come from her summer earnings.

"Look at this. Isn't it awesome?" she asked as she pulled a very small but sweet sundress from the bag. "There's a surprise beach party for my best friend Sunday and I thought this would be just perfect."

As if reading our minds, she continued. "Oh, it's not that I'm afraid of wearing a bathing suit, I have lots of them now; this is for the evening. There's this guy who . . ." The minutes flew by as we listened to every detail of her new infatuation but as she continued, our thoughts flew to Lauren's parents' concerns about the use of rewards.

Some may say that rewards are crutches and contend that we should learn to be strong and that youngsters should do what needs to be done for its own sake. We disagree. Most of us work best when we are rewarded, and until the changes we make accumulate enough to be their own rewards, intentional rewards may help keep us motivated and focused.

To those who might be tempted to refer to the use of rewards as a "crutch," we reply that, as in Lauren's case, and as in the case of many other youngsters, this "crutch" has served an essential purpose—it has helped them to keep going—moving forward—until they have been healed and are strong enough to walk, tall and straight and without assistance, on their own.

Progress Chart Guidelines

To keep track of your youngster's progress:

1. Decide on one long-term goal—an important improvement in behavior or weight, or another change or achievement that can be measured objectively by both you and your youngster. Long-term goals may take some time to reach but it should be clear what they entail. Additional long-term goals can be added, one at a time as appropriate.

   Examples: Lose fifteen pounds, have no "warning notes" sent home from school, get a C or better as a final grade in math. Do not choose changes that cannot be quantified as long-term goals, such as "get thin," "behave at school," or "do well in math."

2. Agree on a short-term goal, an improvement in behavior or other change or achievement that can be quantified that you and your youngster can both measure objectively and one that can be accomplished in a relatively short time; in a

day or week or as a specific incident. Additional short-term
goals can later be added.

Examples: Lose one pound or more each week (based on a
weekly average), get a passing grade or better on the next math
test, or spend two hours on homework each night. Short-term
goals may also include the maintenance of any Choice or
guideline of the program for a given period of time.

3. Decide on the number of Progress Points to be earned for
    the attainment of each short-term goal. The number of
    points awarded is purely subjective and should be agreed on
    by both you and your youngster. The greater the difficulty
    for your youngster, the greater the number of Progress
    Points. In general, keep point awards from 5 to 30.

Examples: Ten points for every pound lost per week; 5
points for every grade above passing on a math test; 5
points for every hour of homework per night, 4 points for
every Swap, and 6 points for every Hold-On per day.
(These are only examples; work out a point system with
your youngster).

4. Record Progress Points by the day, week, or as needed on
    the Progress Chart on page 242.
5. Check off each time a short-term goal has been accomplished.
6. On the Progress Chart, total all Progress Points including
    past and new points earned.
7. Use Progress Points to determine rewards if appropriate.
    Never use rewards to go off the program. When possible,
    connect each reward to your youngster's particular type of
    progress.

Examples: One hundred points earned from weight loss can
be exchanged for a new pair of jeans; 50 points earned
from doing homework can be exchanged for a day at the
mall (all expenses paid); or one week's worth of points
earned from doing homework (25 points) earns the right
to sleep over at a friend's home.

PROGRESS CHART*

Date _____

Long-Term Goal(s) _____
_____
_____

	Progress point value	Check off when completed (✓)
Short-Term Goal(s)_____	_____	_____
_____	_____	_____
_____	_____	_____
_____	_____	_____
_____	_____	_____
_____	_____	_____
_____	_____	_____
_____	_____	_____

New Progress Point Total   _____

Past Progress Point Total   _____

Total Progress Points
  Earned To Date
  (New + Past)   _____

Total Number of Progress
  Points required for Reward
  (fill in if appropriate)   _____

Progress Points Still Needed
  to reach Reward Level   _____

*Copy and customize this Progress Chart as needed for your use.

Which Weight Is the "Right" Weight?

Parents and kids probably disagree about this question more often than any other. If your youngster is "clearly" overweight, in some ways it may be easy for you, for then the problem is defined, the path is clear, and with the guidelines of the program, the end is in sight.

> **If you, as a parent, are in a battle regarding
> whether your youngster is overweight,
> take heart—you are most definitely not alone.**

If, however, there is a question whether your youngster is overweight—if one of you says yes and the other no, or if you, as parent, are in a battle with your spouse or other family member or significant other regarding your youngster's ideal weight, take heart—you are most definitely not alone.

Charts that illustrate "ideal" weight don't help as much as you might think; while they may provide you with weight levels for the "average" youngster, these cold figures are often difficult or even impossible to interpret with your particular youngster in mind. These charts usually do not take into account your youngster's physical build and activity level, the distribution of weight on your child, the child's genetic predisposition, rate of growth and point on the growth continuum, or peer pressure and social demands that today's youngsters experience.

Although you will find a chart detailing "average" heights and weights and Body Mass Index for children and teens on pages 434 and 435, ultimately only you, your youngster, and your youngster's physician can determine the best weight for your child. If there is a question about whether your youngster would benefit by losing weight, we recommend that you make a special appointment to discuss it with your doctor. While we are fully aware of the cost of an appointment, the decision about the best weight for your youngster is of great importance and deserves serious attention.

Deciding on the amount of weight to be lost as well as the rate of weight change in kids, however, is not as simple as it is in adults;

maturing bodies as well as changing heights and bone density in the young call for different decisions from those for adults. Parents need to determine whether their youngsters actually need to lose weight (that is, reduce the number of pounds they weigh) or whether weight maintenance is acceptable, given the fact that height and bone density will be increasing naturally over time and, in proportion, the youngster will end up being slimmer.

> **Youngsters are far more than
> the equivalent of pounds per inch.**

But, as every parent knows, youngsters are far more than the equivalent of pounds per inch. In deciding whether your youngster would benefit by weight loss, consider how your youngster's weight impacts on day-to-day life: Does your child feel self-conscious about weight; do other kids tease or make negative comments on your youngster's appearance; is it affecting your youngster's social life?

While it is important not to get caught up in the "thin is in" pressure that directs too many normal-weight youngsters to deprive themselves of much-needed nutrition, it is also essential to understand the world from your youngster's point of view. Ultimately, we suggest that if your youngster needs to lose weight (with your physician's approval), he or she should follow the guidelines of either The Step-By-Step Plan or The Jump-Start Plan, keeping a balanced eating program and healthy body as the first goal. Then, as the addiction to carbos resolves naturally, the weighty question of what is the best weight for your youngster will usually resolve in the process as well.

Real Gains in Weight Loss

Weighing your youngster is an important part of any eating and weight-loss program. On The Carbohydrate Addict's Program for Children and Teens, keeping track of your youngster's weight loss will help keep motivation high. Whether your youngster is trying to lose weight or is simply attempting to maintain weight so that height increases will help bring about a slimmer appearance, accurate weighing is an essential part of the process.

Many kids (and adults) hate to weigh themselves. Past frustrations and failures can make dieters want to avoid what they have come to assume will be disappointing numbers. Some youngsters will even attempt to convince themselves and their parents that scales aren't necessary. "You don't need to weigh me," they'll argue. "I can tell if I'm losing weight. You'll be able to tell, too," they add.

We totally disagree. Youngsters who are watching their weight do need to be weighed. It provides them with both encouragement and information that may be needed to make any adjustments related to their eating and activity choices. Accurate weighing and the understanding of what these numbers mean are an important part of your youngster's progress.

How often should you weigh your youngster? Youngsters' weights, like the weights of adults, can vary from day to day. Hot weather, salty food, premenstrual changes in the postpubescent girl, and other factors can produce significant changes. Given all these influences, a single once-a-week weighing is not enough. Daily weighings, which are then averaged for the week, are essential in getting a real understanding of your youngster's weight-loss progress. It will help your youngster see how he or she did over the period of the entire week and helps avoid negative reactions based on day-to-day normal variations.

When a researcher measures change, he or she takes as many readings as possible and then averages them and compares the averages over time. To get a real understanding of your youngster's progress, we will help you do the same in just a few easy steps. Averaging your youngster's weight is an important tool, one that will help you keep your youngster on track.

Why Average Your Youngster's Weight?

Most commercial weight-loss programs and physicians measure your youngster's weight loss on the basis of a once-a-week weigh-in. Weekly weigh-ins don't work for two basic reasons. First, youngsters often get the message, as so many of us adults have, that if they are weighed once a week, only the day before the weighing really counts. Weekly weigh-ins fail to teach youngsters that weight loss is the end result of many small changes that add up and that can be maintained for life. Instead, when they are weighed once weekly, kids learn to "cheat" all week, then crash diet the day before the weigh-in. This kind of eating pattern is bad for their health and bad for their addiction, and does not bring about a maintainable weight loss.

Weekly weigh-ins can also frustrate youngsters who are sticking to their program. Since weights naturally vary from day to day, a youngster who has lost weight that week and happens to be weighed on a "heavy day" will find that the weight loss for the week will most probably be negated. It may even appear that the child has gained weight. This youngster now learns the erroneous lesson that he or she has no control over those unwanted pounds. Motivation is almost sure to lag, and what could have been a celebration becomes just another reason to give up.

Here's an example of a youngster's weekly weights—the way the weights would look if the youngster was weighed once a week at a commercial program, for example. If you looked at these figures you would probably conclude that your youngster was making no real progress.

WEEKLY WEIGHTS

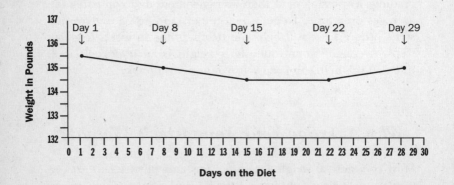

Now look at these same weighings with the addition of all the weights for the days in between the weekly weighings. The addition of the daily weights makes the chart look quite different. The last week of dieting shows that there has been quite a weight loss (Day 23—25) that did not show on the weekly weigh-in. Day 29, taken by itself, looks like weight gain. but it may have been a "heavy" day caused by the eating of salty foods, hot weather, or many other natural causes. If a youngster is weighed only once a week, neither the youngster nor you will ever get to see the whole picture. The low weights that also took place in the last week of the diet may never be seen. Still, many people may be tempted to disregard the weight loss during the second and third days of the last week because of what appears to be a weight gain on the seventh day.

DAILY WEIGHTS

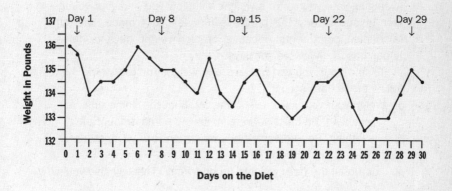

Now consider the same weights, only this time reported as a weekly average of weights. This is the way we have found best represents your youngster's weight loss over time. This one presents a very different picture and, more important, it is a more accurate picture than either of the other two. Averaging your youngster's weight loss will give your child or teen and you a far clearer picture of how well he or she is doing and will help to keep the motivation going as the weight keeps dropping.

WEEKLY WEIGHTS

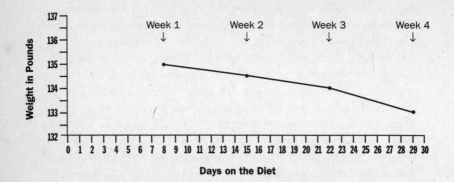

HOW TO AVERAGE
YOUR YOUNGSTER'S WEIGHT

Averaging your youngster's weight will allow you and your young-ster to see clearly the progress that is being made, without false disappointments because of high-weight days or false hopes based on low-weight days.

To find your youngster's average weight for the week, just follow these easy steps:

1. Weigh your youngster every day, at about the same time, and with the child wearing about the same amount of clothing. Record each day's weight on your youngster's Weight Chart (page 436).
2. Add up all the daily weights for one week. This will give you a weekly total.
3. Divide this weekly total by the number of weighings in that week. This will give you your youngster's average daily weight for the week.

Example #1: Your youngster's weights for the week were: 130, 129, 129, 130, 128, 128, 127.

Adding up all the weighings for the one week gives a total of 901.

(continued)

Divide the total by the number of weighings (7).
Use a calculator if you like: 901/7 = 128.7 (round off to 129).
Example #2: Your youngster forgot to get weighed one day, so you have only six daily weights to work from for that week.
Your youngster's weights for the week were: 130, 131, 129, 129, 128, 128.
Adding up all six weighings gives you a total of 775/6 = 129.1 (rounded off to 129).

THE GREAT AMERICAN WEIGH-IN

WHICH SCALE IS BEST?

More important than what kind of scale your youngster uses is making sure that your youngster does indeed use it and that the scale is dependable.

If your youngster is scale-phobic, this is a clear sign that the pain of being overweight, or of being at a weight your youngster thinks is too high, is taking its toll. This distress needs your attention, help, and support. Talk, weigh your youngster, and talk again. As the weight drops, so will the fear. But keep the communication open and the scale in use.

To test the dependability of a scale, test its consistency by weighing yourself (not your youngster) several times in succession. If the weight you see varies by more than a pound or two, get rid of that scale and buy a new one. If you are going to invest in a new scale, we recommend one with a digital quartz readout; we like those that display weights to the half pound so that your youngster can see a change in weight from 130 to 129.5, for instance. Cost for these scales runs anywhere from $40 to $60, but they but they are worth it if they can give accurate readings and keep your youngster motivated.

IS THERE A "CORRECT" WAY TO WEIGH MY YOUNGSTER?
Absolutely. Weigh your youngster at about the same time every day. The best time is first thing in the morning after he or she has gone to the bathroom and before breakfast. Do not weigh your youngster at different times during the day or when he or she is wearing different kinds of clothing and then compare weights. These are false comparisons and can unduly encourage or discourage your youngster. Weigh your youngster once in the morning, on an accurate scale placed on a flat surface. Avoid the "weighing ballet," that is, positioning one's body this way or that to get the lowest weight possible. Have your youngster step on the scale, then record the weight on the Weight Chart (page 436). From then on your youngster's job is to focus on the program, and the weight loss will follow.

The Essential Environment

Your youngster's overrelease of insulin and the blood sugar swings that can result constitute a powerful physical force that pushes your youngster toward an addictive state.

The eating and activity portions of this program (in both The Step-By-Step Plan and The Jump-Start Plan) can help normalize blood sugar levels in your youngster's body and help counter the insulin imbalance that lies at the base of your child's addiction to carbohydrates.

With a body free of the physical drives that have dictated cravings in the past, your youngster's motivation can be strengthened by your praise and recognition of his or her efforts, by the use of Progress Points and the charting of your youngster's progress, by the use of rewards, and, most of all, by your youngster's personal experiences of weight loss, behavior and mood control, and increased ease in learning. External and internal reinforcements can work wonders in keeping motivation high. When combined with changes in your youngster's physical response to carbohydrates, a boost in motivation becomes easier and even more powerful of a motivator of success, but ideally, for the strongest addiction reversal, a supportive environment is important.

An ideally supportive environment for your youngster should include what your youngster needs and should exclude those things that may prove detrimental to your child's success. Taking into account your own financial and time limitations, try to provide the foods your youngster needs and enjoys, both high-carbo foods for appropriate meals and snacks and exciting low-carbo, high-fiber, and protein-rich foods.

Discuss food options with your youngster; perhaps one special treat can be chosen this week and others selected in the weeks to come. Most important, the basic foods needed for your youngster's eating program need to be available at all times; salad makings, for instance, vegetables and protein for Hold-Ons or Add-Ons and Insulin-Balancing Meals as well as rice cakes, popcorn, pretzels, and other complex carbos snacks for Swap Choices.

Ideally, the essential environment also includes the support of a loving family, and a knowledgeable and effective teacher or school counselor whom your youngster trusts. In many cases, however, neither of these helpful support systems is available. That's not necessarily a problem. While additional support is always helpful, we have found that as long as your youngster has one person to confide in, to count on for understanding and advice, trust, and to talk to, the environment can support your child's changes and success.

**Even if you cannot give your youngster
the "ideal" environment, you can provide what
he or she needs to succeed.**

Even if you cannot give your youngster the "ideal" environment, even if some family members may be less than supportive, even if siblings tease or other family members attempt to sabotage your hard work,[4] your caring can make all the difference. We would hope that every carbohydrate-addicted kid, and every youngster in general, could be in a completely encouraging environment, but

---

[4] If family conflict calls for professional intervention or resolution of problems, seek appropriate help.

for so many youngsters the reality is less than perfect. You will find specific advice in Chapter 8, "Getting Ready: Strategies for Success Before You Begin," and Chapter 13, "Straight Talk: Questions, Answers, and Real-Life Help," but for now, trust yourself, do your best, and give your youngster all the love and encouragement you can muster; keep focused on what you can do to help rather than on what others are doing to dissuade.

A major part of your youngster's environment may involve time away from home— when you have little, if any, control.

In addition to time at home, depending on the child's age, your youngster's environment may involve time outside the home: at camp, school, or day care, or in the care of a baby-sitter or relative. A major part of the older youngster's environment involves time spent away from home with friends.

While, in general, you will not want to interfere with personal relationships that your youngster has with peers (unless they are destructive relationships), you should do your best to gain cooperation and support from your youngster's teachers, counselors, or caretakers. The food that your youngster needs must be available when, and in the ways, it is needed; when possible, teachers, counselors, and caretakers can be involved in reinforcing the positive behavioral changes this program can bring about.

In today's world, however, it is very difficult to maintain a united front both at home and away. You may be confronted by teachers, counselors, caretakers, or an administration that is not sympathetic, because of personal prejudices, policy restrictions, or time and energy demands, or, even worse, because of a simple lack of interest.

Each situation is different, but we have found that the best approach is to describe what you want in simple and direct terms. For instance, instead of saying that you want your youngster to have low-carbohydrate foods available at snacks, you are more likely to meet with success if you say that your youngster should have one of the following items for snacks. Then present a list of acceptable foods. If you cannot get the cooperation that you and your youngster require, bring in the food yourself.

Don't get stuck on principle.

Do not stand on ceremony or be distracted by what you think is "fair." You may be paying for a snack at day care, for instance, but if you want your youngster to get the food he or she needs, you may, in addition, have to supply Insulin-Balancing Foods for the day care teacher to give to your child. You may be perfectly correct in your argument that you should not be forced to pay twice (once to the school, once in the store) for the same snack; you may be justified in feeling that your youngster's needs should be attended to, but in the end it is your youngster's welfare that counts, and unless the money involved truly presents a hardship, it might be best to just concentrate on making sure your youngster gets what he or she needs.

If your youngster is unable to get the confirmation and reinforcement that is needed at school, at camp, or from caretakers, you can try one or both of two approaches. First, you might find that a note from your youngster's physician works wonders. A letter that explains that your youngster may suffer from a blood sugar problem and is working with a program designed to correct the problem can help a great deal in breaking down resistances. You might also try describing the problem yourself, in simple terms.

When asking for help, explain the problem, then be specific.

Remember, you can't expect a teacher or counselor or caretaker to read this entire book. Explain what you have learned in a few sentences, then, again, be specific about what you are requesting in terms of help. Rather than using vague terms and asking a teacher to "recognize" or to "encourage" your youngster's progress, for example, you might ask for a weekly note summarizing any changes that the teacher notices. In fulfilling your request for a note, the teacher will naturally become aware of the improvements that your youngster makes.

Still, no matter how hard you try, at home or outside the house, there will be times when you cannot seem to get what is needed to encourage your youngster's success. One of the major barriers you may come across is what we have come to call the Battle for Control.

The Battle for Control

The battle for control is, at best, an unpleasant experience. At worst, it can undermine a great deal of hard work. Potentially it can contribute to your youngster's abandonment of the program as well as of his or her hopes and goals. How you deal with control issues, however, can make the difference between your youngster's success and failure.

Power Plays

When teachers, counselors, or caretakers remain unresponsive to your youngster's needs or when there emerges a battle for control, a very personal decision is called for. You can try to get them to cooperate, but in the end, if they refuse, you have to decide whether to try to compensate for their uncooperativeness by giving your youngster added help at home or, if possible, to "vacate the battlefield." It's a hard choice, and certainly only you can make the decision, but rather than being pulled into a war of wills, you may choose to seek out a different caretaker or request a different teacher or counselor. If vacating is either impossible or impractical, you might try to enlist the help of a co-worker or superior of the person in contention. Most of us have been trained to remain, to continue to try and persuade others by using logic or appealing to their sense of right or duty. Battles for control, however, have little to do with either logic or fairness, and sometimes the best direction in which to move is out.

Rebel Without a Carbo

When youngsters themselves present resistance, you do not have the luxury of vacating the field. Most youngsters, as well as adults, walk a thin line between a desire for approval and a desire for independence. Many youngsters consider most adults—and in particular parents—to be a ready "wall" against which to push in order to help define limits. While the normal boundaries and restrictions that parents typically must enforce offer more than enough room for rebellion, a program that requires changes in eating and activity levels can be fodder for defiance or, at the very least, resistance.

In the face of rebellion, you have three choices.

If you find yourself coming face to face with a rebel in search of an excuse to consume carbos, you basically have three choices: You can attempt to talk your youngster through his or her rebel stance, you can back off and let the chips (no pun intended) fall where they may—and let your youngster learn from his or her mistakes, or you can take a stand and bring to bear your ability to withhold or grant privileges, and, as result, end up in a battle for control.

We strongly recommend that parents respond in the order above. First, try to get your youngster to communicate his or her feelings. We are not saying that you should preach or nag or even remind your youngster of the impact that going off the Program can have, but, rather, listen to what your youngster has to say. Most important, don't argue! Listen. Gather information. Get your youngster to reveal feelings of frustration, fear, and difficulties.

Never argue feelings.

Remember that feelings aren't facts. If your teen tells you that she feels fat, for instance, and she might as well go off the program because she'll never lose weight, it is useless to tell her that she is not fat or that she is losing more weight with each passing week. She cannot, at that moment, hear that if she just "hangs in there," she'll be slim before she knows it. She said she "feels" fat, even if she didn't use those words, and that is something with which you cannot argue. Respond to her feelings by letting her reveal the cause and extent of her unhappiness. Don't respond, "Well, if you feel so fat that's even more reason to stay on the Program"; rather, you might say, "That's a lousy feeling, I know." And you might encourage her to reveal more by adding, "Is the weight loss slowing a bit or are you just feeling heavy today?" Notice that in both choices you are neither validating her perception of reality nor challenging her feelings.

> **Words of rebellion often hide pain,
> frustration, and fear. They may say "go away,"
> but your youngster may need you more than ever.**

It takes some practice to learn how to respond to a youngster's negative emotions, but it gets easier over time. Just remember, when you hear your youngster's words, you are hearing one side of a conflict. The other side wants to lose weight or gain control of blood sugar–related problems. You can best foster the committed side of your youngster's feelings by not challenging the rebellion. Once you are able to nail down the cause of your youngster's feelings, gently offer some solutions or, if none are evident, add some perspective. For instance, if that same teen tells you that someone made a comment about her weight in school, discuss the perpetrator of the insult. Let your youngster take the lead.

Trust the outcome; given half a chance most youngsters will come up with a solution and resolution themselves: "Next time she makes a comment, I'll smile to myself, thinking how jealous she's going to be when I'm slimmer than she is. I'm already prettier."

Perspective helps a great deal. Without doing it directly, help your youngster remember that feelings are fleeting; she felt terrific yesterday and will again tomorrow. The best approach is sympathy and empathy. Give them time to work things out; they'll surprise both you and themselves.

Sometimes you have to stand back and let them swing.

If your youngster is young, unwilling to communicate, or just bent on rebellion, the next best thing you can do is to step back and let them swing. Don't stand in the way. You'll get into an emotional fistfight that will get nobody anywhere. We are not encouraging parents to shrug their shoulders and give up or to vindictively tell their youngsters that they are going to get what they deserve; rather, it is best to stay calm and continue to voice your thoughts in a nonblaming but responsive way. It's not always easy but it really does seem best. To the youngster who says, "I'm going to eat what I want and you can't stop me," you might respond, "It sounds like you're angry and frustrated, and if you are bent on throwing away all the progress you've made, there is nothing I can do about it. If you want to talk about it, though, we can try to figure out how we can work this out so that you get something satisfying to eat right now without feeling that you've made a mess of it."

Sometimes everyone needs a little space and time to cool down; just remember that your job is counselor and guide, adviser, and loving provider—you are not a policeman or guard. You do your best, evaluate whether there is anything you might do better, try to do better when you can. Remember that it takes a desire on your youngster's part to succeed as well.

We often don't know what we've got till it's gone.

Leaving the Program, for a short time or a prolonged period, is not necessarily a sentence of doom, either. Some of our youngsters have quit for a time, returned to old habits and old pain, and come back to the Program more appreciative and more willing than ever. Sometimes we all have to roll in the grass on the other side of the fence before we realize how sweet it is at home.

If you find yourself slipping in terms of empathy and patience, if you find that you no longer have any desire to communicate, then stop talking. Raised voices, threats, and hurtful words remain barriers to future success when the feelings have long since passed. Avoid a battle for control; everyone loses.

Sibling Sabotage
and Family Interference

Challenges to your youngster's success can come from within the family as well as from without. Other youngsters in the family or your spouse (current or ex) as well as relatives may attempt to hinder or directly oppose your youngster's program. Younger siblings may become jealous, older siblings may feel threatened, spouses may vie for your attention, and a variety of relatives and friends may all know "better than you" what is best for your youngster.

Just when you would welcome a bit of support, you may find you get the most conflicting information and the least support, both at the same time.

But take heart. As with any change, for every action you can expect a reaction, equal in force and opposite in direction. Stay focused and help your youngster to do the same. For those who are open to communication, communicate. For those who are not, do not waste your time and energy. Your child needs both right now; invest it where it will do the most good.

If your other youngsters have difficulty with this child's special needs on the Program or with their sibling's success, try to discuss the situation, of course, but, in the end, do not compromise one youngster's success for another youngster's comfort. If cookies tempt your carbo-addicted youngster so much that he or she cannot have them in your home, then by all means—at his or her request—ban them from the house. Your other youngsters can certainly have them outside the home, but the truth is, they won't *die* if they don't have them in the kitchen cabinet at all times. More often, sibling complaints and the noncooperation of spouse are manifestations of jealousy and rivalry.

Don't be fooled. If family members care more for their own convenience and indulgences than they do for the ultimate good of your carbo-addicted youngster, they need to have their self-centeredness pointed out rather than indulged.

Relatives and friends who know "best" may likewise need to be reminded that sometimes the best thing they can do to "help" is to allow your youngster and you work on the problem, together, and without interference.

So stand strong and focus on your youngster; success is the best convincer. Work with your child or teen and help him or her handle any opposition that may be encountered with strength and fortitude. Turn negatives into resolve and watch your youngster emerge victorious.

twelve

Fats: Facts and Myths, A New Look at Health

Most of us would like to find simple solutions to complex questions. The desire for the one-size-fits-all approach may be seen in low-fat recommendations that are sweeping this country. Americans are told that fat makes fat, or, even worse, they are told that dietary fat—and dietary fat alone—kills.

Indeed, although current conventional medical wisdom dictates that too much dietary fat can compromise ideal weight and good health, what most Americans are not being told is that carbohydrates—eaten too frequently, eaten in excess, or eaten without balance—can be just as harmful or, in many cases, far worse for the health of a great portion of the population. While some people may be "fat-sensitive," others, it appears, may be "carbohydrate-sensitive."

> The carbohydrate-addicted body turns
> carbohydrates in the diet
> into fat in the blood
> and then stores it as fat in the body.

For the carbohydrate-sensitive individual, carbohydrates in the diet are turned readily into fat in the blood and then stored in the body in the form of fat. The impact of frequent and excess carbos in the diet, especially simple sugars, may well lead to increased risk for heart disease, high blood pressure, adult-onset diabetes, and stroke, and may even encourage the growth of some forms of cancer.

It seems so odd that while health agencies would never presume to recommend one eyeglass prescription for an entire nation, they are indeed saying that everyone should follow a single eating prescription. This simplistic thinking may be easy to follow but, in reality, the results are often less than positive.

While in recent years the number of deaths attributed to heart disease has dropped dramatically, according to a recent study published in the *Journal of the American Medical Association*, this reduction has been due, for the most part, to the fine technological advances in diagnosing as well as pharmaceutical and surgical interventions. In addition, according to data from the National Institutes of Health and the American Heart Association, the *incidence* of heart disease itself has not decreased. In other words, with all the dietary changes that have been made, the number of people suffering from heart disease in this country has not dropped, and much of the credit for the increased longevity you hear about is due not to dietary changes, but to technological advances.

Indeed, as carbohydrate intake has increased and protein intake has decreased, a great portion of the population is getting sicker:

The incidence of adult-onset diabetes has skyrocketed.
The rate of obesity has almost doubled among our younger
    women.
Breast cancer now takes a far greater toll. A far greater
    number of women are developing breast cancer (odds have
    greatly increased as well) and a greater number of women
    are dying of it.
A variety of other disease have thrived and grown.

And while all these diseases and disorders have been linked to high levels of insulin, most people still go on believing in the media's pro-carbo push, encouraging the public to indulge in high-carbo diets without providing them with an understanding of the other side of the research.

High Blood Fat Levels

It is almost impossible to turn on the television or to open a magazine without being warned about the horrors of high blood fat levels. The message may seem simple and clear, but the truth, in fact, is neither.

While some researchers have linked high fat in the blood to atherosclerosis, heart attacks, strokes, and some forms of cancer in some people, an equal or greater number of scientists have linked high insulin levels to the same diseases—and more.

Most parents are left feeling guilty for almost anything they do, or fail to do, to keep their youngsters healthy.

Now the last thing that most people in this country need to hear is that there is yet another cause for concern in their diets, or in their youngsters' diets. The media has terrified parents, leaving them feeling guilty about almost anything they do, or fail to do, to keep their youngsters healthy. But overgeneralizations and simplifications that do not stand up to intelligent scrutiny can do even more harm than good.

What is the best diet for youngsters? The answer is that there is no "best" diet or "best" anything else for any group of people. What is best for *your* youngster to eat depends on *your* youngster's physical makeup. Just as you wouldn't expect your child to be able to see well through eyeglasses prescribed for a friend, you cannot possibly expect your youngster to thrive on an eating program that it is supposed to be right for everyone.

While nationwide eating recommendations may seem comforting and appear to provide a sense of well-being for a while, they may, in the end, do little to increase your youngster's chances for good health and long life.

At best, following one-size-fits-all dietary recommendations can unnecessarily limit your youngster's choices; at worst, you may be directing your youngster into an eating program that will provide the poorest choices for your youngster's particular health risk profile.

> **What matters is what is right for**
> ***your* youngster's particular health profile.**

Finding the right nutritional balance for your youngster is, in some ways, like buying your child a new outfit of clothes. It doesn't matter how good the clothes look while they are still on the hanger; what counts is how well they fit *your* child. In the same way, while low-fat diets may be right for some kids, if your youngster is carbohydrate-addicted (and therefore overreleases insulin when consuming carbohydrate-rich foods frequently or in an unbalanced way), a low-fat diet that is usually high in carbohydrates may bring on the very health problems you are seeking to avoid.

In the classification of different types of blood fat problems that medical laboratories use, the most common type in the United States today is Type IV hyperlipidemia (excess fat in blood). Though your doctor may know it by its scientific name, chances are that in your laboratory report it will show up only as a combination of numbers indicating high levels of "undesirable" blood fats and low levels of "desirable" blood fats.

> **The most common form of blood fat problem in this country**
> **is nicknamed "carbohydrate-induced high blood fat."**

This most prevalent blood fat problem is *not,* that's right, is *not* caused by dietary fat but rather is caused by the consumption of carbohydrate-rich foods. In fact, this type of blood fat problem is nicknamed "carbohydrate-induced high blood fat," and, remember, it is the most common form of blood fat problem in this country today.

Though scientific study after study has connected blood sugar swings, excess weight gain, and many risk factors for heart disease and other medical problems to a single common link—that is, to high levels of insulin—the most powerful study to date documents the influence of high insulin levels in determining the future health of children.

In 1996, in the medical journal *Circulation*, of the American Heart Association, Drs. Weihang, Srinivasan, and Berenson in the Bogalusa Heart Study revealed what so many researchers had been witnessing for so many years: the deadly impact of excess insulin on youngsters' health. Studying over sixteen hundred youngsters, ages five to twenty-three, these scientists measured insulin levels to understand this hormone's powerful connection to health-risk factors in children and teens.

During the first eight years of the study, the scientists found that youngsters with consistently high levels of insulin were, unfortunately, far more likely to have:

> Higher levels of triglycerides.
> Higher levels of LDL (undesirable) cholesterol.
> Higher levels of VLDL (undesirable) cholesterol.
> Higher levels of blood pressure.
> Lower levels of HDL (desirable) cholesterol.

In addition, they were consistently more likely to be overweight (by body-mass index).

These scientists continued to follow the youngsters' progress and discovered that insulin's health-threatening effects were even more powerful than other researchers had realized.

As adults, former "persistently high insulin youngsters" were found to be thirty-six times more likely to become obese, two and one-half times more likely to have high blood pressure, and three times more likely to have blood fat problems than those with persistently low insulin levels—all, we would add, may be attributable to insulin's devastatingly powerful influence.

What is most impressive to us as scientists, and distressing to us as well, is that all the health problems these young adults had endured had occurred by the time they were only twenty to thirty-one years of age. One can only imagine the health problems that young adults with high insulin levels are likely to develop by their forties or fifties. In the final words of the study, Drs. Weihàng, Srinivasan, and Berenson call for preventive measures to be taken early in life. This study, and the youngsters who participated in it as well as their parents—all of whom we very likely will never meet—have made us even more committed to getting our program to you and to your youngster, now.

So why are parents continuing to be told that dietary fats are the bad guys and that dietary carbohydrates—which bring on consistently high levels of insulin—are the good foods to choose for youngsters? If you are a believer in the good of mankind, you might assume that the overstatement of the benefit of low-fat diets comes from a simple misunderstanding.

The original low-fat research combined a low-fat diet with high fiber. It now appears that the high fiber (not the low fat) may well have been the positive influence in early test results. Initial reports, however, may not have separated the two influences, though much of the follow-up research clearly indicated that high fiber was the "good guy." Big business may have had a hand in continuing the push for low-fat recommendations long after opposing research revealed that low fat alone did not bring about the expected health benefits that are so often expounded.

At first big business tried to cash in on the positive effects of high fiber. If you remember, not too many years ago, fiber was "in." From muffins to crackers, from cookies to cereals, everyone was pushing fiber. At that point, the research was being interpreted correctly and the benefit of a high-fiber diet was pretty impressive. There remained, however, one major problem. Fiber didn't sell. It wasn't attractive in concept and it was even less appealing in taste. Furthermore, there were limitations on which foods could be made to incorporate high-fiber additions, and most of all, the public wasn't buying it, in more ways than one.

Fat, on the other hand, had a great deal going for it commercially. Fat phobia tied into the prejudices already dwelling within many people's minds and, if the advertisements of food producers sometimes blurred the lines between body fat and dietary fat, so much the better for sales.

> **Though fat is often *not* the culprit,
> it does make for great sales.**

So what was good for business was what we were told was good for us, all of us. Americans moved onto the low-fat bandwagon, and although scientists by the score are still disproving the universal good that low-fat diets are supposed to ensure, and though high-carbo diets have been shown repeatedly to cause more harm than good to those who are carbohydrate-sensitive, the hype goes on, and so do the sales.

The frequent intake of carbohydrates (in particular, simple sugars) *in combination* with a high level of saturated dietary fat (that is, a high–saturated fat, high-carbo diet) certainly can do double duty in setting up some carbo-addicted youngsters for future heart problems. For some carbo-addicted youngsters, this combination can spell real problems, and we agree that breaking the fat-carbo connection may help protect some youngsters from the hazards of this deadly duo, but for the carbohydrate-addicted youngster, a high-carbo, low-fat diet can be a major step in the wrong direction

You may choose to incorporate a low-fat version of this program by using some of the recommendations on page 417, but be aware that low-fat diets may not be appropriate for all youngsters. As always, check with your youngster's physician first, and in deciding the level of dietary fat that is right for your youngster, discuss your family's medical history as well as your youngster's addiction to carbohydrates.

Many parents have been happily surprised to find that, as their youngsters continue on the program, their youngsters' blood fat levels improve naturally. This welcome improvement is not surprising, however, when you consider that these youngsters' bodies were literally built to turn carbohydrates into fat. Normalizing their bodies' metabolic imbalance can help correct the root cause of potential blood fat problems that almost certainly might otherwise haunt them and harm them in the years to come.

An Exciting Breakthrough

Researchers have actively debated the influence of diet on breast cancer. While the television reports continue to spread the word that a high-fat diet contributes to the incidence or growth of breast cancer (often based on the assumption of the "evils" of dietary fat), well-designed scientific studies generally fail to link dietary fat to breast cancer. The largest study of its kind, however, has put together a most relevant link for the carbohydrate-addicted young woman—that is, the connection between a carbohydrate-rich diet and breast cancer risk.

In May 1996, in the well-respected medical journal the *Lancet*, Dr. Silvia Franceschi and her fellow researchers analyzed the diets of over twenty-five hundred women. This well-designed study revealed that, contrary to "popular" wisdom, *un*saturated fatty acids protected against breast cancer, and, not surprising to those familiar with the scientific facts, the greatest health risk factor for breast cancer was a high-carbohydrate diet.

This carbohydrate-insulin-cancer connection is not unexpected when one considers that insulin, released in response to the intake of carbohydrates, has been described as a "powerful fertilizer" to tumor cells or that, as reported by Dr. F. Kakar and colleagues from their work on animals, in the journal *Clinical Nutrition,* insulin injections significantly accelerated the growth of cancerous tumors of the breast.

If your youngster is female, decreasing the frequency and intensity of her insulin response may very well not only make her life better, it could quite possibly save it as well.

Taking It to Heart
and a Whole Lot More

We are not going to fill you with forebodings and fear. We are not about to make you feel guilty or helpless, or both. The facts are simple and positive: Although, as they enter adulthood, high insulin levels can make carbo-addicted youngsters far more prone to cardiovascular and other heart-related problems, the great news is that—with the balanced insulin levels this program can bring—your child or teen can reverse the odds. And you can take heart in the gift of health you are providing for your youngster.

While we hear a great deal about what raises our youngsters' risk for heart problems later in life, we rarely are told *why*. Lack of exercise, excess weight, stress, high-fat diets—all, we are told, lead to increased health risk. But of greater importance, all these health risks have one thing in common: All are linked to excess levels of insulin in the blood, the same high levels of insulin that stimulate your youngster's carbo cravings.

Wouldn't it be great if the same program that was designed to reduce your youngster's cravings for carbohydrates also reduced your youngster's insulin levels and, likewise, your youngster's risk for insulin-related heart problems? As you may have already guessed, on The Carbohydrate Addict's Program for Children and Teens, as insulin levels drop, so does your youngster's insulin-related heart risk.

How important is insulin to your youngster's health risk? Take a look at what the scientists are saying. In 1990 Dr. D. C. Simonson began to inform fellow scientists that although excess levels of insulin had been tied to cardiovascular disease for over twenty years, researchers were just beginning to fully understand the connection. He added that excess levels of insulin were "characteristic of a number of common human disease states including obesity, adult-onset diabetes, high blood pressure, and atherosclerotic heart disease." These discoveries have led scientists to declare that excess insulin is "now recognized to be the hallmark of several common disease states."

Under Pressure

The most prevalent form of high blood pressure is called essential hypertension. For years this term designated high blood pressure that had neither clear nor certain cause. Until recently the bad news, as reported by Dr. Norman M. Kaplan in the *Archives of Internal Medicine,* had been that over the past fifteen years the average blood pressure for the population at large had changed

little and, in fact, had risen for some. Old "truths" and treat-
ments had failed time and time again. Most adults were left to
take the same old medications with no assurance that their lives
would not be ruined by a stroke or cut short by a heart attack.

The good news is that scientists appear to have discovered a
vital link—the connection between high blood pressure and high
insulin levels. In 1990 a French research team headed by Dr. E.
Feraille pointed to the body's inability to handle insulin normally
as the most important cause of weight-related high blood pressure. Only one year later, in 1991, Drs. Landin, Tengborn, and
Smith published their research findings in the *Journal of Internal
Medicine.* In this important paper, they called for fellow scientists
and physicians to be aware that excess levels of insulin could play
an important role in the development of high blood pressure. In
their research summary, these well-respected scientists concluded
that the insulin connection to high blood pressure may open up a
whole new field for the treatment of cardiovascular disease.

**The Carbohydrate Addict's Program for Children and
Teens can help your youngster avoid the "deadly quartet."**

Other scientists have detailed four different ways in which
excess insulin can raise blood pressure, and Dr. Norman Kaplan,
in the medical journal *Archives of Internal Medicine,* notes that,
taken together, insulin's four pathways to high blood pressure
form a "deadly quartet," a quartet that could be avoided, one
may presume, by eliminating the lethal source.

Similar Opposites

Hypoglycemia,[1] which is characterized by low blood sugar levels,
may seem at first to be the opposite of adult-onset diabetes,

---

[1]Unless otherwise indicated, the term "hypoglycemia" will be used to indicate
the condition reactive hypoglycemia only.

which is characterized by high blood sugar levels, but clearly, it is not! Many adult-onset diabetics go through a period of being hypoglycemic early in their lives. Indeed, for many people, hypoglycemia may be the first step in a staircase that leads to adult-onset diabetes. (For a description of the physical changes that lead to low blood sugar levels, see page 118.)

> **Hypoglycemia and adult-onset diabetes**
> **may be opposite sides of the same coin.**

A common link to carbohydrate addiction, to many forms of reactive hypoglycemia, and to adult-onset diabetes is an excess of insulin. We believe that all three of these disorders are, in many cases, progressive stages of a single physical disorder.

Often the first to appear is an addiction to carbohydrates. High insulin levels lead to intense carbohydrate cravings, which lead to more frequent and/or more concentrated intake of carbohydrates (in particular, simple sugars), which, in turn, lead to high insulin levels. The carbo cycle repeats.

In time, if a youngster's carbohydrate craving/insulin release cycle is not broken, high levels of insulin may begin to rush too much blood sugar out of the bloodstream too quickly, channeling wherever it can, into the muscle, organ, or fat cells. Blood sugar levels can spike quickly, then may drop even more quickly and, as they drop, bring on some of the typical signs of hypoglycemia (sweating, irritability, lack of focus, inability to concentrate, mood swings, headache).

If the influx of carbos continues, insulin levels stay abnormally high and, depending on the youngster's genetics, the cells of the muscles and organs can be forced to protect themselves from high blood insulin levels by "closing down" their doors or receptor sites. The youngster, and the cells themselves, are said to have become "insulin resistant" and, because much of the blood sugar is now being channeled into the fat cells, weight gain is often the result.

As time goes on, especially in those youngsters who gain weight easily and/or have a family history of adult-onset diabetes, as blood insulin levels remain too high for too long, even the fat cells become resistant or "shut down." The result: Too much sugar remains in the bloodstream and brings on the condition called adult-onset diabetes (Type II).

For the slim carbohydrate addict and the youngster with no family history of adult-onset diabetes, the Carbohydrate Addict's Diet for Children and Teens can help stabilize insulin and blood sugar levels, reduce or eliminate insulin-related hypoglycemic episodes, and channel vital food energy where it is needed most.

For the youngster whose family history does include adult-onset diabetes, The Carbohydrate Addict's Diet for Children and Teens may relieve a great deal more than behavioral, learning, mood, and weight problems. By reducing insulin levels, you may be helping your youngster avoid the ravages of adult-onset diabetes and the heartache and ill health it brings.

CARBO ADDICTION AND DIABETES: ESSENTIAL DIFFERENCES

Diabetes is a disorder in which too much blood sugar (glucose) remains in the bloodstream. This excess blood sugar may be the result of:
1. the body's ability to make enough insulin, or
2. the body's inability to use the insulin it makes.

In Type I diabetes, not enough insulin (or no insulin) is available to help remove blood sugar from the bloodstream.

In Type II diabetes, too much insulin may cause some of the cells to close down in the face of an insulin overload. The body becomes unable to use insulin (insulin-resistant), and blood sugar has no way to leave the bloodstream. The body may compensate by producing greater and greater quantities of insulin until the pancreas is "exhausted" and can no longer produce insulin at all.

Although Type II diabetes is often referred to as adult-onset diabetes, it can occur in youngsters, usually adolescents, often those who have weight problems and family histories of the disorder. Because of a youngster's age, many physicians assume these kids do not produce enough insulin (Type I) when, in fact, they are producing so much excess insulin that their bodies have become resistant to it.

Carbohydrate addiction is defined by chronically high insulin levels and the cravings it produces. While many carbohydrate addicts may never become diabetic (Type II), depending on one's genetics, a long-standing carbohydrate addiction that is neither controlled nor corrected can, for many, be a first step in becoming a Type II diabetic.

A Blessing in Disguise

If high blood pressure, heart disease, high blood fat levels, or adult-onset diabetes runs in your family, your youngster's carbohydrate addiction may be a blessing in disguise; it well may signal how essential it is to change the way your youngster takes in carbohydrates for health and for life.

thirteen

Straight Talk: Questions, Answers, and Real-Life Help

Starting Off Right: Breakfast Alternatives

I am not sure what to give my youngster for his Insulin-Balancing Breakfasts. Do you have any suggestions?

In many ways, Insulin-Balancing Breakfasts can be tailored to your youngster's needs and preferences as well as to yours. Keep in mind that the only rules that apply when it comes to Insulin-Balancing Breakfasts are that these meals must contain Insulin-Balancing Foods only, and that you should incorporate nutritional recommendations (if any) of your youngster's physician into your choice of foods.

If your youngster prefers more conventional breakfasts, you can always rely on a variety of omelettes that may include any combination of Insulin-Balancing Foods; a cheese omelette made from real eggs or egg substitutes and regular or low-fat cheese, for instance, can start your youngster's day right. Mushroom, green pepper, and other combinations can add variety. Cottage cheese is a favorite for some youngsters as well. Do not rely on eggs or cottage cheese all the time (though cottage cheese is listed as a Insulin-Balancing Food, carbo contents vary, and it can be borderline high in carbos).

Look over the Insulin-Balancing Food List on page 183 and remember that all the foods listed there (in both regular and low-fat varieties) are available to be included your youngster's breakfasts; no other limits exist except the ones you and youngster set.

If your youngster misses muffins, french toast, pancakes, or a nice serving of hearty hash, you will find Insulin-Balancing varieties of these typically high-carbo foods beginning on page 308. If the high-carbohydrate versions of these breakfast treats are craved and coveted, they can still be enjoyed. Simply turn a Combo Meal into a real reward by having an old-fashioned breakfast at dinnertime!

If your youngster is open to broadening the conception of breakfast foods, he or she need not be restricted to typical breakfast choices; suddenly, all those favorite high-protein, low-carbohydrate foods can be enjoyed at breakfast time. Chicken salad, made the night before from chicken, celery, and mayonnaise, served with cool sliced cucumbers, can be delicious; a slice of leftover meat or poultry (roast beef or chicken, for instance) from last night's dinner wrapped with mustard in lettuce leaves, or tuna salad made with celery and mayonnaise (with or without sliced or chopped hard-boiled egg), made the night before, can offer a surprisingly tasty and quick Insulin-Balancing Breakfast. Some kids like steak and eggs as an occasional alternative, or a grab-and-run treat of celery stuffed with cream cheese. If appropriate, choose low-fat alternatives for breakfast in all foods except mayonnaise (low-fat mayo usually contains mostly sugar and water, so use a smaller portion of real mayonnaise, rather than a low-fat substitute).

Remember that Insulin-Balancing Meals cannot include high-carbohydrate beverages, so make certain that your youngster steers clear of juices and milk during Insulin-Balancing Meals and offer some cool bottled water, seltzer, or perhaps some herbal tea (regular or iced, without sweetener) instead. Milk and whole fruit can still be enjoyed at all Combo Meals.

Avoiding Lunchtime Challenges

What do I do about my youngster's lunches?

Lunches should be planned for ahead of time (when possible), packed, and dealt with, but sometimes lunchtime challenges are difficult to avoid. Lunchtime challenges fall into two categories: first, getting the food to your youngster, and second, getting your youngster to eat the food.

Getting the food to your youngster is relatively simple. It is usually pretty easy for youngsters on The Step-By-Step Plan to bring Add-On Insulin-Balancing Foods to school. Finger salads can be made up of raw celery sticks (not carrots), cucumber coins, and other Insulin-Balancing Vegetables. Keep them cool and crisp and seal them in a zipper-sealed plastic bag. These Add-Ons can supplement the school lunch purchased in the cafeteria or can be part of the lunch your youngster brown-bags to school. Look over the recipe section in Chapter 14. You will find lots of recipes in the Insulin-Balancing section that will give you some good take-along suggestions for Add-Ons.

If your youngster is on The Jump-Start Plan, some planning and packing are going to be necessary. If lunch is purchased in the school cafeteria and it is very important to your youngster to buy lunch, check with the chief dietitian each month for a list of planned menus. Keep in mind that when the cafeteria says "hamburger" or "tuna fish salad," these foods and others may contain carbohydrate-rich fillers such as bread and may even have added sweeteners as well. Still, you can try to plan so that, as much as possible, your youngster can get meals from the cafeteria. Depending on what is being served that day, you will want to supplement the fare with Insulin-Balancing Foods from home. You will find some good suggestions by looking over the recipe section in Chapter 14. Many of the Insulin-Balancing recipes are suited for lunchtime take-alongs on The Jump-Start Plan.

On The Jump-Start Plan, getting Insulin-Balancing Food at lunchtime will be your first challenge; making sure that your child or teen is eating Insulin-Balancing Foods, and only Insulin-Balancing Foods at lunch, is the second challenge. If your youngster is highly motivated; if weight loss is a goal or if changes in behavior, mood, or learning are greatly desired, your youngster is more likely to be able to resist the temptations of a typical schooltime lunch.

If, on the other hand, on The Jump-Start Plan your youngster has a difficult time saying no to carbohydrate-rich lunchtime offerings, or if peer pressure is putting too great a demand on your child, we have found that we bypass all lunchtime challenges by considering lunch the daily Combo Meal.[1] In that way, your youngster is free to enjoy Carbohydrate-Rich Foods with classmates. If your youngster is in Phase One of The Jump-Start Plan, you should try to make sure that all other daily meals (including breakfast, dinner, and snacks) are made up of Insulin-Balancing Foods only. (You will find fun recipes in Chapter 14; see page 308 for some breakfast suggestions.)

Do keep in mind how important an encouraging environment is to your youngster's success. You will find some helpful suggestions in Chapter 11, "Strategies for Success," and you will find the love and commitment and strength you need deep inside yourself. When the challenges seem great, keep the goal in mind.

A Matter of Trust

Can't I just avoid talking about the Program with my youngster and simply begin making some of the small changes involved in The Step-By-Step Plan unobtrusively and on my own?

Instead of discussing whether your youngster is willing to start the Program, a parent might think about just inconspicuously adding salad to one meal for a week, and then some protein-rich foods the next. We strongly discourage this approach. While you may be getting the food you want into your youngster, you are not making the changes the youngster needs to make to incorporate new eating habits for life. By sneaking your youngster into the Program, you are making temporary changes in the body but failing to make permanent ones in your child's mind. Change comes not only from doing things differently, but from understanding what you are doing and why you are doing it. When your child decides, with you, to follow the program, he or she will gain much more than more healthful eating habits.

---

[1] Combo Meals may be switched to a breakfast, dinner, or snacktime as desired, but only one Combo Meal per day on Phase One of The Jump-Start Plan.

Most of our youngsters not only lose their cravings, lose excess weight, and gain control of their behavior, mood swings, or attention problems, they also gain a greater sense of pride, a feeling of accomplishment, and the experience of successfully dealing with their problems. All these experiences will help carry them into adulthood with confidence, and they all stem from choosing to make change, working for the change, then reaping the rewards and feeling the accomplishment of a job well done.

The Radical Approach

Wouldn't it be easier just to eliminate all carbohydrates, especially sugars?

The person who is an alcoholic may choose to avoid alcohol; the adult or youngster who is addicted to carbohydrates, however, cannot and should not avoid carbohydrates. Carbohydrates are essential to good health, to life itself. Your youngster *cannot* survive indefinitely without carbohydrates in his or her diet. Foods rich in complex carbohydrates, like potatoes, corn, peas, and other starchy vegetables, as well as whole grains, are absolutely vital to your youngster's (and your) continued health. A small portion of simple sugars, on the other hand, while not necessarily essential, are important to many youngsters (and adults) as well. None of us should ever try to do without complex carbos in our diets, and few of us are willing to do without any simple sugars.

The good news, however, is that balancing your youngster's carbohydrate-rich meals and snacks with protein-rich and high-fiber foods, and decreasing the number of times each day your youngster eats Carbohydrate-Rich Foods, will vastly decrease the carbo cravings and hunger. Researchers such as Dr. T. W. Jones and colleagues, reporting in the medical journal *Pediatrics,* have examined the effects of dietary carbohydrates on youngsters' insulin, adrenaline, and blood sugar levels and have concluded that balanced meals, which include, among other foods, protein, complex carbohydrates, and fiber, will help limit hormonal and blood sugar swings.

> **On this program, your youngster
> does not have to give up favorite foods.**

Whether your youngster (on The Step-By-Step Plan) moves slowly and steadily, decreasing the number of times each day that Carbohydrate-Rich Foods are enjoyed and balancing them with Insulin-Balancing Foods, or (on The Jump-Start Plan) moves more quickly, both plans will help your youngster break free of the addiction without asking your youngster to give up essential (and much-loved) foods.

Fat Facts

Shouldn't I be concerned about fat in my youngster's diet?

The Carbohydrate Addict's Diet for Children and Teens may be adapted to be low-fat or very-low-fat, depending on your physician's recommendations. Each child is different, and advice may vary accordingly. No one prescription, whether it is for eyeglasses or for general nutrition, is right for everyone. Carbohydrate-addicted youngsters have difficulty handling the carbohydrates in their food; their bodies turn the starches and sugars in their foods into fat in their blood and then store it as fat in their bodies. Although many parents find that concerns about their youngster's weight and blood fat levels are no longer a problem once their youngsters have been following the guidelines of the Carbohydrate Addict's Diet for Children and Teens, only your doctor can make the final decision.

If your doctor wants your youngster to follow a low-fat diet, you will find guidelines on page 417 and a complete chapter detailing important fat facts and myths beginning on page 260. The choices are up to you. You can substitute low-fat cheese and meat alternatives along with chicken and turkey in place of fat-drenched meats. Most recipes will offer you low-fat alternatives for dairy foods (do make sure your youngster gets the calcium he or she needs). High-fiber additions will come naturally with the Add-On vegetables or salad Choices your youngster selects.

As in all things, nutritional and not, one size does not fit all. Talk to your doctor, talk to your youngster, and listen to your own good sense.

Healthy Hype

I've been feeding my youngster as much "healthy" food as I can get. Shouldn't that be enough?

What is touted as "healthy" food or what is assumed to be "healthy" food may be far from healthy for *your* youngster. Food producers have managed to find amazingly creative ways around the labeling laws. Packaged turkey that flashes the words "only 2 percent fat" actually can contain as much as 25 percent fat when you know how to do the calculations. How do they get away with it? On the front of the package they may use weight as their method of comparison. If the item contains a great deal of water, the percentage of fat by weight is very little; by caloric comparison the percentage of fat may be much higher. The most common example of percentage subterfuge can be seen in "2 percent milk," which actually is 36 percent fat!

Food producers are allowed to call it "2 percent milk," but it actually contains 36 percent fat!

For carbohydrate-addicted youngsters, vital information must include the amount of carbohydrates—in particular, simple sugars in foods—because carbohydrates will often trigger an insulin release and then the cravings, weight, and other problems with which carbo-addicted youngsters and their parents must cope. Once again, labels can mislead. Although simple sugars may differ greatly from complex carbos in the ways they impact on your youngster's body and behavior, sugars are listed under the heading "carbohydrates" according to the nutritional labeling laws now in place. To make matters worse, consumers may be unaware that the percentages of carbohydrates that appear on labels contain in these calculations sugars as well as complex carbohydrates.

If you rely on the nutrition label alone to provide you with essential information, a food item that provides mostly sugar as its source of carbohydrates could wrongly appear to be a "healthy" food.

Instead, look at the list of ingredients as well. Most important: Ingredients that end in the suffix "ose" are, in fact, sugars, including sucrose, fructose, dextrose, maltose, lactose, and galactose. In addition, because they are much cheaper than table sugar, food producers include a great deal of corn syrup and high-fructose corn syrup (which may contain very little fructose and a great deal more of blood sugar–disturbing glucose).

Ingredients are listed from greatest to least, with the ingredients that contribute most to the food listed first, but here again, if they want to, food producers can mislead. By using several different ingredients that are high in sugar but that have different names, food producers can include a great deal of sugar in a food without it appearing as the first, second, or third ingredient.

Look at the following list of ingredients, for instance: enriched white flour, brown sugar, low-fat milk products, corn syrup, high-fructose corn syrup. Because these manufacturers have split their high-sugar ingredients into different products with different names, the consumer may be unaware that, in actuality, if you grouped the sugars together, they would far outweigh the flour and milk products, and the sugars would appear as the first and primary ingredient instead of further down in the list.

Parents of carbohydrate-addicted youngsters need to read the list of ingredients and learn to recognize "ose" words in the list, and to be aware that corn syrups and high-fructose corn syrups are sugars as well. Other additives like monosodium glutamate (MSG) can appear under these names: hydrolyzed food starch, hydrolyzed vegetable protein, flavor enhancer, or natural ingredients, or, even worse, as more than one of these. (By the way, monosodium glutamate is used by laboratories to make experimental animals become fat!).

So reading the list of ingredients and knowing what it is really saying is very helpful in your quest to give your youngster health-building nutrition, but keep an important rule in mind: Do not focus only on what is *in* the food; stay aware of what the food does in your youngster's body. What is "healthy" food for one child or teen may be less than "healthy" in another. Read the ingredients to understand what is in the food and then watch and see how the food affects *your* youngster.

Not-So-Sweet Rewards

I thought fructose was okay. After all, it comes from fruit.

Sometimes we jokingly wonder if fructose, or fruit sugar, employs its own public relations person. This type of sugar has somehow managed to get a great reputation, and many people falsely believe it is a "safe" sugar, different from other sugars and far better for you.

> ### Don't be fooled by fructose fantasies.

Let's get one thing straight—sugar is sugar. Whether or not it is found in the fruit or on your table, it is sugar. It is true that when fruit sugar is combined with fibrous material as it occurs in nature, that is, when you eat the whole fruit, the fiber helps slow down some of the blood sugar swings that will often occur when the fiber is not present. But as Dr. John Bantle and his colleagues reported in their article in the *New England Journal of Medicine*, the fructose-related blood sugar leveling effect appears to come from the fiber rather than from the fructose itself, and there appears to be no significant differences in blood sugar swings when table sugar (sucrose) is used as a sweetener versus fructose (fruit sugar). So if you are feeding your youngster fruit juice or foods that are sweetened with fruit juice or fructose in the belief that you have found a way around sugar-related blood sugar swings, you may be fooling yourself. The idea that "fruit juice is better than sucrose as a sweetener" appears to be far more fantasy than fact.

By the way, fructose (fruit sugar) is *not*, we repeat, is *not* a complex carbohydrate. It is a simple sugar, actually "simpler" than table sugar. Glucose, on the other hand, appears to bring on greater blood sugar spikes than either sucrose or fructose. Amazingly, the food industry is allowed to refer to some high-glucose sweeteners as "high-fructose corn syrup." If this sounds confusing to you, we agree. So, in addition to sucrose and fructose, be on the lookout for glucose, the sugar we have come to call the "blood sugar tyrant."

One thing for sure, if your youngster is set on eating sugar-rich foods, making them part of a well-rounded meal and decreasing how many times each day these foods are eaten can greatly help to keep blood sugar swings under control. Both The Jump-Start Plan and The Step-By-Step Plan that make up The Carbohydrate Addict's Diet for Children and Teens will help you, and your youngster, to do both.

Nature Versus Nurture

If carbohydrate addiction is inherited, how can an eating program help?

This program is designed to do one thing and one thing alone: to reduce excess levels of insulin that are the trademark of carbohydrate addiction.

This tendency to release too much insulin is inherited, but it can still remain a tendency, rather than a full-blown problem, if the frequent intake of carbohydrates and the unbalanced way in which most youngsters take in their carbos is changed. With less frequent intake and more balance in their meals, youngsters can experience a freedom from the cravings, blood sugar swings, and weight, behavior, mood, and motivation problems that often result. If your youngster has been sedentary, an increased level of activity can help in balancing insulin levels as well.

Though the genetics your youngster inherited cannot be changed, their effect on your youngster can be controlled—for life.

Glycemic Indications

Does this program use the glycemic index?

You may have heard of the glycemic index as reported by the media in relation to nutritional research, or as it has been referred to by several authors in their books on weight loss or diabetes. The glycemic index measures blood sugar responses to different foods prepared in different ways. It has several failings. First, as far as we have seen, it doesn't measure insulin responses to these foods, and how much insulin is released will determine how much of a drive your youngster experiences to go back and eat the food again. So let's say you find that a particular food has a low glycemic index, that is, it doesn't cause too much of a blood sugar peak after it has been eaten. Unfortunately, that tells you nothing about how strongly your youngster is going to crave more of the same foods or, even worse, foods that have a higher glycemic index. Foods with a low glycemic index, then, could in themselves not cause blood sugar swings but could be a sort of "priming" type of food that brings your youngster back for more . . . and more.

Real-life kids don't eat like adults do in the laboratory.

A second failing of the glycemic index is that each food was measured in a meal made up only of that food. As far as we have seen, no foods were mixed to see if their combined effect might be different. Evaluations based on this untested assumption could be likened to looking at a single lit match and a gallon of gasoline separately and assuming that because each by itself could not cause an explosion, in combination the match and gasoline were safe.

The other foods your youngster eats in combination with carbos, or the lack of other foods, can have a powerful effect in increasing or decreasing the impact of that carbo on your youngster's blood sugar levels, yet these researchers appeared to examine each carbo as if it existed in isolation.

The last failing of the glycemic index is the most important. Blood sugar responses indicate the responses of "normal" subjects and may tell you nothing about how your youngster will respond. Not only do we know that youngsters and adults respond differently to the same foods, we know that carbohydrate-addicted kids respond differently from nonaddicted youngsters. Though no single chart or index can tell you how *your* youngster responds to the food, you may start by looking at the list of Carbohydrate-Rich Foods beginning on page 184. With this list in mind, see which changes take place within two hours of your youngster's consumption of these foods. Stop, look, and listen; most of all, trust the truth you see right before your own eyes.

Fat Facts

Which is more important to avoid: fats or carbos in my youngster's diet?

Neither; no healthy program of eating should ever exclude either fats or carbohydrates. Certainly your own youngster's physician must guide you, but it is your task as a parent to make sure that your physician understands the impact that carbohydrates may be having on your youngster. Physicians have been trained to focus on fats; help your health professional pay attention to *your* youngster's sensitivity to carbohydrates.

You will find vital information about dietary fats versus carbohydrates beginning on page 260 (in Chapter 12), and some real-life help on lowering fat intake while keeping your youngster on The Carbohydrate Addict's Program for Children and Teens on page 417.

Remember, fats in the diet may become fat in the blood and may then be stored as fat in the body, but the same happens when your youngster eats carbohydrates too often or without balance and, in the carbohydrate-addicted youngster, carbos may be the prime culprit.

So talk over fat issues with your physician but make sure that both of you have all the "fat facts." If your doctor feels that lowering dietary fat is necessary, your youngster can do that, most certainly, while following this program, but for your youngster's well-being, remember that the way in which he or she takes in carbos may be critical.

Vegetable Phobic

My child will not look at, much less eat, anything that remotely resembles a vegetable. What can I do?

Many youngsters hate the *category* vegetables, but almost all of them will eat at least one or two (or maybe three?) vegetables when you consider vegetables one by one. For Insulin-Balancing Meals, look over the list of Insulin-Balancing Foods (page 183) and consider each vegetable. Would your youngster eat *any* of these vegetables if they were served raw with a dip? If they were sautéed or stir-fried with protein and turned into a homemade Chinese-like meal? If they were served occasionally topped with cheese or bacon chips? Many parents with vegetable-hating kids are surprised to find that there are a few vegetables, prepared in a special way, that a youngster is willing to eat. When it comes to Combo Meals, a great many additional vegetables are open to you (see page 185 for a list of Carbohydrate-Rich Vegetables and pages 362–373 for Carbohydrate-Rich vegetable and dip recipes) but try to balance high-carbo vegetables with some fiber-rich Insulin-Balancing Vegetables, even at Combo Meals. Make sure you do not overcook the vegetables (a typical problem), and check out our recipe section beginning on page 316 for special Insulin-Balancing dip and vegetable ideas. If your youngster still staunchly refuses to eat even a single vegetable, he or she can still stay on the program. With the approval of your youngster's physician, have your youngster continue to follow the steps or guidelines of the plan as closely as possible, being certain to eat Insulin-Balancing Foods as they are called for. In time, as your youngster's insulin release is reduced, the dislike of all things vegetable will most likely fade.

Remember that cucumber slices and celery sticks are low-carbohydrate, Insulin-Balancing Vegetables and can be enjoyed in any meal, and that carrots are high in carbohydrates and should be included in Combo Meals only.

The Prescription Decision

What about drugs?

Many medications may not be recommended for, or may not have been tested on, children; some may carry the risk of long-term, serious, or possibly life-threatening side effects. In addition, since these medications do not correct the cause of the problem, they must be taken for life, or, if they are discontinued, the problem can return.

While the prescription decision is one that must be made in consultation with your youngster's physician, we believe that whenever possible, it is best to correct the cause of a problem without the use of medications.

Everyday Celebrations

When can I allow my child to "cheat" a little on the Program? Can my youngster temporarily go off the diet during vacations or holidays?

It is essential that you, as a parent, keep in mind that your youngster's carbohydrate addiction is the result of a physical imbalance, an imbalance that will return every time your child or teen goes off his or her eating and activity program. If you yield to your youngster's requests to cheat a little during vacations, holidays, parties, or celebrations, for instance, you will see a result that reflects far more than a simple backsliding in weight or attention or mood problems.

First, you will be giving your youngster the message that it is acceptable to give in to the addiction at socially sanctioned times. Soon the frequency of these events will increase and, almost without fail, you can expect there will be more cheating than following of the Program.

Second, your youngster will stop seeing the Program as a way of life that corrects a physical imbalance but will view it as a temporary Band-Aid that can be removed at will. Excess levels of insulin are no small matter, and your youngster needs to realize that just as there is no vacation from this physical imbalance, there is no vacation from the treatment for the problem.

We tell parents to deal with cheating issues as if they were dealing with a youngster with diabetes. You would never think of telling a diabetic youngster it was acceptable to stop taking insulin injections or to cheat on a diabetic diet because of a holiday or vacation or celebration. In the same way, eating and activity Choices that are designed to reduce your youngster's excess levels of insulin should not be abandoned, even for special events or for limited times.

If you stay constant, your youngster will find that staying on the Program, and the feelings of victory as well as the avoidance of weight, mood, motivation, and behavior problems, more than make up for a chance to give in to temptation. To make it even more compelling, remember that staying on the Program is a great deal easier than trying to get back on it. And, of course, the Program itself allows a great deal of latitude and enjoyment of your youngster's favorite foods during Combo (Reward) Meals.

> **There are a whole host of treats your youngster can enjoy without going off the Program.**

On the other hand, there is a great deal you can do to add to your youngster's enjoyment of the Program while supporting his or her involvement in it. If you are going on vacation, look for restaurants where your youngster can get meals in keeping with his or her meal plans, especially restaurants that include salad bars or offer buffets, where the choices are wider than typical menu fare. Consider special treats, perhaps those that might be a little too expensive for everyday meals. In all cases, keep balance and other guidelines in mind, but for special times, consider special treats.

Remember that this program allows the enjoyment of Carbohydrate-Rich Foods every day; there is no need to go off the Program to enjoy the foods that are most loved. This program is not one of deprivation, and the old "but it's my birthday" or "but we're on vacation" excuse doesn't hold water here. Vacations and birthdays and other celebrations pass quickly; if you hold your ground and work within the Program, you youngster will learn to respect that the Program and the benefits it brings can be constant and dependable and still rewarding, for life.

PART IV

When Things Get Cookin'

fourteen

Gourmet Delights and Recipes on the Run

Cooking is absolutely *not* a requirement on The Carbohydrate Addict's Program for Children and Teens. Absolutely not. Our lives today are filled with impossible demands on our time and attention. The last thing most parents need to be told is that, to help their youngsters, they are suddenly going to have to become gourmet cooks.

On the other hand, if you are one of those special and (we hope) well-appreciated parents who cook, your talents, skill, and interest will find a special place in this program.

For the "cook," for the "can't cook," and for the "can't cook right now" parent, the pages that follow will provide new and exciting choices:

> Real-life suggestions for incorporating occasional heat-and-eat meals into your youngster's program.
> QuickFix breakfasts, lunches, dinners, and snacks.
> Gourmet recipes of all kinds.

While keeping the Program's guidelines in mind, you can choose meal preparation suggestions that meet your youngster's preferences and needs but also fit well into the demands of your lifestyle.

A WIDE VARIETY OF MEALTIME CHOICES

Where to Find What's Good to Eat

Eating Out:
Tips in the Face of Temptation

Eating outside the home can present unique challenges for any youngster on a special eating program, or for any youngster who is trying to eat healthily, for that matter.

You will find school lunchtime suggestions beginning on page 275 and suggestions for fast food and restaurant choices, as well as tips that will help your child enjoy eating at other people's homes in the pages that follow.

Fast-Food Victories[2]

Most fast-food restaurants have opened their menus to a wider variety of "healthier" choices, and the youngster on The Carbohydrate Addict's Program for Children and Teens has a much easier time than he or she might have had a few years ago. For Combo Meals, for instance, youngsters may choose a balanced lunch or dinner that includes salad or coleslaw as well as chicken patties or burgers. Most fast-food restaurants offer bottled water and plain iced tea (without sugar or artificial sweetener). A special treat or a nice piece of fruit can top off the meal.

For Insulin-Balancing Meals and Snacks, salads (with carrots and croutons removed) and chicken breast (broiled not breaded and fried, with bun removed), make for tasty choices within the Program's guidelines.

> **Important Note:** Fast-food rotisserie chicken may be marinated in sugar as well as monosodium glutamate before it is cooked, and for those who are concerned about fat, it may actually be higher in fat content than its fried counterpart. If your child chooses rotisserie chicken, be aware that it is not necessarily a low-fat food, and if it is consumed, it should be eaten at Combo Meals or Snacks only.

Restaurant Recommendations

When eating out, your child can enjoy a well-balanced Combo Meal at almost any restaurant. You may need to call first to make certain that your youngster will be able to complete the meal within the sixty-minute limit. In addition, make certain that appropriate vegetables are available.

For Insulin-Balancing Meals and Snacks, you can encourage your youngster to make the same choices as he or she would make at home. Again, you may need to call the restaurant first to make sure that the foods your child needs are available.

---

[2]Eating at fast-food restaurants is neither condoned nor recommended.

Do not allow your youngster to go to a restaurant without being certain that the foods he or she needs will be available.

Do not allow your child to go to a restaurant without being certain that the entire meal or snack can be served within the one-hour time limit.

Do encourage your youngster to order first, so that other people's orders do not present unnecessary temptation.

Do plan and offer suggestions and troubleshooting alternatives as appropriate.

Do choose restaurants that offer special treats that your child especially enjoys at appropriate meals or snacks.

Special tips:

Ask that salad be brought immediately so that your youngster has something to eat other than bread and butter.

Make certain that the server knows that the one-hour time limit is important to your child's health and well-being; you might even explain that this request is necessary because of a "medical condition."

Never take a food server's word that a food does not contain "sugar," "filler," or monosodium glutamate. You are fooling yourself if you think you can truly rely on the answer. Many people who do not know, do not say that they do not know. So whenever possible, ask to see the label (especially at deli counters) or, if you are unsure, skip it for the time being.

Other Homes, Other Challenges

Use the same tips as recommended for restaurant eating. Family members and friends may sometimes prove less cooperative than strangers. Do not allow yourself to be swayed by implied guilt, intimidation, or vague promises. Your child's health and well-being is at stake. Act as if your youngster were allergic to a certain type of food (which he or she essentially is), and above all, never allow your child's needs, or your concerns, to be devalued or ignored.

Incorporating Heat-and-Eat Food Choices into Your Youngster's Program

Here are some suggestions for balancing heat-and-eat foods so that they may be included as part of your youngster's balanced Combo Meals.

Although packaged foods tend to be higher in fat and more sugar-laden than home-cooked alternatives, these appear to be some of the best in terms of balance.

Note: Heat-and-eat foods are almost always too high in carbohydrate content to be included in Insulin-Balancing Meals or Snacks, or in Combo Snacks. Include them in Combo Meals only.

HEAT-AND-EAT MEAL	ADD FOR COMBO MEAL BALANCE
Stouffer's® Lean Cuisine® Entrees	
Angel Hair Pasta	Meat, poultry, fish, or meat alternative; salad and vegetables; dessert, if desired, including fruit.
Baked Chicken and Whipped Potatoes and Stuffing	Salad and vegetables; dessert, if desired, including fruit.
Beef Pot Roast and Whipped Potatoes	Salad and vegetables; dessert, if desired, including fruit.
Cafe Classics Cheese Lasagne with Chicken Scaloppine	Salad and vegetables; dessert, if desired, including fruit.
Cafe Classics Chicken Parmigiana	Starch or grain products (pasta, potato, rice, noodles, or bread); salad and vegetables; dessert, if desired, including fruit.
Chicken and Vegetables	Starch or grain products (pasta, potato, rice, noodles, or bread); salad and some additional vegetables; dessert, if desired, including fruit.
Chicken Chow Mein with Rice*	Salad and vegetables; dessert, if desired, including fruit.
Chicken Oriental with Vegetables and Vermicelli	Salad and some additional vegetables; dessert, if desired, including fruit.
French Bread Pizzas (all varieties)	Meat, poultry, fish or meat alternative; salad and vegetables; dessert, if desired, including fruit.

*Item may exceed dietary fat recommendations. As always, follow the advice of your youngster's physician.

HEAT-AND-EAT MEAL (*continued*)	**ADD FOR COMBO MEAL BALANCE** (*continued*)
Glazed Chicken with Vegetable Rice	Salad and some additional vegetables; dessert, if desired, including fruit.
Meatloaf and Whipped Potatoes	Salad and vegetables; dessert, if desired, including fruit.
Rigatoni	Meat, poultry, fish, or meat alternative; salad and vegetables; dessert, if desired, including fruit.
Salisbury Steak with Macaroni & Cheese	Salad and vegetables; dessert, if desired, including fruit.
Stuffed Cabbage with Whipped Potatoes	Some additional meat, poultry, fish, or meat alternative; salad; dessert, if desired, including fruit.

Stouffer's® Entrees

Homestyle Baked Chicken & Gravy and Whipped Potatoes*	Salad and vegetables; dessert, if desired, including fruit.
Homestyle Beef Pot Roast and Browned Potatoes*	Salad and vegetables; dessert, if desired, including fruit.
Homestyle Chicken and Noodles*	Salad and vegetables; dessert, if desired, including fruit.
Homestyle Chicken Parmigiana with Spaghetti*	Salad and vegetables; dessert, if desired, including fruit.
Homestyle Meat Loaf with Whipped Potatoes*	Salad and vegetables; dessert, if desired, including fruit.
Homestyle Roast Turkey and Homestyle Stuffing*	Salad and vegetables; dessert, if desired, including fruit.
Lasagne with Meat Sauce*	Meat, chicken, fish, or meat alternative; salad and vegetables; dessert, if desired, including fruit.
Stuffed Peppers	Additional meat, poultry, fish or meat alternative; salad; dessert, if desired, including fruit.

Kid Cuisine®

Big League Hamburger Pizza*	Meat, poultry, fish, or meat alternative; salad and vegetables; dessert, if desired, including fruit.
Futuristic Fish Sticks	Starch or grain products (pasta, potato, rice, noodles, or bread); salad and vegetables; dessert, if desired, including fruit.
Magical Macaroni and Cheese	Meat, poultry, fish, or meat alternative; salad and vegetables; dessert, if desired, including fruit.
Pirate Pizza with Cheese*	Meat, poultry, fish, or meat alternative; salad and vegetables; dessert, if desired, including fruit.
Rip-Roaring Macaroni and Beef*	Additional meat, poultry, fish, or meat alternative; salad and vegetables; dessert, if desired, including fruit.

*Item may exceed dietary fat recommendations. As always, follow the advice of your youngster's physician.

HEAT-AND-EAT MEAL (*continued*)   ADD FOR COMBO MEAL BALANCE (*continued*)

Smart Ones®

Angel Hair Pasta	Meat, poultry, fish, or meat alternative; salad and vegetables; dessert, if desired, including fruit.
Chicken Marsala	Starch or grain products (pasta, potato, rice, noodles, or bread); salad and vegetables; dessert, if desired, including fruit.
Chicken Mirabella	Starch or grain products (pasta, potato, rice, noodles, or bread); salad and vegetables; dessert, if desired, including fruit.
Grilled Salisbury Steak	Starch or grain products (pasta, potato, rice, noodles, or bread); salad and vegetables; dessert, if desired, including fruit.
Roast Glazed Chicken	Starch or grain products (pasta, potato, rice, noodles, or bread); salad and vegetables; dessert, if desired, including fruit.
Stuffed Turkey Breast	Salad and vegetables; dessert, if desired, including fruit.

Weight Watcher's®

Paella Rice and Vegetables	Meat, poultry, fish, or meat alternative; salad; dessert, if desired, including fruit.

Hot Pockets®

All varieties*	Additional meat, poultry, fish, or meat alternative; salad and vegetables; dessert, if desired, including fruit.

Lean Pockets®

All varieties*	Additional meat, poultry, fish, or meat alternative; salad and vegetables; dessert, if desired, including fruit.

*Item may exceed dietary fat recommendations. As always, follow the advice of your youngster's physician.

RECIPES FOR SWAP CHOICES

Offer any of these treats in place of your youngster's typical sugary snacks. For each repeated daily replacement, consider that a Swap has been successfully completed.

QuickFix Recipes are marked with the logo in the upper right corners.

LOONIE TOONIES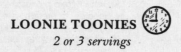
2 or 3 servings

A zesty tuna treat that is a delight to eat.

> 1 can (6½ ounces) chunk tuna, packed
>   in oil or water*
> 2 stalks celery, diced
> ½ cup black ripe olives,* pitted and
>   quartered
> 2 tablespoons prepared Italian dressing
> 1 cup sour cream*
> ½ teaspoon garlic powder
> ½ teaspoon paprika
> 8 medium-sized lettuce leaves

Drain the tuna, rinse in cold water, and place it in a large mixing bowl. Add the celery, olives, dressing, sour cream, garlic powder, and paprika and mix thoroughly. Spoon a small portion of mixture into each lettuce leaf, roll up, and place seam side down on platter. Serve with crackers if desired.

Choose low-fat varieties or alternatives and/or low-salt varieties, as appropriate.

**Egg substitutes cannot be used in this recipe. If fat content is inappropriate, select a more appropriate recipe.*

RAINBOW VEGETABLE DIP AND SPREAD
4 servings

A colorful blend of "crunchies" that are fun to eat when transformed into a delicious dip. Serve with cut-up raw vegetables or on whole-grain crackers in place of typical snacks that are packed with simple sugars or crowded with carbohydrates.

> ½ medium head of red cabbage, cored
>   and cut into wedges
> 3 large carrots, peeled and cut into
>   chunks
> 1 cucumber, peeled
> 1 bunch red radishes, trimmed
> ½ small red Bermuda onion, cut into
>   chunks
> 1 stalk celery, trimmed and cut into
>   chunks
> ¼ cup olive oil*
> 2 tablespoons vinegar
> ¼ teaspoon salt
> ⅛ teaspoon dry mustard
> ⅛ teaspoon sugar

Fit a food processor with a shredding disk and feed in the cabbage wedges and carrot chunks. Empty the container into a medium mixing bowl as it becomes full.

Slice the cucumber lengthwise and remove the seeds. Insert the slicing disk into the processor and feed in the radishes, onion, celery, and cucumber. Remove sliced vegetables and rinse and dry the processor bowl.

Lock the steel blade into the processor. With the motor running, add the oil, vinegar, and seasonings through the feed tube. Slowly add all the sliced and shredded vegetables, processing until all the vegetables are well puréed.

---

†*Low-fat mayonnaise often contains a high proportion of sugar. Use only regular mayonnaise (not a low-fat variety) at all Insulin-Balancing Meals and Snacks. If regular mayonnaise is an inappropriate choice, select a different recipe or dressing.*

GREEN AND WHITE MUNCHABLES
3 to 4 servings

Bursting with fiber to help balance the carbohydrates, this offers a bonus of vitamins and minerals as well.

> 1/2 pound broccoli, cut into florets
> 1/2 pound cauliflower, cut into florets
> 1 teaspoon olive oil
> 2 garlic cloves, flattened
> 2 tablespoons pine nuts
> 1/2 cup seedless grapes, halved
> Salt
> Ground black pepper

Place 1/4 inch water, broccoli, and cauliflower in a large skillet. Cook over high heat until the vegetables are crisp-tender, about 5 minutes.

Drain the vegetables in a colander, dry out the skillet, and add the oil.

Warm the oil over medium heat, then return the vegetables to the skillet, browning them for 5 to 7 minutes. Add the garlic, pine nuts, and grapes, and cook, tossing gently, until the grapes begin to soften and the garlic is golden brown. Sprinkle with salt and pepper.

Cool, remove and discard the garlic cloves, and serve.

*Choose low-fat varieties or alternatives and/or low-salt varieties, as appropriate.

**Egg substitutes cannot be used in this recipe. If fat content is inappropriate, select a more appropriate recipe.

FRESH FRUIT SWAP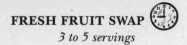
3 to 5 servings

A quick, easy, and refreshing Swap.

> 1 medium tart apple, cut in wedges
> 2 medium ripe pears, cut in wedges
> 2 oranges, peeled and divided into
>   segments
> Fresh orange juice or lemon juice
> 3 ounces each of several of your young-
>   ster's favorite cheeses*, cut into
>   cubes: regular or low-fat varieties of
>   any semisoft cheese such as Brie,
>   Cheddar, Swiss

On a large platter, arrange the apple, pear, and orange segments. Sprinkle the apples and pears with orange or lemon juice to prevent discoloration. Scatter the cheese cubes randomly over the fruit. Cover the platter with plastic wrap and chill before serving.

Serve as is or add crackers around the edges of the platter.

†*Low-fat mayonnaise often contains a high proportion of sugar. Use only regular mayonnaise (not a low-fat variety) at all Insulin-Balancing Meals and Snacks. If regular mayonnaise is an inappropriate choice, select a different recipe or dressing.*

STUFFED MUSHROOMS
3 or 4 servings

A outstanding Swap, easy to prepare and fun to eat.

> 8 medium-sized fresh mushroom caps
> 1 tablespoon butter or margarine
> 2 ounces cream cheese*
> 1/2 tablespoon heavy cream (or milk)*
> 1/2 tablespoon teriyaki sauce
> 1/2 teaspoon fresh chives, minced
>   (optional)
> 1/2 teaspoon fresh lemon juice
> Salt
> Ground black pepper
> Paprika
> Lettuce leaves, for garnish

Preheat the oven to 350 degrees.

Wipe the mushroom caps with damp paper towel.

Melt the butter in a shallow baking pan just large enough to hold the caps in one layer.

In a medium bowl, combine the cream cheese, cream, teriyaki sauce, chives, lemon juice, and salt and pepper. Mix until smooth. Spoon a generous amount of the mixture into each inverted mushroom cap and sprinkle lightly with paprika to taste.

Arrange the stuffed caps in the prepared baking dish and bake until tender, 10 to 15 minutes.

Place on serving tray with a garnish of lettuce leaves.

Choose low-fat varieties or alternatives and/or low-salt varieties, as appropriate.

**Egg substitutes cannot be used in this recipe. If fat content is inappropriate, select a more appropriate recipe.*

CLAM IT UP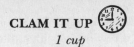
1 cup

An exciting dip for raw vegetables or whole-grain crackers.

> 8 ounces cream cheese*
> 2 teaspoons Worcestershire sauce
> 1 teaspoon mayonnaise
> 1 teaspoon fresh lemon juice
> 2 ounces mild prepared horseradish
> 1 can (6 ounces) canned clams,
>   minced, and juice*
> Parsley flakes

Blend the cream cheese, Worcestershire sauce, mayonnaise, horseradish, and lemon juice. Thoroughly stir in the clams and juice. Place in a serving dish. Garnish with parsley flakes.

POPEYE'S FAVORITE DIP
1¹/₂ cups

Wonderful warm or cold. Good today, even better when left to blend until tomorrow.

> 8 ounces frozen spinach, chopped,
>   cooked, and drained (retain ¹/₄ cup
>   spinach liquid)
> 1 tablespoon chives or onion, chopped
> 2 tablespoons butter or margarine*
> 2 ounces Parmesan cheese,* grated
> ¹/₄ cup sour cream*
> ¹/₂ teaspoon garlic, minced
> ¹/₂ teaspoon teriyaki sauce
> 1 teaspoon celery, minced
> Ground black pepper

†Low-fat mayonnaise often contains a high proportion of sugar. Use only regular mayonnaise (not a low-fat variety) at all Insulin-Balancing Meals and Snacks. If regular mayonnaise is an inappropriate choice, select a different recipe or dressing.

Squeeze as much water as possible out of the cooked spinach according to package directions, drain, and retain liquid.

In a medium saucepan, sauté the chives or onion in the butter until wilted. Cool slightly. Add the spinach, Parmesan cheese, sour cream, garlic, teriyaki sauce, spinach liquid, celery, and black pepper to taste. Heat slowly over low heat, stirring occasionally until mixture is creamy.

Pour into a serving dish, chill, and serve with your youngster's favorite sliced raw vegetables or whole-grain crackers, or as a topping for cooked vegetables.

SNOW PEAS, PLEASE
4 servings

A gratifying and readily available Swap to satisfy the fussiest vegetable hater.

> 2 tablespoons olive oil*
> 1 onion, finely chopped
> 1 garlic clove, finely chopped
> $1/4$ cup water chestnuts, sliced
> $1/2$ pound snow pea pods, trimmed
> 1 tablespoon teriyaki sauce
> $1/4$ cup chicken broth

Heat the oil in a medium skillet over medium heat. Add the onion and sauté until golden brown. Add remaining ingredients, cover, and continue to cook for 4 minutes exactly.

Remove from heat immediately. Refrigerate, drained or undrained, and serve anytime a quick Swap is needed.

Choose low-fat varieties or alternatives and/or low-salt varieties, as appropriate.

**Egg substitutes cannot be used in this recipe. If fat content is inappropriate, select a more appropriate recipe.*

TANGY VINAIGRETTE DIP AND DRESSING
Approximately ⅓ cup

A great dip for cool, fresh vegetables or a delightful dressing for your youngster's favorite tossed salad. For a special Swap salad, sprinkle some real or low-fat bacon chips and croutons on top.

> ¼ cup olive oil*
> 2 tablespoons vinegar
> 1 tablespoon onion, minced
> ¼ teaspoon salt
> ⅛ teaspoon dry mustard
> ⅛ teaspoon sugar

Place all ingredients in a jar or small bottle with a lid. Shake well and serve.

Store leftovers in the refrigerator.

---

†*Low-fat mayonnaise often contains a high proportion of sugar. Use only regular mayonnaise (not a low-fat variety) at all Insulin-Balancing Meals and Snacks. If regular mayonnaise is an inappropriate choice, select a different recipe or dressing.*

ALL ABOUT VEGETARIAN CHOICES: NONMEAT ALTERNATIVES

QuickFix Recipes are marked with the 🕓 logo in the upper right corners.

A wide variety of nonmeat-based alternatives to meat, poultry, and fish are widely available at supermarket and health food stores. Each day, new vegetarian items continue to make their way to store shelves.

Here are some of the many vegetarian alternatives currently on the market, although not all products are available at all stores. If you cannot find the product you want, ask the store manager to order the item for you. If the store manager cannot help you, write to or call the manufacturers and distributors listed below or check your business telephone listings for the name of the store or distributor nearest you.

Important Note: Nonmeat alternatives qualify as Insulin-Balancing Foods only if they contain 0–4 grams of carbohydrates per average serving. These alternatives can be used as Add-Ons or during Hold-On or Insulin-Balancing Meals or Snacks. Other items are higher in carbohydrate content (5 grams or more of carbohydrates per average serving) and should be included only in Combo Meals or Snacks. Check labels for carbohydrate levels.

NONMEAT ALTERNATIVES
"Burgers"
Better'n Burgers® (Morningstar Farms)
Fri-Pats® (Worthington Foods)
Garden Vege Patties™ (Morningstar Farms and Natural Touch)
Granburger (Worthington Foods)
Grillers® (Morningstar Farms)
Ground Meatless™ Burger (Worthington Foods)
Okara Pattie (Natural Touch)
Patty Mix (Loma Linda)
Prime Patties™ (Morningstar Farms)
Redi-Burger® (Morningstar Farms)
Sizzle Burgers (Loma Linda)
Vege Burgers (Natural Touch and Loma Linda)
Vegan Burgers (Worthington Foods and Natural Touch)
Vegetarian Burger™ (Worthington Foods)
Vita-Burger® (Loma Linda)

"Chops" and "Cutlets"
Choplets® (Worthington Foods)
Cutlets (Worthington Foods)
Multigrain Cutlets (Worthington Foods)
Veelets® (Worthington Foods)

"Steaks"
Griddle Steaks (Loma Linda)
Prime Stakes™ (Worthington Foods)
Swiss Stake with Gravy (Loma Linda)
Stakelets® (Worthington Foods)
Vegetable Stakes™ (Worthington Foods)
Vegetarian Steaks (Worthington Foods)

"Roasts," "Meat Loaf," and "Meat" Dinners
Country Stew (Worthington Foods)
Dinner Cuts (Worthington Foods)
Dinner Entrée (Natural Touch)
Dinner Roast (Worthington Foods)
Savory Dinner Loaf (Loma Linda)
Savory Slices (Worthington Foods)
Pot Pie—Beef Style (Worthington Foods)

"Hot Dogs," "Sausage," and "Bacon"
Big Franks (Loma Linda)
Breakfast Links® (Morningstar Farms)
Breakfast Patties® (Morningstar Farms)
Breakfast Strips® (Morningstar Farms)
Deli Franks® (Morningstar Farms)
Ground Meatless™ Sausage (Worthington Foods)
Leanies® (Worthington Foods)
Linkettes™ (Loma Linda)
Little Links (Loma Linda)
Prosage®, patties and links (Worthington Foods)
Saucettes® (Morningstar Farms)
Stripples® (Worthington Foods)
Superlinks™ (Worthington Foods)
Vege Franks® (Natural Touch)
Veja-links® (Worthington Foods)

Sandwich "Meats"
Bologno™ (Worthington Foods)
Corned Beef (Worthington Foods)
Salami (Worthington Foods)
Sandwich Spread (Loma Linda)
Smoked Beef (Worthington Foods)
Wham™ (Worthington Foods)

"POULTRY" ALTERNATIVES
Chik-Nuggets (Loma Linda)
Chick Patties™ (Morningstar Farms)
Chicken Supreme (Loma Linda)
Chic-ketts® (Worthington Foods)
ChikStiks™ (Worthington Foods)
Crispy Chik Patties (Worthington Foods)
Diced Chik (Worthington Foods)
FriChik® (Worthington Foods)
Fried Chicken with Gravy (Loma Linda)
Golden Croquettes (Worthington Foods)
Pot Pie Chicken-Style (Worthington Foods)
Sliced Chik™ (Worthington Foods)
Smoked Turkey (Worthington Foods)
Turkee Slices™ (Worthington Foods)

"FISH" ALTERNATIVES
Fillets™ (Worthington Foods)
Ocean Platter (Loma Linda)
Tuno® (Worthington Foods)
Vegetable Skallops™ (Worthington Foods)

For more information write or call for the name of the store nearest you.
Morningstar Farms, Natural Touch, or Worthington Foods:
  Consumer Affairs, 900 Proprietors Road, Worthington, OH 43085

Tree of Life Distributors:
  Northeast Division:
    (800) 735–5175
  Northwest Division:
    (800) 366–3986
  Western Division:
    (800) 827–2803
  Midwest Division:
    (800) 999–4200
  Southeast Division:
    (800) 874–0851
  Southwest Division:
    (800) 800–2175

INSULIN-BALANCING MEAL AND SNACK RECIPES

Do not substitute more common high-carbohydrate variations for these recipes during Insulin-Balancing Meals or Snacks.

QuickFix Recipes are marked with the  logo in the upper right corners.

Breakfasts

These special Insulin-Balancing variations of breakfast favorites are great for Jump-Start Plan Insulin-Balancing Meals or Snacks or for Step-By-Step Plan Hold-On Choices.

MORNING MUFFINS
4 muffins

A delicate muffin that is surprisingly satisfying.

>   1 teaspoon polyunsaturated vegetable oil
>   2 eggs,** separated
>   ¼ teaspoon cream of tartar
>   ¼ cup cottage cheese*
>   ¼ teaspoon vanilla
>   3 tablespoons soy flour†

Preheat the oven to 300 degrees. Coat the muffin cups with the oil.

Beat the egg whites until frothy. Add cream of tartar and beat until stiff peaks form.

Choose low-fat varieties or alternatives and/or low-salt varieties, as appropriate.

**Egg substitutes cannot be used in this recipe. If fat content is inappropriate, select a more appropriate recipe.*

In a medium bowl, combine the egg yolks, cottage cheese, vanilla, and soy flour. Mix well. Add the mixture to the beaten egg whites and fold in gently. Fill each muffin cup ⅔ full with batter.

Bake the muffins until they are golden brown and spring back at the touch of the back end of a fork, 25 to 30 minutes.

Turn out the muffins and serve warm.

POWERHOUSE PANCAKES
2 servings

A great way to start a busy day.

> 2 eggs,** separated
> 1 cup small-curd cottage cheese*
> ¼ cup soy flour†
> Salt
> Dash of cinnamon
> ⅛ teaspoon cream of tartar
> 1 tablespoon vegetable oil
> 2 or 3 tablespoons sour cream*
>   (optional)

In a medium bowl, combine the egg yolks, cottage cheese, soy flour, salt to taste, and a dash of cinnamon.

In a separate bowl, beat the egg whites and cream of tartar until stiff but not dry. Fold the beaten whites into the yolk-cheese mixture.

Heat a large oiled skillet or square griddle and drop the batter by large spoonfuls onto hot surface. Fry the pancakes until golden brown on one side; turn each and brown the other side.

Serve at once, with or without sour cream topping.

---

†*Low-fat mayonnaise often contains a high proportion of sugar. Use only regular mayonnaise (not a low-fat variety) at all Insulin-Balancing Meals and Snacks. If regular mayonnaise is an inappropriate choice, select a different recipe or dressing.*

‡*Soy flour is much lower in carbohydrate content than regular flour; do not use all-purpose flour as a substitute for soy flour in Insulin-Balancing recipes. Soy flour is available in most health food stores.*

DOUBLE DECKER DUO
2 servings

A wonderful combination of proteins; warm and robust for a cold winter morning.

> ½ tablespoon olive oil
> ¼ tablespoon Worcestershire sauce
> Salt
> Ground black pepper
> ¼ pound lean hamburger or ground
>   turkey
> 2 eggs,** poached
> Parsley, chopped, for garnish

Heat the olive oil in a large frying pan over medium-high heat. Meanwhile, add Worcestershire and salt and pepper to taste to the ground meat. Form into 2 patties.

Fry the patties until brown on one side and then brown the other side. Lower the heat and continue to cook to desired doneness.

Top each patty with a warm poached egg and serve garnished with parsley.

*Choose low-fat varieties or alternatives and/or low-salt varieties, as appropriate.

**Egg substitutes cannot be used in this recipe. If fat content is inappropriate, select a more appropriate recipe.

MOUSE OMELET
2 or 3 servings

A wonderful treat for the cheese lover in all of us.

> 4 eggs*
> Salt
> Ground black pepper, to taste
> 1/3 cup Parmesan cheese,* freshly
>   grated
> 2 tablespoons butter*
> 3 ounces Gruyère cheese,* grated
> 1/2 green bell pepper, seeded and thinly
>   sliced

Preheat the broiler.

In a small bowl, beat the eggs lightly and add salt and pepper to taste. Stir in the Parmesan cheese.

Melt the butter in an ovenproof omelet pan, add the beaten eggs, and stir with a whisk as the eggs cook.

When the omelet is nearly set but still moist on top, add the Gruyère and sliced bell peppers. Slide the omelet under the broiler until the cheese is bubbly, about 2 to 3 minutes.

Fold the omelet once, slide it onto a serving plate, and serve.

†*Low-fat mayonnaise often contains a high proportion of sugar. Use only regular mayonnaise (not a low-fat variety) at all Insulin-Balancing Meals and Snacks. If regular mayonnaise is an inappropriate choice, select a different recipe or dressing.*

MUSHROOM OMELET
2 or 3 servings

A tasty alternative to meat entrées.

> 2 tablespoons butter*
> 2 scallions, sliced
> 10 fresh medium-sized mushrooms,
>   sliced
> 4 eggs*
> 2 tablespoons cream*
> Salt
> Ground black pepper

Melt 1 tablespoon of the butter in a deep skillet. Add the scallions and mushrooms, and sauté until the scallions are tender and the mushrooms begin to brown. Set aside.

In a small bowl, combine the eggs and cream and whisk until smooth. Add salt and pepper to taste.

Heat an omelet pan over medium heat and add the remaining 1 tablespoon of butter.

Pour the egg mixture into the pan. Do not touch until the eggs form large bubbles. Then, using a spatula, gently push the cooked portion of the eggs to the center, tilting the pan to allow the uncooked portions to spread out.

When the omelet base is set (in 30 to 40 seconds), place mushroom and scallion mixture on one side of the omelet. Using a spatula, fold the omelet so that the plain side covers the filled side.

Gently transfer omelet to warmed plates and serve immediately.

Choose low-fat varieties or alternatives and/or low-salt varieties, as appropriate.

**Egg substitutes cannot be used in this recipe. If fat content is inappropriate, select a more appropriate recipe.*

NEW MORNING OMELET
2 servings

A special twist on an old favorite.

> 1/2 cup mushrooms, sliced, canned or
>   sautéed in olive oil* until tender
> 1/3 cup sour cream*
> Dried or fresh dill weed
> 3 eggs*
> Salt
> Ground black pepper
> 1 tablespoon butter or margarine

In a small bowl, combine the mushrooms, sour cream, and dill weed to taste. Set the mixture aside for filling the omelet.

In a medium bowl, combine the eggs, 2 tablespoons of water, and salt and pepper to taste.

In an omelet pan over medium heat, melt the butter, and add the egg mixture.

Do not touch until eggs form large bubbles. Then, using the spatula, gently push the cooked portion of the eggs to the center, tilting the pan to allow uncooked portions to spread out.

When the omelet base is set in 30 to 40 seconds, arrange the mushroom filling on one side only. Using the spatula, fold the omelet so that the plain side covers the filled side. Remove the pan from the heat and let set for 20 to 30 seconds.

Gently transfer the omelet to warmed plates and serve immediately.

---

†*Low-fat mayonnaise often contains a high proportion of sugar. Use only regular mayonnaise (not a low-fat variety) at all Insulin-Balancing Meals and Snacks. If regular mayonnaise is an inappropriate choice, select a different recipe or dressing.*

HIGH-PROTEIN CINNAMON BREAD
2 servings

A beautiful bread that is low in carbohydrates.

> 1 teaspoon butter*
> 3 eggs,** separated
> 1/2 teaspoon cream of tartar
> 1/4 cup cottage cheese*
> 1/2 teaspoon powdered cinnamon
> 1/4 teaspoon vanilla
> 3 tablespoons soy flour†

Preheat oven to 300 degrees. Grease the bottom and sides of a 4 x 7-inch loaf pan with the butter.

Beat the egg whites until frothy. Add the cream of tartar and continue to beat until stiff but moist peaks form.

In a medium bowl, combine the cottage cheese, cinnamon, vanilla, egg yolks, and soy flour. Mix well but do not overmix. Add to the beaten egg whites and fold in gently.

Pour the mixture into the prepared pan and bake until the loaf is brown and springs back when touched with the back of a fork, 40 to 45 minutes.

Choose low-fat varieties or alternatives and/or low-salt varieties, as appropriate.

**Egg substitutes cannot be used in this recipe. If fat content is inappropriate, select a more appropriate recipe.*

MOCK FRENCH TOAST
1 serving

This low-carbohydrate version of an old-favorite will please your youngster, and you as well.

> Butter, oil, appropriate low-fat substi-
> tute, or spray
> 1 teaspoon cream*
> 1 egg*
> 2 slices High-Protein Cinnamon Bread
> (page 314)

Grease a griddle or pan.

In a medium bowl, lightly beat the cream and egg. Dip bread slices into the cream and egg mixture and fry until both sides are brown.

Serve warm.

†Low-fat mayonnaise often contains a high proportion of sugar. Use only regular mayonnaise (not a low-fat variety) at all Insulin-Balancing Meals and Snacks. If regular mayonnaise is an inappropriate choice, select a different recipe or dressing.

‡Soy flour is much lower in carbohydrate content than regular flour; do not use all-purpose flour as a substitute for soy flour in Insulin-Balancing recipes. Soy flour is available in most health food stores.

Dips, Dressings, Salads, and Vegetables

These special Insulin-Balancing recipes will help add zest and fun to any meal or snack.

CREAMY GREEN DIP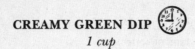
1 cup

A perfect dip for any crisp fresh vegetable. Serve with Insulin-Balancing Vegetables anytime.

> 1 cup sour cream*
> 1 teaspoon dried sweet basil
> 2 tablespoons fresh chives, chopped
> 1 teaspoon garlic, minced
> Dash of curry powder
> Paprika, to taste

In a medium bowl, combine all ingredients until well blended. Chill and serve with your youngster's favorite fresh vegetables.

SAVORY SOUR CREAM DIP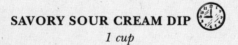
1 cup

A tangy change of taste to add spice to any Insulin-Balancing Vegetable.

> 1 cup sour cream*
> 1 teaspoon prepared horseradish
> Paprika
> Oregano

In a medium bowl, combine the sour cream, horseradish, and paprika and oregano to taste. Chill and serve with cold fresh vegetables for dipping.

Choose low-fat varieties or alternatives and/or low-salt varieties, as appropriate.

DIPPITY DIP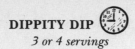
3 or 4 servings

A smooth yet spicy dip that can be enjoyed as a fun salad dressing, too. Serve at Insulin-Balancing Meals or Snacks with lots of fresh, Insulin-Balancing Vegetables.

> 8-ounce package cream cheese,* soft-
>   ened
> 1 tablespoon mayonnaise†
> 1 tablespoon cream*
> 1 tablespoon chives, chopped
> Teriyaki sauce, to taste
> Sesame oil, to taste

In a medium bowl, combine the cream cheese, mayonnaise, cream, and chives until blended. Add teriyaki and sesame oil to taste. Chill and serve with fresh Insulin-Balancing Vegetables for dipping, or as a topping on a tossed salad.

**Egg substitutes cannot be used in this recipe. If fat content is inappropriate, select a more appropriate recipe.

†Low-fat mayonnaise often contains a high proportion of sugar. Use only regular mayonnaise (not a low-fat variety) at all Insulin-Balancing Meals and Snacks. If regular mayonnaise is an inappropriate choice, select a different recipe or dressing.

GREEN GARDEN MAYONNAISE
About 1 cup

A tempting dressing with a mild flavor and creamy texture.

> 1 stalk celery with leaves, roughly
>   chopped
> 5 spinach leaves, torn up
> 5 scallions, finely chopped
> 1/2 teaspoon dried sweet basil
> 1/2 teaspoon fresh lemon juice
> 1/2 cup mayonnaise†

In a food processor, chop the celery, spinach, and scallions. Add the basil, lemon juice, and mayonnaise. Blend well. Serve on Insulin-Balancing Vegetables or fish, or as a wonderful addition to tuna or chicken salad.

SAUCY VINAIGRETTE
About 3/4 cup

A surprisingly delicious and simple dressing to top off any salad.

> 6 tablespoons olive oil*
> 2 tablespoons white vinegar
> 1/4 teaspoon ground black pepper
> 1/4 teaspoon salt
> 1 garlic clove, peeled and cut in half
>   lengthwise

Choose low-fat varieties or alternatives and/or low-salt varieties, as appropriate.

**Egg substitutes cannot be used in this recipe. If fat content is inappropriate, select a more appropriate recipe.*

In a small mixing bowl, combine 1 tablespoon of the olive oil, 1 tablespoon of the vinegar, pepper, and salt. Mix well. Continue whisking while adding 2 additional tablespoons of olive oil. Add the remaining vinegar and olive oil and blend until smooth.

Place the mixture in a jar, add the garlic halves, cover, and refrigerate for 24 hours. Shake well before using.

BASIC ITALIAN DRESSING

About 1 cup

Basically delicious as a dressing or as a fun and tangy dip.

> 1/2 cup olive oil*
> 1/4 cup white vinegar
> 1 garlic clove, minced
> 1/2 teaspoon salt
> Ground black pepper, to taste

In a small bowl blend all the ingredients until smooth. Transfer to an appropriate container and refrigerate for at least 2 hours. Shake well before using.

---

†*Low-fat mayonnaise often contains a high proportion of sugar. Use only regular mayonnaise (not a low-fat variety) at all Insulin-Balancing Meals and Snacks. If regular mayonnaise is an inappropriate choice, select a different recipe or dressing.*

SPROUT 'N' CHEF SALAD
2 or 3 servings

Surprise your youngster with this simple but satisfying salad topped off with any Insulin-Balancing dip or dressing that appeals.

2 cups fresh bean or alfalfa sprouts
1/4 cup green pepper, chopped
1/4 cup celery, chopped
1/2 cup cucumber, thinly sliced
4 ounces chicken breast, cut in julienne
   strips
2 ounces hard cheese,* such as Swiss
   or Cheddar, cut in julienne strips
1 hard-boiled egg, sliced (optional)

In a large bowl, gently combine the sprouts, green pepper, celery, and cucumber. Top with chicken, cheese strips, and egg slices, if desired. Toss with dip or dressing of choice and serve.

*Choose low-fat varieties or alternatives and/or low-salt varieties, as appropriate.

**Egg substitutes cannot be used in this recipe. If fat content is inappropriate, select a more appropriate recipe.

CAESAR SALAD
3 or 4 servings

An old standby with a brand-new twist.

> Salt, a few dashes
> 1 garlic clove, peeled and halved
> 1 teaspoon dry mustard
> 1 tablespoon fresh lemon juice
> Hot sauce
> 2 tablespoons olive oil*
> 2 bunches romaine lettuce
> 1 tablespoon Swiss cheese,* grated
> 2/3 can drained anchovies
> 1 egg, minimally boiled for safe
>   consumption

Sprinkle salt in the bottom of a large wooden bowl and thoroughly rub the bottom and sides of the bowl with the garlic clove. Add the mustard, lemon juice, and hot sauce to taste, and stir until the salt dissolves. Whisk in the olive oil until blended.

Tear the lettuce into bite-sized pieces and place in the bowl.

Sprinkle with grated Swiss cheese and stir in the anchovies. Break the egg and empty its contents over the salad. Thoroughly mix by tossing gently until the ingredients are distributed uniformly. Serve chilled.

---

†*Low-fat mayonnaise often contains a high proportion of sugar. Use only regular mayonnaise (not a low-fat variety) at all Insulin-Balancing Meals and Snacks. If regular mayonnaise is an inappropriate choice, select a different recipe or dressing.*

CREAMY CUCUMBER SALAD
3 or 4 servings

An easy dish that tastes as if should be served for special occasions.

1 cup sour cream*
1 teaspoon scallions, chopped
1/2 teaspoon salt
Ground black pepper
1 tablespoon white vinegar
2 medium cucumbers, peeled and thinly
  sliced
4 large romaine lettuce or cabbage
  leaves
1/4 teaspoon dried basil
1/4 tablespoon paprika

Mix the sour cream, scallions, salt, pepper to taste, and vinegar. Add the cucumber slices and toss lightly.

Serve on lettuce or raw cabbage leaves, garnished with basil and paprika.

Choose low-fat varieties or alternatives and/or low-salt varieties, as appropriate.

**Egg substitutes cannot be used in this recipe. If fat content is inappropriate, select a more appropriate recipe.*

SEA SALAD
3 or 4 servings

A wonderful blend of the "fruits" of the sea.

> 1/4 pound bay or sea scallops
> 1/4 pound fresh fish of choice, diced
> 2 tablespoons olive oil*
> 1 tablespoon teriyaki sauce
> 2/3 pound medium boiled shrimp,
>   shelled, deveined, and diced
> 1/2 cup cucumber, coarsely chopped
> 1/2 cup celery, chopped
> 1/2 cup scallions, chopped
> Coarsely ground black pepper
> Mayonnaise,† Basic Italian Dressing
>   (page 319), or Saucy Vinaigrette
>   (page 318)
> 4 large lettuce leaves

In a large pan, sauté the scallops and fish in the olive oil and teriyaki sauce until they are tender; do not overcook.

In a large bowl, combine the diced shrimp with the scallops and fish. Add the cucumber, celery, scallions, and pepper to taste. Add mayonnaise or your youngster's favorite Insulin-Balancing dressing or dip to taste and toss lightly.

Cover and chill for 2 hours.

Line a plate with lettuce leaves, spoon the salad into the center, and serve.

---

†*Low-fat mayonnaise often contains a high proportion of sugar. Use only regular mayonnaise (not a low-fat variety) at all Insulin-Balancing Meals and Snacks. If regular mayonnaise is an inappropriate choice, select a different recipe or dressing.*

TENDER, CHEESY CAULIFLOWER 🕐
3 or 4 servings

A simple and quick dish to prepare.

> 4 cups cauliflower florets
> 1 cup shredded Cheddar cheese*

In a deep skillet over the highest possible heat, add ½ cup of water to the cauliflower florets. Cover and heat for 4 minutes. Turn off heat, remove skillet from heat immediately, drain, and return the florets to the pan. Sprinkle the cheese over cauliflower. Cover and let stand for 3 minutes.

Serve immediately with a salad and protein to make a delicious, well-balanced Insulin-Balancing Meal, or as is for a satisfying Insulin-Balancing Snack.

GREEN BEAN STIR FRY
3 to 4 servings

This vegetable side dish will disappear in no time.

> ¼ cup olive oil*
> 2 tablespoons teriyaki sauce
> 2 stalks celery, diced
> 2 garlic cloves, minced
> 1 pound green beans, cut or broken into
>   1- or 2-inch lengths

In a deep skillet over medium-high heat, mix the olive oil and teriyaki sauce thoroughly. Add the celery and sauté over medium heat until it softens. Add the garlic and stir well. Add the green beans and sauté, tossing until they are barely tender.

Place the mixture in a serving dish. Serve immediately, or chill and serve cold.

Choose low-fat varieties or alternatives and/or low-salt varieties, as appropriate.

**Egg substitutes cannot be used in this recipe. If fat content is inappropriate, select a more appropriate recipe.*

SAUTÉED CABBAGE
3 or 4 servings

Strong smell, great taste.

> 2 pounds green cabbage
> 2 shallots, minced
> 1 tablespoon fresh parsley, minced
> Ground black pepper
> ½ cup homemade chicken broth
> ½ teaspoon fennel seeds

Core the cabbage from the base to keep the head together. Slice into wedges about 1½ inches thick.

In a large skillet, combine the cabbage, shallots, parsley, pepper to taste, and broth. Cover and cook over moderate heat for 10 to 12 minutes, basting with broth several times. Just before the cabbage is done, sprinkle the fennel seeds on top.

Serve hot or cold.

†*Low-fat mayonnaise often contains a high proportion of sugar. Use only regular mayonnaise (not a low-fat variety) at all Insulin-Balancing Meals and Snacks. If regular mayonnaise is an inappropriate choice, select a different recipe or dressing.*

Snacks and Finger Foods

These special Insulin-Balancing easy-to-pack and fun-to-eat recipes will delight and satisfy your youngster. Best of all, they keep craving-triggering carbohydrates low.

MEATBALL "POPS"
3 to 4 servings

A neat little snack or finger food that satisfies.

> ¼ pound ground beef*
> ¼ pound ground pork*
> 3 tablespoons Italian salad dressing*
> 1 large egg
> ½ cup chives, chopped
> Salt
> Garlic powder, if desired
> Coarsely ground pepper
> 3 tablespoons olive oil*
> Lettuce leaves

In a medium bowl combine the beef, pork, salad dressing, egg, chives, salt to taste, garlic powder, and pepper to taste. Shape the mixture into 15 to 20 little meatballs.

Add the oil to a medium skillet and set over medium heat. Brown the meatballs on all sides in the hot oil.

Remove the meatballs and place them on a bed of lettuce. Serve warm or cold with mustard for dipping and with some celery sticks or other fresh Insulin-Balancing Vegetables for a complete and satisfying snack.

*Choose low-fat varieties or alternatives and/or low-salt varieties, as appropriate.

**Egg substitutes cannot be used in this recipe. If fat content is inappropriate, select a more appropriate recipe.

SALAMI CUBES‡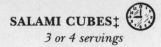
3 or 4 servings

A wonderful snack that travels well.

> ½ cup olive oil, for frying
> 1 egg
> ¼ cup Parmesan cheese, grated
> ¾ pound salami, cubed
> 4 large lettuce leaves

Heat the oil in a medium frying pan.

Break the eggs in a medium bowl and beat well. Put the Parmesan cheese into another medium bowl. Dip salami cubes, one at a time, into the eggs and then coat with Parmesan cheese.

Fry the cubes for 20 to 30 seconds in the hot oil, turning to fry all sides.

Place on a bed of lettuce and serve warm, or chill and pack for a snack. These can be used as finger food alone, or with a small container of mustard for dipping; cucumber slices or other Insulin-Balancing Vegetables are good on the side.

SNACKS "ON THE WING"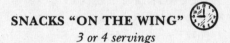
3 or 4 servings

A simple recipe that is fun to prepare and fun to eat.

> 8 chicken wings*
> 2 tablespoons teriyaki sauce
> 1 tablespoon olive oil
> ½ teaspoon powdered garlic
> 1 tablespoon dried sweet basil

†Low-fat mayonnaise often contains a high proportion of sugar. Use only regular mayonnaise (not a low-fat variety) at all Insulin-Balancing Meals and Snacks. If regular mayonnaise is an inappropriate choice, select a different recipe or dressing.

‡This recipe contains ingredients that are particularly high in fat content. If fat content makes this an inappropriate recipe for your youngster, serve only on occasion, as a special treat as recommended by your child's physician, or choose a more appropriate recipe.

Preheat oven to 350 degrees. Rinse and pat dry the chicken wings.

Line a large baking tray with aluminum foil, lay the wings on the tray so that they are evenly spaced, and sprinkle each wing with teriyaki sauce.

Brush olive oil on each wing and sprinkle with garlic and basil.

Place in the oven and bake for 30 to 35 minutes or until golden brown.

Remove from the oven, cool, and refrigerate until ready to serve as an on-the-spot snack or to pack for a snack away from home. These may be used as finger food alone or with a small container of mustard for dipping. Add some crisp Insulin-Balancing Vegetables for a complete snack.

STUFFED CELERY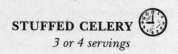
3 or 4 servings

A high-fiber, protein-rich snack that will keep carbohydrate cravings low.

> 8 large stalks of celery, rinsed and
>   trimmed of leaves
> ½ cup green pepper, chopped
> 8-ounce package cream cheese,* soft-
>   ened
> 4 drops teriyaki sauce
> Ground black pepper
> Garlic powder

Cut the celery stalks into 4-inch sticks and set aside.

In a medium mixing bowl, combine green pepper, cream cheese, teriyaki sauce, and pepper and garlic powder to taste, until thoroughly mixed. Using a butter knife, fill the hollow of each celery stick with the cheese mixture.

Pack for lunch or keep for late day or evening snacks.

*Choose low-fat varieties or alternatives and/or low-salt varieties, as appropriate.

**Egg substitutes cannot be used in this recipe. If fat content is inappropriate, select a more appropriate recipe.

NEW-WAVE CHICKEN NUGGETS
3 or 4 servings

A superb standby.

> ³⁄₄ pound skinless, boneless chicken
>   breast
> 1 tablespoon fresh lemon juice
> 1 tablespoon olive oil
> ½ teaspoon powdered garlic
> 1 tablespoon dried sweet basil
> 3 tablespoons Parmesan cheese,*
>   grated

Preheat the oven to 350 degrees. Rinse and pat dry the chicken breasts. Cut the chicken into lengthwise strips approximately ½ inch wide.

Line a large baking tray with aluminum foil. Lay the strips on the tray so that they are evenly spaced, and sprinkle each with lemon juice. Brush olive oil on each strip and sprinkle with garlic powder and basil. Dip each strip in grated Parmesan cheese and return to the baking tray.

Bake for 30 to 35 minutes or until golden brown.

Remove from the oven, cool, and refrigerate until ready to serve. These may be used as a finger food alone, or with a small container of mustard for dipping and some fresh green beans or other crunchy Insulin-Balancing Vegetables.

---

†Low-fat mayonnaise often contains a high proportion of sugar. Use only regular mayonnaise (not a low-fat variety) at all Insulin-Balancing Meals and Snacks. If regular mayonnaise is an inappropriate choice, select a different recipe or dressing.

CHICKEN COINS
3 to 4 servings

These are delicious as finger food alone or with mustard for dipping, and some crisp fresh Insulin-Balancing Vegetables.

> 4 medium chicken breast halves,
>   pounded or sliced medium-thin
> 1/4 pound mozzarella cheese,* thinly
>   sliced
> 4 strips of cooked bacon*
> 1 tablespoon teriyaki sauce
> 1 tablespoon olive oil
> 1 teaspoon garlic, minced

Preheat the oven to 350 degrees.

Place one pounded chicken breast flat on a platter. Lay a strip of bacon on top of a slice of mozzarella cheese and roll them up together. Set the cheese/bacon roll at one end of the chicken breast and roll into the breast lengthwise, forming a log. Repeat with the remaining chicken, cheese, and bacon.

Arrange the rolls in a baking pan, sprinkle each with teriyaki sauce, olive oil, and garlic, and put the pan in the oven. Bake for 35 to 40 minutes or until golden brown.

Remove from the oven, cool, and refrigerate in a suitable container.

When ready to prepare as a home snack or a pack-and-take snack, cut each log into 1/2-inch-thick "coins."

Choose low-fat varieties or alternatives and/or low-salt varieties, as appropriate.

**Egg substitutes cannot be used in this recipe. If fat content is inappropriate, select a more appropriate recipe.*

GREEN "WORMS"
3 or 4 servings

These can be enjoyed alone as finger food, or with any meat, chicken, or other protein-rich finger food or snack.

> 1 tablespoon olive oil
> ³/₄ pound green beans, washed and
>   trimmed
> 1 teaspoon teriyaki sauce
> ¹/₂ teaspoon garlic, minced
> 1 teaspoon dried basil
> ¹/₄ cup Parmesan cheese,* grated

Put the oil and 1 tablespoon water in a saucepan, mix, and set on a high heat. Lower the heat and add the beans. Add teriyaki sauce, basil, and garlic, and stir well.

Cover tightly and simmer until the beans are barely tender, about 20 minutes. Drain, cool, and sprinkle with Parmesan cheese. Refrigerate.

CHEESE BALL SURPRISE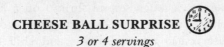
3 or 4 servings

This little treat can be especially nice when your youngster asks for something different.

> 4 ounces cheddar cheese,* cut in
>   chunks
> 1 teaspoon dried basil
> 1 teaspoon prepared mustard
> 16 small black or green olives,* pitted,
>   without pimiento

---

†*Low-fat mayonnaise often contains a high proportion of sugar. Use only regular mayonnaise (not a low-fat variety) at all Insulin-Balancing Meals and Snacks. If regular mayonnaise is an inappropriate choice, select a different recipe or dressing.*

Bring the cheese to room temperature. Mash and blend the chunks with basil and mustard.

Form the mixture into 16 small balls, shaping an olive into the center of each ball.

Pack for lunch or refrigerate for a late day or evening snack.

SHRIMP WITH SPECIAL HERB SAUCE
3 or 4 servings

Always a successful start for any dinner, or as an at-home snack.

> 20 shrimp, boiled, shelled, and
>   deveined
> 4 large lettuce leaves
> ¼ cup mayonnaise†
> 1 teaspoon dried basil
> 1 teaspoon chives, chopped
> 1 teaspoon cucumber, chopped
> Juice of 1 small lemon

For each person, arrange several shrimp on a large lettuce leaf. Cover each with waxed paper or plastic wrap and chill.

Combine the remaining ingredients and chill for 1 hour. Spoon the mayonnaise sauce over the shrimp and serve.

---

*Choose low-fat varieties or alternatives and/or low-salt varieties, as appropriate.

**Egg substitutes cannot be used in this recipe. If fat content is inappropriate, select a more appropriate recipe.

BEDEVILED EGGS
3 or 4 servings

Great for them to grab "on the run" or to take along.

> 4 hard-boiled eggs, cooled
> ¼ cup chicken, cooked and chopped,
>   or canned tuna, drained
> 1 tablespoon mayonnaise†
> ½ teaspoon teriyaki sauce
> Ground black pepper
> Lettuce leaves

Cut the eggs lengthwise and remove yolks. Arrange the egg whites on a cake rack on aluminum foil.

Mash the yolks, then combine them with the chicken or tuna, mayonnaise, and teriyaki sauce. Mix well, and add pepper to taste.

Spoon the yolk mixture into the cavities of the egg whites.

Place on a serving tray lined with large lettuce leaves and serve chilled.

---

†*Low-fat mayonnaise often contains a high proportion of sugar. Use only regular mayonnaise (not a low-fat variety) at all Insulin-Balancing Meals and Snacks. If regular mayonnaise is an inappropriate choice, select a different recipe or dressing.*

Meat, Poultry, and Fish

These exciting protein-rich recipes add flavor and satisfaction to any Insulin-Balancing Meal or Snack.

QUICKIE STEAKS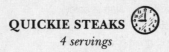
4 servings

This hearty lunch choice is fast and easy to prepare.

> ¼ cup olive oil*
> 1 teaspoon teriyaki sauce
> 2 large stalks celery including leaves,
>   chopped
> 8 minute steaks*

In a medium skillet, combine the olive oil and teriyaki sauce. Sauté the chopped celery until wilted.

Add the steaks and brown on one side, about 2 minutes, then turn and brown on the other side, about 1 minute.

Serve warm.

Variation: Layer slices of your youngster's favorite cheese* on top of the steaks after removing from heat; cover and let melt for 2 or 3 minutes.

Choose low-fat varieties or alternatives and/or low-salt varieties, as appropriate.

**Egg substitutes cannot be used in this recipe. If fat content is inappropriate, select a more appropriate recipe.*

PEPPERED BEEF
4 to 8 servings

A tempting and delectable dish to satisfy the fussiest eater. Serve for the whole family and guests, or save the leftovers to serve cold for tomorrow's Insulin-Balancing Meals and Snacks.

> 1 lean beef fillet,* about 2 pounds,
>   rolled and tied
> 2 garlic cloves, slivered
> 2 tablespoons teriyaki sauce
> 1 tablespoon paprika
> 1 tablespoon coarsely ground black
>   pepper
> 1 teaspoon dried sweet basil

Preheat the oven to 425 degrees.

Using a sharp pointed knife tip, poke 1-inch slits into the surface of the beef and insert a garlic sliver into each until all the slivers are used. (Try to distribute them evenly over surface.)

Pour teriyaki sauce over the roast and sprinkle with paprika, pepper, and basil.

Put the fillet in a shallow roasting pan, insert a meat thermometer into the thickest part of roast, and place in the oven. After 15 minutes reduce the heat to 350 degrees and continue roasting until desired doneness (using the meat thermometer as your guide).

---

†*Low-fat mayonnaise often contains a high proportion of sugar. Use only regular mayonnaise (not a low-fat variety) at all Insulin-Balancing Meals and Snacks. If regular mayonnaise is an inappropriate choice, select a different recipe or dressing.*

SAUCY SIRLOIN STEAK
6 to 8 servings

A hearty dish with a saucy twist.

> 3 tablespoons olive oil*
> 1 tablespoon butter*
> 1 lean sirloin steak,* 1½ to 2 pounds
> ½ cup scallion bulbs, chopped
> 2 tablespoons onion, chopped
> 1 tablespoon white vinegar
> Coarsely ground black pepper, to taste
> Parsley sprigs

In a deep skillet combine the olive oil and butter and set over medium heat. When the skillet is hot, add the steak and cook for 8 to 10 minutes per side, depending on desired doneness.

Put the cooked steak on a platter and keep warm. Raise the heat to medium-high. Add the scallions, onion, and vinegar to the oil in the skillet and stir for 20 seconds, scraping up any brown bits; then simmer for 1 minute.

Return heat to medium and return the steak to the skillet. Cook 1 minute on each side and remove from heat.

Slice the steak crosswise (against the grain) into thin pieces, pour on the sauce in the skillet and serve garnished with parsley sprigs.

*Choose low-fat varieties or alternatives and/or low-salt varieties, as appropriate.

**Egg substitutes cannot be used in this recipe. If fat content is inappropriate, select a more appropriate recipe.

LEMON VEAL
4 to 6 servings

A marvelous combination of flavors; something new and different.

1/4 cup olive oil*
1/2 cup scallions, chopped
1 1/2 pounds boneless veal, cubed
1/2 cup chicken broth
1/2 cup large green olives,* pitted
2 stalks celery, diced
1 teaspoon lemon zest, grated
1/4 cup sour cream*
1/2 teaspoon dried tarragon
1 tablespoon fresh lemon juice
Ground black pepper
Salt

In flameproof casserole, heat 2 tablespoons of oil over medium heat, add scallions, and sauté until tender (about 3 minutes). Add the veal cubes and brown quickly over medium-high heat. Turn off the heat and set aside.

In a small bowl, combine the broth, olives, celery, lemon zest, remaining olive oil, sour cream, tarragon, and lemon juice. Add the mixture to the casserole, cover, and simmer until the veal is tender (about 1 hour). Add pepper and salt to taste and serve at once.

†*Low-fat mayonnaise often contains a high proportion of sugar. Use only regular mayonnaise (not a low-fat variety) at all Insulin-Balancing Meals and Snacks. If regular mayonnaise is an inappropriate choice, select a different recipe or dressing.*

DILLY BURGERS
3 or 4 servings

New twist on an old favorite. Good cold for snacks.

> 1 pound lean ground round steak*
> ½ tablespoon garlic, minced
> ½ tablespoon fresh or dried dill, chopped
> Salt
> Ground black pepper
> Teriyaki sauce
> Hot sauce (optional)

Combine the ground round with the garlic and dill and divide into equal burgers.

Heat a deep skillet over medium heat until quite hot (about 3 to 5 minutes). Sprinkle salt to taste on the bottom of pan and add the patties.

Sear both sides of the burgers, reduce the heat, and continue to cook to desired doneness (rare, medium, well).

Sprinkle each burger with black pepper and teriyaki sauce to taste. Add hot sauce as desired. Serve immediately.

SPICY STEAK
3 or 4 servings

A special spicy treat.

> Coarsely ground black pepper
> 1 pound lean sirloin strip steak*
> 1 tablespoon olive oil
> 1 teaspoon salt
> 4 tablespoons (½ stick) butter*
> 1 teaspoon teriyaki sauce
> Fresh lemon juice
> Parsley sprigs

Choose low-fat varieties or alternatives and/or low-salt varieties, as appropriate.

**Egg substitutes cannot be used in this recipe. If fat content is inappropriate, select a more appropriate recipe.*

Sprinkle pepper to taste on a cutting board or similar flat surface, press the steak into the pepper, and work into both sides, using the palms of your hands.

Put the oil in a large skillet, sprinkle with salt, and heat. When the oil begins to brown, place the steaks in the skillet and brown over high heat. Reduce the heat and cook to desired doneness, turning once.

In a small pan, combine the butter, teriyaki sauce, and lemon juice, and heat.

Remove the steak from the skillet and slice against the grain. Pour the butter sauce over slices. Garnish with parsley sprigs and serve at once.

PORK ROAST
8 servings

Serve this wonderful dish to your whole family or to guests, or save the delicious leftovers for hot or cold snacks.

> 1 lean boneless pork roast, 2 pounds
> 1 tablespoon teriyaki sauce
> 3 tablespoons olive oil*
> 2 tablespoons sesame oil*
> 2 garlic cloves, minced

Preheat the oven to 350 degrees.

Insert a meat thermometer into the thickest part of the pork roast and set the roast on a rack in a deep baking pan with 1 inch of water in the bottom of the pan. Pour teriyaki sauce over the top of the roast. Combine olive and sesame oils, mix, and pour over the top of the roast. Sprinkle on the garlic.

Roast about 2½ hours, or to the desired temperature on the meat thermometer.

Serve warm for the first Insulin-Balancing Meal or Snack, then serve cold slices or use in salads for the next day or two.

†Low-fat mayonnaise often contains a high proportion of sugar. Use only regular mayonnaise (not a low-fat variety) at all Insulin-Balancing Meals and Snacks. If regular mayonnaise is an inappropriate choice, select a different recipe or dressing.

FENCE POSTS AND BEEF‡
4 servings

A quick recipe for using those leftovers that you hate to see go to waste.

> 8 fresh asparagus spears
> 1 pound cooked beef from a lean roast
>   or steak, sliced
> 1 tablespoon butter
> 2 tablespoons sour cream
> 1 cup Swiss cheese,* grated
> ½ teaspoon salt
> 2 teaspoons fresh lemon or lime juice
> 1 tablespoon Dijon mustard

Preheat the oven to 350 degrees.

Pour 1 inch of water into a deep skillet, add the asparagus spears, and turn heat to high. Cover and cook for 4 minutes. Turn off the heat and drain the asparagus. Keep covered. Arrange the beef slices in a medium casserole dish and lay an asparagus spear over each slice.

Melt the butter in small saucepan. Reduce the heat and add the remaining ingredients, stirring until completely mixed. Pour the sauce over the asparagus and beef.

Place in the oven and bake until hot, 8 to 10 minutes. Serve warm.

Choose low-fat varieties or alternatives and/or low-salt varieties, as appropriate.

**Egg substitutes cannot be used in this recipe. If fat content is inappropriate, select a more appropriate recipe.*

HERBY LAMB LOINS
4 servings

Great with crisp cucumbers or green beans.

> 1 pound boneless lean lamb loins*
> 1 tablespoon ground black pepper
> 2 garlic cloves, minced
> 1/4 teaspoon thyme
> 1 tablespoon dried sweet basil
> 1/2 cup celery, chopped
> 2 tablespoons teriyaki sauce
> 1 cup cauliflower florets

Put the lamb pieces in a medium bowl.

In a small bowl combine the black pepper, garlic, thyme, basil, celery, and teriyaki sauce. Mix well. Immediately pour the mixture over the lamb, cover, and refrigerate overnight.

When ready to cook, pour 1 inch of water into a large, deep skillet, add the cauliflower florets, and set the heat at high. Steam for 4 minutes. Remove from heat and set aside.

Remove the lamb from its marinade and broil (or grill over hot coals) for 2 to 3 minutes on a side until done.

Slice the lamb thin, add the cauliflower florets, and serve immediately.

---

†*Low-fat mayonnaise often contains a high proportion of sugar. Use only regular mayonnaise (not a low-fat variety) at all Insulin-Balancing Meals and Snacks. If regular mayonnaise is an inappropriate choice, select a different recipe or dressing.*

‡*This recipe contains ingredients that are particularly high in fat content. If fat content makes this an inappropriate recipe for your youngster, serve only on occasion, as a special treat as recommended by your child's physician, or choose a more appropriate recipe.*

MEDITERRANEAN LAMB
6 to 8 or more servings

Make this for a family feast and save the leftovers for Insulin-Balancing Meals and Snacks.

> 1 lean lamb roast, 3 pounds
> 1 garlic clove, crushed
> 1 teaspoon salt
> 2 tablespoons coarsely ground black
>   pepper
> 1 teaspoon sweet dried basil
> 1/2 teaspoon powdered ginger
> 1 bay leaf
> 1/2 teaspoon dried thyme
> 1/2 teaspoon dried sage
> 1/2 teaspoon dried marjoram
> 1 tablespoon teriyaki sauce
> 1 tablespoon olive oil

Preheat oven to 350 degrees. Place the lamb on a rack in a roasting pan.

In a small bowl combine the remaining ingredients and mix thoroughly. Make slits in the lamb and rub the mixture into the slits and over the entire surface of the lamb.

Insert a meat thermometer into the thick part of the roast and set the lamb in the oven. After 10 minutes reduce the heat to 300 degrees. Roast until desired doneness.

Remove the bay leaf, slice the meat, and serve it warm with pan drippings or cold as a delicious leftover.

*Choose low-fat varieties or alternatives and/or low-salt varieties, as appropriate.

**Egg substitutes cannot be used in this recipe. If fat content is inappropriate, select a more appropriate recipe.

NEW AGE TURKEY BURGERS
3 or 4 servings

A nice switch from an old favorite.

> 1 tablespoon olive oil
> 1 pound ground turkey
> 1 garlic clove
> 1 tablespoon fresh lemon juice
> Dash of curry powder
> Dash of dry mustard
> Dash of marjoram
> Ground black pepper

Heat the oil over medium heat in a medium skillet.

Mix all the remaining ingredients in a medium bowl. Form into patties and brown on both sides in the hot skillet until cooked through to the center.

Serve warm or cold. (If you serve the burgers warm, you might wish to melt some of your youngster's favorite cheese* on top.)

SULTRY LEMON CHICKEN
2 to 4 servings

A wonderful summer delight, but it can be enjoyed in the winter as well. This dish is great cold and you can also use any leftovers for chicken salad.

> 4 large boneless, skinless chicken
>   breasts
> 2 tablespoons fresh lemon juice
> 2 teaspoons olive oil
> 2 garlic cloves, minced
> ¼ teaspoon dried sweet basil
> ¼ teaspoon cayenne pepper
> ¼ teaspoon teriyaki sauce

†*Low-fat mayonnaise often contains a high proportion of sugar. Use only regular mayonnaise (not a low-fat variety) at all Insulin-Balancing Meals and Snacks. If regular mayonnaise is an inappropriate choice, select a different recipe or dressing.*

Rinse the chicken breasts thoroughly, pat dry, and arrange in a single layer in a shallow baking dish.

In a small bowl, combine the remaining ingredients and mix well.

Pour the mixture over the chicken and turn to distribute on both sides. Cover and refrigerate overnight for best results.

Grill the chicken breasts on a greased grill over hot coals or broil at least 6 minutes per side until cooked through.

OLIVE CHICKEN
3 or 4 servings

A sure taste delight for family and guests alike.

> 1 tablespoon olive oil
> 4 boneless, skinless chicken breasts
> 1 tablespoon fresh lime juice
> 1 tablespoon white vinegar
> 1 garlic clove, minced
> 4 black olives, pitted and sliced
> 4 green olives, sliced, without pimiento
> 2 tablespoons dried basil
> 4 green pepper rings
> Ground black pepper

In a large skillet, heat the olive oil and brown the chicken over medium-high heat. Lower the heat, cover, and cook until it is tender, 8 to 10 minutes. Remove the chicken to a serving plate and keep warm.

Combine the lime juice, vinegar, garlic, black and green olives, and basil, and toss in the skillet used for the chicken, heating gently.

Slice the chicken and arrange on plates. Pour the olive sauce over the slices, garnish with green pepper rings, and sprinkle on black pepper to taste.

*Choose low-fat varieties or alternatives and/or low-salt varieties, as appropriate.

**Egg substitutes cannot be used in this recipe. If fat content is inappropriate, select a more appropriate recipe.

CHICKEN AND GREEN BEANS
6 to 8 servings

A stir-fry that is easily prepared in advance yet served up on the spot.

 2 pounds boneless, skinless chicken
   breasts
 2 tablespoons olive oil*
 2 tablespoons gingerroot, minced
 2 cups green beans, trimmed, in 2-inch
   pieces
 ½ pound mushrooms, cleaned and
   sliced
 ¾ cup chicken stock
 1 tablespoon teriyaki
 1 tablespoon mayonnaise†
 1 cup red or white cabbage, sliced
 Ground black pepper

Cut the chicken into strips the size of your little finger. Set aside.

In a large heavy skillet, heat the oil very hot. Slowly add chicken and 1 tablespoon of the gingerroot to the skillet. If the chicken sticks, add a bit more oil. Stir slowly and constantly for about 2 minutes. Remove from the skillet and set aside.

In the hot skillet, combine the green beans, mushrooms, and remaining gingerroot and stir continually for 2 minutes. Add a little water if sticking occurs.

Mix the chicken stock and teriyaki sauce and pour the liquid over the green bean mixture in the skillet. Cover and let steam for 2 minutes.

Stir in the chicken mixture, mayonnaise, and 1 tablespoon of water and bring to a boil. Add the cabbage and stir for 1 minute or until cabbage is crisp-tender. Sprinkle with pepper to taste and serve warm.

---

†*Low-fat mayonnaise often contains a high proportion of sugar. Use only regular mayonnaise (not a low-fat variety) at all Insulin-Balancing Meals and Snacks. If regular mayonnaise is an inappropriate choice, select a different recipe or dressing.*

SPICY SHRIMP‡
4 servings

A sure winner, but this dish must chill for 24 hours, so plan ahead.

> 2 tablespoons celery leaves
> 1 tablespoon mixed pickling spices
> 1 teaspoon salt
> 1 pound medium shrimp
> 1 bay leaf
> 1/3 cup salad oil*
> 1/4 cup white vinegar
> 1 tablespoon capers and juice
> 2 teaspoons celery seeds
> 1 or 2 drops hot sauce

Fill a medium saucepan partway with water. Add the celery leaves, pickling spices, and 1/2 teaspoon of the salt. Bring to a boil and add the shrimp. Reduce the heat to a simmer, cover the pan, and heat for 5 minutes, then drain. Peel and devein the shrimp under cold water.

In a shallow dish, layer the shrimp.

Place the remaining ingredients, including the remaining 1/2 teaspoon of salt, in a small bowl, combine well, pour over the shrimp, and cover the dish. Chill at least 24 hours, occasionally spooning marinade over the shrimp. Remove the bay leaf and serve cold on a bed of lettuce.

Choose low-fat varieties or alternatives and/or low-salt varieties, as appropriate.

**Egg substitutes cannot be used in this recipe. If fat content is inappropriate, select a more appropriate recipe.*

BROILED SWORDFISH
4 to 6 servings

A treat that fish-loving kids and parents can all enjoy.

> 1½ pounds swordfish steaks
> Salt
> Ground black pepper
> ⅛ teaspoon paprika
> ¼ cup olive oil*
> 2 tablespoons sweet basil
> 2 tablespoons fresh lemon juice
> Watercress

Grease the broiler rack, set the rack at a level about 2 inches below the heat source, and preheat.

Wash the swordfish steaks, dry on paper towels, and sprinkle with salt and pepper to taste, and the paprika.

Place the steaks on the preheated broiler rack. Coat the tops of the steaks with 2 tablespoons of the olive oil and broil for 3 minutes.

Carefully turn the steaks, coat with the remaining olive oil, sprinkle with sweet basil, and broil for 4 or 5 more minutes longer or until done all the way through.

Sprinkle with lemon juice and garnish with watercress. Serve warm.

---

†*Low-fat mayonnaise often contains a high proportion of sugar. Use only regular mayonnaise (not a low-fat variety) at all Insulin-Balancing Meals and Snacks. If regular mayonnaise is an inappropriate choice, select a different recipe or dressing.*

‡*This recipe contains ingredients that are particularly high in fat content. If fat content makes this an inappropriate recipe for your youngster, serve only on occasion, as a special treat as recommended by your child's physician, or choose a more appropriate recipe.*

BAKED FISH AND SOUR CREAM
4 to 6 servings

This mouth-watering preparation is a sumptuous choice for a quick Insulin-Balancing Lunch or Dinner.

> 1 garlic clove
> 1½ pounds whitefish or flounder fillets
> 1 tablespoon butter*
> ½ teaspoon paprika
> 1 cup sour cream*
> ½ teaspoon parsley, chopped
> ¼ teaspoon fresh dill

Preheat the oven to 350 degrees.

Cut the garlic clove in half lengthwise and rub both sides of each fillet with the cut sides of the halves.

Make a paste of the butter and paprika and rub it on both sides of each fillet.

Place the fillets in an ovenproof dish and spread on the sour cream.

Cover the dish and bake 40 to 50 minutes, or until fillets flake with fork.

Remove from the oven, uncover, and sprinkle with parsley and dill. Serve immediately.

Choose low-fat varieties or alternatives and/or low-salt varieties, as appropriate.

**Egg substitutes cannot be used in this recipe. If fat content is inappropriate, select a more appropriate recipe.*

BAKED BLUEFISH
8 servings

Humble but luscious. Great for family meals, or serve it for lunch and enjoy the wonderful cold leftovers.

> 2-pound bluefish, cleaned and split
> 2 tablespoons olive oil*
> 1 teaspoon sesame oil*
> 2 garlic cloves, finely minced
> 1 tablespoon fresh lemon juice
> 1/4 cup parsley, chopped
> Lemon wedges

Preheat the oven to 425 degrees.

Spread 1 tablespoon of the olive oil over the surface of a large, shallow baking pan (microwavable or conventional). Place fish, cut sides up, in the pan and sprinkle the surfaces uniformly with a mixture of the remaining olive oil and the sesame oil. Sprinkle on the garlic and lemon juice.

Bake, uncovered, until the flesh flakes with fork, 20 to 25 minutes.

Garnish with parsley and serve with lemon wedges.

SOLE TRIUMPH
4 servings

Quick preparation, tantalizing presentation.

> 1-pound sole fillet
> 1 tablespoon fresh lemon juice
> 2 teaspoons olive oil
> 1/2 teaspoon dried sweet basil
> 1/4 cup mushrooms, sliced
> Coarsely ground black pepper

†Low-fat mayonnaise often contains a high proportion of sugar. Use only regular mayonnaise (not a low-fat variety) at all Insulin-Balancing Meals and Snacks. If regular mayonnaise is an inappropriate choice, select a different recipe or dressing.

Preheat the oven to 425 degrees.

Arrange the fillets in a single layer, in a suitable baking dish (microwavable or conventional).

In a small bowl, combine the lemon juice, olive oil, basil, and mushroom slices. Mix thoroughly and sprinkle over the fillets. Add pepper to taste.

Bake uncovered for 10 to 12 minutes, or until the flesh flakes easily with a fork. Serve immediately.

HEARTY HALIBUT STEAKS
4 servings

A robust dish to satisfy the finicky fish eater.

>2 halibut steaks, about 1½ inches
>   thick
>Salt
>2 stalks celery, diced
>½ cup mushrooms, sliced
>1 tablespoon teriyaki sauce
>Ground black pepper
>½ teaspoon dried, crumbled thyme
>   leaves
>¼ cup melted butter*

Preheat the oven to 350 degrees.

Arrange the fish steaks in a shallow buttered baking pan (microwavable or conventional). Add salt to taste. Combine the remaining ingredients and sprinkle half the mixture on each steak.

Bake, uncovered, about 25 to 30 minutes or until the fish flakes easily with a fork. Serve at once.

Choose low-fat varieties or alternatives and/or low-salt varieties, as appropriate.

**Egg substitutes cannot be used in this recipe. If fat content is inappropriate, select a more appropriate recipe.*

POACHED SALMON STEAK
3 or 4 servings

So good. Delicious warm for lunch, or as a new taste treat served cold for breakfast.

> 2 tablespoons butter*
> ¼ cup onion, chopped
> ¼ cup green pepper, chopped
> ¼ cup celery, chopped
> ¼ cup white vinegar
> Salt
> White or black peppercorns
> 1 salmon steak, about 1 pound

In a large skillet melt the butter, add the onion, green pepper, and celery. Cook mixture 5 to 8 minutes. Add 1 quart of water, the vinegar, and salt and peppercorns to taste, and simmer for 5 minutes.

Bring the liquid to a full boil. Meanwhile, wrap the salmon steak in coarse cheesecloth. Submerge the wrapped salmon in the boiling liquid. Immediately lower the heat and allow the fish to simmer for 25 to 30 minutes.

Remove the salmon steak, carefully unwrap it, and serve warm with mustard or an Insulin-Balancing dip.

---

†*Low-fat mayonnaise often contains a high proportion of sugar. Use only regular mayonnaise (not a low-fat variety) at all Insulin-Balancing Meals and Snacks. If regular mayonnaise is an inappropriate choice, select a different recipe or dressing.*

HERBY CRABMEAT SALAD
3 or 4 servings

A luncheon taste treat with almost no prep time.

> 2 tablespoons olive oil*
> 1 pound raw or cooked crabmeat
> Salt
> Coarsely ground black pepper
> 1 tablespoon fresh lemon juice
> 1/2 tablespoon dried sweet basil
> 1/2 tablespoon scallions, chopped
> 1/2 teaspoon dried tarragon
> Fresh parsley sprigs

If the crabmeat is raw, carefully remove all bits of nonedible material.

In a skillet, heat the olive oil until hot, add the crabmeat, and stir constantly until cooked thoroughly and warm (1 to 2 minutes for cooked crabmeat, 2 to 4 minutes for raw crabmeat).

Remove from heat and add salt and black pepper to taste, the lemon juice, basil, scallions, and tarragon; mix thoroughly. Garnish with parsley and serve warm or cold.

Choose low-fat varieties or alternatives and/or low-salt varieties, as appropriate.

**Egg substitutes cannot be used in this recipe. If fat content is inappropriate, select a more appropriate recipe.*

POPEYE CASSEROLE
3 or 4 servings

A tasty dish that will give your youngster strength and energy for the day's activities. This makes great use of leftover meat or poultry.

1½ cups raw spinach, torn
2 tablespoons olive oil*
2 tablespoons butter*
1 tablespoon garlic, minced
2 thick slices cooked chicken, turkey,
   beef, lamb, or pork, diced
2 medium eggs
2 tablespoons heavy cream*
Ground black pepper
3 tablespoons Parmesan cheese,*
   grated

Preheat the oven to 350 degrees.

Wash the spinach well. Place the spinach in a large skillet in ½ inch of water, cover, and steam for 4 to 6 minutes. Drain. Return the spinach to the skillet and set aside.

In a small skillet or frying pan, heat the olive oil and butter for 2 or 3 minutes. Add the garlic and cook over medium-low heat until it browns. Add the garlic mixture to the skillet containing the spinach. Add diced meat or poultry and simmer, stirring occasionally, for 5 minutes.

In a large bowl, mix eggs, cream, and pepper to taste. Add the spinach mixture and the Parmesan cheese to the egg mixture.

Oil an 8-inch-square baking dish, pour in the mixture, and bake for 30 minutes. Serve warm or cold.

†*Low-fat mayonnaise often contains a high proportion of sugar. Use only regular mayonnaise (not a low-fat variety) at all Insulin-Balancing Meals and Snacks. If regular mayonnaise is an inappropriate choice, select a different recipe or dressing.*

Vegetarian Style: Nonmeat Alternatives

These exciting protein-rich recipes can be included in any Insulin-Balancing Meal or Snack.

CLAMSHELL EGGS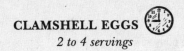
2 to 4 servings

A high-protein dish that is easy and quick.

> 4 hard-boiled eggs**
> ¼ cup cottage cheese*
> ¼ teaspoon garlic, minced
> ¼ tablespoon dried basil
> ½ tablespoon prepared mustard
> Hot sauce, to taste

Cut the eggs in half lengthwise. Scoop out the yolks and place them in a small bowl. Set the whites aside. Add remaining ingredients to the yolks and mash together thoroughly.

Use the mixture to fill the hollows in the whites.

Choose low-fat varieties or alternatives and/or low-salt varieties, as appropriate.

**Egg substitutes cannot be used in this recipe. If fat content is inappropriate, select a more appropriate recipe.*

FLOWERS AND "CHICKEN"
Serves 3 or 4

An unusual combination that is truly delicious.

> 1/2 head of cauliflower
> 4 teaspoons butter*
> 1 cup sour cream*
> 1/2 cup Parmesan cheese,* grated
> 1/4 cup fresh basil, chopped
> Ground black pepper
> 1 cup vegetarian "chicken,"† diced and
>   browned
> 1 cup green pepper, chopped

Preheat the oven to 350 degrees.

Cut cauliflower into 2-inch florets. Place 1 inch of water in a deep skillet, add the florets, and turn on the burner heat to full. Cover and simmer for 4 minutes. Turn off heat, drain, and keep covered.

In a large skillet, melt the butter and add the sour cream, Parmesan cheese, basil, and pepper to taste. Stir until cheese is melted.

Lightly grease a shallow baking dish (conventional or microwavable). Arrange "chicken" and cauliflower in the dish; sprinkle with chopped green pepper, and pour the sour cream sauce over all. Top with a dash of ground black pepper to taste. Bake for 20 minutes.

---

†*Low-fat mayonnaise often contains a high proportion of sugar. Use only regular mayonnaise (not a low-fat variety) at all Insulin-Balancing Meals and Snacks. If regular mayonnaise is an inappropriate choice, select a different recipe or dressing.*

‡*For Insulin-Balancing Meals and Snacks, nonmeat alternatives should contain 4 grams of carbohydrate or less per average serving. Check nutritional label. For a discussion on meat substitutes, see page 306.*

VEGETARIAN "BURGERS"
4 to 6 servings

A tasty, easy-to-prepare dish for the non-meat-eater and the carnivore alike.

1 tablespoon olive oil*
3 tablespoons butter*
1 garlic clove, minced
6 vegetarian "burgers"†
6 stalks celery, chopped
2 bay leaves
3 tablespoons fresh parsley, chopped
Salt
Ground black pepper
1 teaspoon dried thyme
1½ cups sour cream*
1 teaspoon paprika
2 tablespoons teriyaki sauce

Preheat the oven to 375 degrees. Coat a deep casserole dish with the olive oil.

In a small saucepan melt the butter and sauté the garlic. Brown the "burgers" on both sides, at least 3 minutes per side. Place them in the casserole dish.

Sauté the celery in the hot oil from the "burgers" for 5 minutes. Add 1 cup of water, the bay leaves, parsley, salt and pepper to taste, and thyme, and heat for 5 minutes, stirring constantly. Pour the mixture over the "burgers," cover, and bake 1 hour. Remove bay leaves.

Immediately before serving, stir sour cream, paprika, and teriyaki sauce well and top casserole with mixture.

Choose low-fat varieties or alternatives and/or low-salt varieties, as appropriate.

**Egg substitutes cannot be used in this recipe. If fat content is inappropriate, select a more appropriate recipe.*

CREAMY CAULIFLOWER "BURGERS"
2 to 4 servings

A tasty dish that will tickle the taste buds of kids of any age.

> 3 tablespoons olive oil*
> 2 medium garlic cloves, minced
> 4 vegetarian "burgers"†
> 4 ounces sour cream*
> 1 head of cauliflower, cut into 1-inch
>   pieces
> 1 tablespoon fresh parsley, chopped
> ¼ cup Parmesan cheese*
> 1 teaspoon dried oregano
> 4 ounces mozzarella cheese,* sliced
>   not too thin

Preheat the oven to 350 degrees.

In a large skillet over medium heat, combine 2 tablespoons of the olive oil with the minced garlic and brown lightly. Add the vegetarian "burger" slices and sauté for 3 or 4 minutes. Add the sour cream and ½ cup of water, and simmer for 12 to 15 minutes.

In a large skillet over medium heat, sauté the cauliflower in the remaining tablespoon of oil, several pieces at a time, until golden brown. (Additional oil may be needed.)

Arrange half of the cauliflower in the bottom of a well-oiled baking dish. Cover with half of the sour cream and "burger" mixture. Sprinkle half of the Parmesan cheese and add half of the mozzarella slices. Arrange the remaining cauliflower, sour cream mixture, and cheeses as above.

Bake until golden brown on top, 25 to 30 minutes.

---

†*Low-fat mayonnaise often contains a high proportion of sugar. Use only regular mayonnaise (not a low-fat variety) at all Insulin-Balancing Meals and Snacks. If regular mayonnaise is an inappropriate choice, select a different recipe or dressing.*

‡*For Insulin-Balancing Meals and Snacks, nonmeat alternatives should contain 4 grams of carbohydrate or less per average serving. Check nutritional label. For a discussion on meat substitutes, see page 306.*

ASPARAGUS AND EGG CASSEROLE
2 or 3 servings

This quick and easy casserole dish is a wonderful way to sneak vegetables into your youngster's meals.

> $\frac{1}{2}$ tablespoon butter*
> 1 (14-ounce) can asparagus spears
> 3 hard-boiled eggs,** sliced
> Salt
> Ground black pepper
> $\frac{1}{4}$ cup Cheddar cheese,* grated
> $\frac{1}{2}$ cup fresh mushrooms, sliced
> 2 ounces imported Swiss cheese,*
>   sliced

Preheat oven to 350 degrees. Use the butter to grease the bottom and sides of a medium casserole.

Arrange half the asparagus spears in the bottom of the casserole. Cover with half the egg slices and salt and pepper to taste. Sprinkle with half the Cheddar cheese. Top with the remainder of the asparagus spears, cover with the remaining egg slices, season with salt and pepper to taste, and add remainder of the Cheddar cheese. Arrange the Swiss cheese slices over all and bake for 30 minutes.

Serve warm.

Choose low-fat varieties or alternatives and/or low-salt varieties, as appropriate.

**Egg substitutes cannot be used in this recipe. If fat content is inappropriate, select a more appropriate recipe.*

TOFU CAN DO
2 to 4 servings

An intriguing combination of vegetables and quality protein.

1 teaspoon sesame oil*
1 tablespoon olive oil*
1 (2-inch) lengthwise slice of gingerroot
3 garlic cloves, minced
2 scallions, chopped finely
1 cup mushrooms, sliced
1½ cups firm tofu, sliced
1 cup green pepper, thinly sliced
1 head of bok choy, washed and sliced
1 cup fresh sprouts, any variety
1 tablespoon teriyaki sauce
4 large Romaine lettuce leaves

To a heated wok add the sesame oil, olive oil, ginger, garlic, and scallions and sauté for 7 or 8 minutes. Add the mushrooms, tofu, green pepper, and bok choy. Sauté for another 5 minutes, then add sprouts and teriyaki sauce. Stir well and simmer for 3 more minutes. Remove the slice of gingerroot.

Serve warm on a bed of lettuce leaves.

†Low-fat mayonnaise often contains a high proportion of sugar. Use only regular mayonnaise (not a low-fat variety) at all Insulin-Balancing Meals and Snacks. If regular mayonnaise is an inappropriate choice, select a different recipe or dressing.

CURRIED TOFU AND GREEN BEANS
3 or 4 servings

A vegetarian curry that satisfies.

1½ cups small squares of drained tofu
1½ pounds green beans, washed and
    trimmed
2 tablespoons olive oil*
½ teaspoon gingerroot, minced
Salt
½ teaspoon cayenne
½ teaspoon ground turmeric
¼ teaspoon cinnamon
¼ teaspoon ground coriander
¼ teaspoon mustard seeds
¼ teaspoon cumin seeds
1 garlic clove, minced

Wash the green beans and cut them into bite-sized pieces. Add the tofu squares. Set aside.

In a large skillet heat the olive oil and add all the seasonings. Stir the mixture around until everything in the skillet is thoroughly warmed, then add green beans, tofu, and ¼ cup of water. Stir again, cover tightly, and let the green beans and tofu steam for 3 or 4 minutes.

Serve warm.

Choose low-fat varieties or alternatives and/or low-salt varieties, as appropriate.

**Egg substitutes cannot be used in this recipe. If fat content is inappropriate, select a more appropriate recipe.*

CHEESE MOUSSE

3 or 4 servings

This special treat is high in fat so, with your physician's okay, save it for your special kid for special occasions.

> ⅔ cup light cream*
> 1⅓ envelopes unflavored gelatin
>   powder
> 2 eggs,** separated
> 8 ounces Roquefort cheese*
> ⅔ cup heavy cream*
> Pinch of cream of tartar

Put the light cream in a small saucepan and sprinkle the gelatin on top. When gelatin has softened, heat gently, stirring often, until the gelatin is completely dissolved and the cream is hot.

Beat the egg yolks until lemon-colored and fluffy. Continue beating as you add half of the hot cream, a little at a time. Return the mixture into the pot containing the remaining cream, stirring gently and heating carefully until the mixture begins to thicken.

Mash the Roquefort until there are no large lumps. Mix in some of the hot cream and egg yolk mixture and work the cheese until it forms a smooth paste. Add the remaining cream and egg yolk mixture and stir well. Set aside to cool.

Beat the heavy cream until peaks form. In a separate bowl, with clean beaters, add a pinch of cream of tartar to the egg whites to help firm them up, then beat the whites until they are stiff but not dry.

Carefully fold first the whipped cream and then the beaten egg whites into the cooled cheese mixture.

Transfer the mixture into a well-oiled mold of about 4-cup capacity, and chill for several hours or until set.

When ready to serve, invert the mold on a platter and garnish the mousse with a variety of crunchy Insulin-Balancing Vegetables including cucumber slices, celery strips, mushrooms, cauliflower florets, and green pepper slices.

---

†Low-fat mayonnaise often contains a high proportion of sugar. Use only regular mayonnaise (not a low-fat variety) at all Insulin-Balancing Meals and Snacks. If regular mayonnaise is an inappropriate choice, select a different recipe or dressing.

COMBO MEAL AND SNACK RECIPES

QuickFix Recipes are marked with the 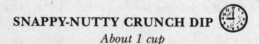 logo in the upper right corners.

Dips, Dressings, Salads, and Vegetables

These exciting recipes may be included as part of any Combo Meal or Snack.

Keep Combo Meals in balance by including, in addition to a salad, equal portions of protein, vegetables, and carbohydrates. Keep Combo Snacks in balance as well.

Remember, Combo Meal and Snack recipes usually include carbohydrate-rich ingredients, and these recipes should never be included in your youngster's Insulin-Balancing Meals or Snacks.

SNAPPY-NUTTY CRUNCH DIP
About 1 cup

If your kid loves peanut butter, this dip will be a hit.

> ½ cup crunchy peanut butter*
> 2 teaspoons brown sugar
> ¼ cup fresh lemon juice
> 2 tablespoons chili sauce
> ½ teaspoon teriyaki sauce
> Cayenne pepper

In a medium bowl, combine the peanut butter, brown sugar, lemon juice, chili sauce, and teriyaki sauce. Mix until thoroughly blended.

Taste first and then add cayenne pepper, one dash followed by blending and tasting until the desired "bite" is reached.

Serve with your youngster's favorite crackers, fresh fruit, or crisp sliced vegetables as appropriate.

MEAN BEAN DIP
About 2¹/₂ cups

A flavorful companion to chips,* crackers, or vegetables.

¹/₂ can (14-ounce) red kidney beans
¹/₂ can (14-ounce) white kidney beans
¹/₂ cup tomato puree
¹/₂ cup seasoned or unseasoned
   tomato sauce
¹/₄ cup honey
2 tablespoons molasses
1 medium tomato, chopped
1 tablespoon teriyaki sauce

In a large saucepan, combine the red and white beans, tomato puree, tomato sauce, honey, and molasses. Place the saucepan over medium heat and stir constantly until the mixture is hot and looks "saucy," about 8 to 10 minutes. Do not allow the mixture to stick to the pot.

Pour the hot contents into a blender. Add the chopped tomato and teriyaki sauce and blend until smooth.

Place the mixture in a bowl, cover, and chill before serving.

---

*Choose low-fat varieties or alternatives and/or low-salt varieties, as appropriate.

**Egg substitutes cannot be used in this recipe. If fat content is inappropriate, select a more appropriate recipe.

†Low-fat mayonnaise often contains a high proportion of sugar. Use only regular mayonnaise (not a low-fat variety) at all Insulin-Balancing Meals and Snacks. If regular mayonnaise is an inappropriate choice, select a different recipe or dressing.

GREEN SPICED DIP

About 1¹/₂ cups

An unusual combination that would tickle Popeye's taste buds. For best results, prepare at least 2 hours ahead.

> 10 ounces fresh spinach, rinsed well
>   and trimmed
> 1 teaspoon cider or white vinegar
> 1 garlic clove, coarsely minced
> ¹/₂ teaspoon dried cumin
> ¹/₂ teaspoon dried coriander
> ¹/₂ teaspoon powdered ginger
> Salt
> Ground black pepper
> ¹/₄ cup plain yogurt*
> 1 teaspoon dried paprika

In a large frying pan filled with ¹/₄ inch of water and placed over high heat, blanch the spinach until it just wilts. Drain immediately and cool in a colander. Press gently to remove as much liquid as possible.

In a food processor, combine the spinach, vinegar, garlic, cumin, coriander, ginger, and salt and pepper to taste. Blend 5 to 10 seconds. Add the yogurt and blend until smooth. Chill for 2 hours to allow flavors to meld.

Transfer the dip to a serving bowl, sprinkle with paprika, and serve with your youngster's favorite chips,* fresh fruit, or crisp vegetables as appropriate.

Choose low-fat varieties or alternatives and/or low-salt varieties, as appropriate.

**Egg substitutes cannot be used in this recipe. If fat content is inappropriate, select a more appropriate recipe.*

SOUR CREAM DRESSING

About 1¹/₂ cups

A creamy white topping for salads at Combo Meals or Snacks.

¹/₄ teaspoon salt

2 tablespoons sugar

1 tablespoon flour

¹/₂ teaspoon dry mustard

1 egg,** slightly beaten

2 tablespoons butter,* melted

1 cup light cream*

¹/₄ cup cider or wine vinegar

1 cup sour cream*

In the top of a double boiler, off heat, combine the salt, sugar, flour, and mustard.

In a medium bowl, mix the egg, butter, cream, and vinegar until smooth. Add to contents of double boiler very slowly, stirring constantly. Cook over boiling water, stirring constantly, until mixture begins to thicken.

Strain, cool, and fold in the sour cream until smooth.

†*Low-fat mayonnaise often contains a high proportion of sugar. Use only regular mayonnaise (not a low-fat variety) at all Insulin-Balancing Meals and Snacks. If regular mayonnaise is an inappropriate choice, select a different recipe or dressing.*

SOMETHIN' HONEY DRESSING
About 1½ cups

A sweet and tangy treat for salads at Combo Meals or Snacks.

2 tablespoons honey
1 cup sour cream*
¼ cup pineapple juice
½ teaspoon lemon zest, grated
¼ teaspoon powdered cinnamon
Dash salt

In a medium bowl, combine all the ingredients. Mix well until smooth and creamy.

Serve with your youngster's favorite green salad.

MYSTERY SALAD DRESSING
About 1½ cups

An unusual blend of ingredients that offers a surprising change for Combo Meals and Snacks.

6 ounces condensed tomato soup
½ cup tarragon vinegar
½ cup white vinegar
½ teaspoon salt
½ teaspoon paprika
1 tablespoon Worcestershire sauce
¼ cup sugar
½ teaspoon ground black pepper
1 teaspoon dry mustard
1 teaspoon raw onion, grated

Mix all the ingredients together in a quart jar and shake well. Let set for at least 2 hours. Chill well before serving on salads at Combo Meals and Snacks.

Choose low-fat varieties or alternatives and/or low-salt varieties, as appropriate.

TUTTI-FRUTTI DRESSING
About 1¹/₂ cups

A wonderful combination of the fruits of nature.

> ¹/₄ teaspoon salt
> 2 tablespoons sugar
> 1 tablespoon flour
> ¹/₂ teaspoon dry mustard
> 1 egg,** slightly beaten
> 2 tablespoons butter,* melted
> ¹/₄ cup cider vinegar
> 1 cup fresh orange juice
> ¹/₄ cup slivered almonds
> 1 banana, diced

In the top of a double boiler, combine the salt, sugar, flour, and mustard.

In a medium bowl, combine the egg, butter, vinegar, and orange juice and whisk until smooth. Add very slowly to the contents of double boiler, stirring constantly.

Cook over boiling water, stirring constantly, until the mixture begins to thicken.

Strain and cool.

Stir in the almonds and banana. Serve on fruit salads at Combo Meals or Snacks.

**Egg substitutes cannot be used in this recipe. If fat content is inappropriate, select a more appropriate recipe.*

†Low-fat mayonnaise often contains a high proportion of sugar. Use only regular mayonnaise (not a low-fat variety) at all Insulin-Balancing Meals and Snacks. If regular mayonnaise is an inappropriate choice, select a different recipe or dressing.

CARROT-RAISIN SALAD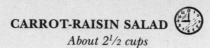
About 2½ cups

A tasty combination of root and fruit.

> 4 large carrots, washed and cut into
>   chunks
> ⅓ cup raisins
> ⅓ cup mayonnaise*
> ⅛ teaspoon salt

Using the shredding disk in the food processor, shred carrots. Empty the container into a large bowl as it fills. Add the raisins, mayonnaise, and salt to the carrots and mix well.

Chill and serve with meal.

CUCUMBER COINS
3 or 4 servings

A simple, tasty starter that is best prepared at least 2 hours ahead.

> 3 tablespoons cider or white vinegar
> 1 tablespoon water
> 1½ teaspoons sugar
> ½ teaspoon salt
> 1 sprig fresh dill
> 2 scallions, diced
> 3 cucumbers, peeled and thinly sliced

In a medium bowl, combine the vinegar with 1 tablespoon of water, the sugar, salt, dill, and scallions. Add cucumber slices and stir gently to mix well.

Refrigerate at least 2 hours.

*Choose low-fat varieties or alternatives and/or low-salt varieties, as appropriate.

**Egg substitutes cannot be used in this recipe. If fat content is inappropriate, select a more appropriate recipe.

GOING NUTTY
4 or 5 servings

Vegetables with a whole new twist.

> 1/4 head of cauliflower
> 3 large carrots, peeled
> 1 small head of iceberg lettuce
> 1 small green pepper
> 1/2 bunch of radishes
> 1/2 cup walnuts, chopped
> 1/2 cup honey
> 1/3 cup fresh lemon juice
> 1/2 cup evaporated milk*
> 1/2 teaspoon salt

Cut the cauliflower and carrots into chunks. Cut the lettuce into wedges. Remove the stem, seeds, and membranes from the green pepper and cut into quarters. Trim the radishes.

Insert the slicing disk in the food processor and guide cauliflower, carrots, lettuce, green pepper, and radishes through the feed tube to slice fine. As the container becomes full, transfer vegetables to a large serving bowl. When all the vegetables are sliced, stir in the walnuts. (Or slice and chop same ingredients finely by hand.)

To make the dressing, mix the honey and lemon juice well in a blender, mixer, or food processor, or by hand. Add the milk slowly and continue mixing until well blended. Stir in the salt.

Pour the dressing over the salad ingredients and toss to combine.

---

†*Low-fat mayonnaise often contains a high proportion of sugar. Use only regular mayonnaise (not a low-fat variety) at all Insulin-Balancing Meals and Snacks. If regular mayonnaise is an inappropriate choice, select a different recipe or dressing.*

SPICY VEGETABLE BALLS
3 or 4 servings

Serve with your youngster's favorite dip, dressing, or sauce.

> 1/2 cup carrot chunks, lightly steamed
> 1/2 cup broccoli florets, lightly steamed
> 1/2 cup potato chunks, lightly steamed
> 1/2 cup celery chunks, lightly steamed
> 2 egg yolks**
> Salt
> Ground black pepper
> Curry powder
> Chili powder
> Cayenne pepper
> Teriyaki sauce
> Dried basil
> Fresh lemon juice
> Paprika
> 1/4 cup bread crumbs
> 1/4 cup olive oil*

Put the steamed vegetables in a blender or food processor and cover with fresh water. Blend at low speed until finely chopped. Drain in a colander and press hard on the vegetables to remove as much of the liquid as possible.

When the vegetables have cooled, transfer them to a bowl and stir in the egg yolks and salt, pepper, curry powder, chili powder, cayenne, teriyaki sauce, basil, lemon juice, and paprika to taste.

Combine the vegetable purée with enough bread crumbs to make a thick batter. (Add water if necessary.) Chill the mixture for 1 hour.

Using a spoon or spatula, form the mixture into 12 to 15 balls, each about 1 inch in diameter.

Choose low-fat varieties or alternatives and/or low-salt varieties, as appropriate.

**Egg substitutes cannot be used in this recipe. If fat content is inappropriate, select a more appropriate recipe.*

In a large skillet, heat the oil very hot and fry the balls, in batches if necessary, about 5 minutes or until golden brown.

After cooking, the croquettes may be kept warm briefly in a 350-degree oven.

Serve these with your youngster's favorite dip or sauce.

GREEN BEANS AMANDINE
4 to 6 servings

Sounds sophisticated, tastes great.

> ¹/₄ cup olive oil*
> 2 tablespoons teriyaki sauce
> ¹/₄ pound slivered almonds
> 2 garlic cloves, minced
> 1 pound green beans, cut or broken into
>   1-inch lengths

In a deep skillet, combine the olive oil and teriyaki sauce. Add the almonds, mix well, and heat over medium heat until the almonds begin to brown. (Watch them carefully; they burn easily.) Lower the heat immediately and add the garlic, mixing well. Immediately add the green beans and cook until they are barely tender, stirring often.

Put the beans in a serving dish and cover to keep warm, or chill and serve cold.

---

†*Low-fat mayonnaise often contains a high proportion of sugar. Use only regular mayonnaise (not a low-fat variety) at all Insulin-Balancing Meals and Snacks. If regular mayonnaise is an inappropriate choice, select a different recipe or dressing.*

VEGETABLE CHEESE BALLS
3 to 4 servings

A fun grab-and-eat special treat.

2 zucchini, peeled
2 ounces hard cheese (such as Swiss,
    Cheddar or Gouda), cut into chunks
4 sprigs fresh parsley
3/4 cup fine dry bread crumbs
1 egg**
1/2 cup cottage cheese*
1/2 teaspoon oregano
Salt
Ground black pepper

Preheat the oven to 350 degrees.

Cut the zucchini in halves lengthwise. Scoop out the centers and set the pulp aside. Cook the zucchini shells in boiling water until softened but not cooked (about 4 to 5 minutes).

Carefully drop cheese chunks into a blender running on high speed and blend until the cheese is grated.

Add parsley and blend. Reduce speed to low.

Add bread crumbs, egg, cottage cheese, oregano, salt, and pepper, blending until mixture is smooth and thick. Transfer the filling to a bowl.

Finely chop the reserved zucchini pulp and add to the filling mixture.

Pack the filling tightly into the zucchini shells. Arrange the stuffed zucchini in a baking dish containing 1/2 inch of water. Bake at 350 degrees for 45 to 50 minutes, or until the zucchini shells are tender and the filling is cooked.

Serve as is or with your youngster's favorite sauce or gravy.

*Choose low-fat varieties or alternatives and/or low-salt varieties, as appropriate.

**Egg substitutes cannot be used in this recipe. If fat content is inappropriate, select a more appropriate recipe.

CHEESE-STUFFED CABBAGE
3 to 4 servings

A new vegetable dish with an unusual filling.

1 large head of green cabbage (about 5 pounds)

2 ounces hard cheese* (such as Swiss, Cheddar, or Gouda), cut into chunks

4 sprigs fresh parsley

3/4 cup fine dry bread crumbs

1 egg**

1/2 cup cottage cheese*

1/2 teaspoon oregano

Salt

Ground black pepper

3 fresh tomatoes, coarsely chopped

2 cups canned sauerkraut*

Preheat the oven to 350 degrees.

Remove the core from the cabbage. Place the cabbage in a large pot of boiling water and cook until the outer leaves are softened and pliable. Set aside while you prepare the filling.

Drop the cheese chunks into a blender set on a high speed and blend until the cheese is grated. Add the parsley and blend. Reduce the speed to low. Add the bread crumbs, egg, cottage cheese, oregano, and salt and pepper to taste and blend until the filling mixture is smooth and thick.

Line the bottom of a shallow baking dish with the chopped tomatoes mixed with the sauerkraut.

Divide the filling mixture among the large, softened outer cabbage leaves. Roll up each leaf from the stem end, tucking in the sides. Place in a baking dish, seam side down, and pour in 1/2 inch of water. (One large cabbage yields about 10 to 12 cabbage rolls.) Cover and bake for 45 to 50 minutes, or until the filling is cooked.

Serve the cabbage rolls with some of the tomato-sauerkraut mixture spooned over them.

†*Low-fat mayonnaise often contains a high proportion of sugar. Use only regular mayonnaise (not a low-fat variety) at all Insulin-Balancing Meals and Snacks. If regular mayonnaise is an inappropriate choice, select a different recipe or dressing.*

Meat, Poultry, and Fish

These protein-rich dishes can be included in any Combo Meal or Snack. Add vegetables and salad for balance. But remember, use Combo Meal recipes for Combo Meals and Snacks only.

CHEESY MEAT LOAF
3 or 4 servings

A welcome change and a taste delight.

> 2½-inch slice of Italian bread
> ⅓ cup milk*
> 1 Italian sausage link*
> 1 pound ground chuck*
> 1 egg,** beaten
> 1 onion, chopped
> 1 tablespoon parsley, chopped
> ½ garlic clove, chopped
> ¼ cup Parmesan cheese,* grated
> 1 cup mozzarella,* diced
> 1½ tablespoons ketchup
> Salt
> Ground black pepper
> ¼ cup fresh bread crumbs
> Romaine lettuce leaves

Preheat the oven to 350 degrees. In a medium bowl, soak the bread in the milk for 5 minutes and squeeze dry. Tear into small pieces.

Remove the sausage from its casing, break it into small pieces, and put the meat in a large bowl. Add the ground chuck to the sausage; add the egg, onion, parsley, garlic, Parmesan cheese, mozzarella, ketchup, and soaked bread. Add salt and pepper to taste. Mix thoroughly.

*Choose low-fat varieties or alternatives and/or low-salt varieties, as appropriate.

**Egg substitutes cannot be used in this recipe. If fat content is inappropriate, select a more appropriate recipe.

On a large cutting board, shape the meat mixture into a loaf, roll the loaf in the fresh bread crumbs, and put it in a large oiled baking pan.

Bake 60 to 70 minutes, until thoroughly cooked.

Arrange a bed of romaine lettuce leaves on a serving platter and set the meat loaf on top. Serve immediately.

NEW ENGLAND BEEF STEW
4 servings

There is nothing like a hearty beef stew to satisfy a healthy hunger.

> 1 pound lean corned beef brisket
> 1 garlic clove
> 1 whole clove
> 6 whole black peppercorns
> 1 bay leaf
> 4 medium carrots, peeled
> 3 large potatoes, peeled
> 6 small onions, peeled
> 1 small head of cabbage (approximately
> 3 pounds)
> Fresh parsley, minced

Rinse the corned beef and place it in a kettle of cold water deep enough to cover the meat. Add the garlic, clove, peppercorns, and bay leaf. Bring to a boil, reduce the heat, and simmer 5 or 6 minutes. Skim foam from the surface, cover the brisket, and continue to simmer for 3 to 3½ hours until thoroughly cooked.

Add the carrots, potatoes, and onions. Cut the cabbage into 8 wedges, add those to the pot, and simmer for an additional ½ hour.

Remove the meat from the pot and slice thinly across the grain. Remove and discard the bay leaf. Arrange the vegetables on a platter around the brisket slices and serve garnished with parsley. (A nice mustard sauce makes a fine addition.)

---

†*Low-fat mayonnaise often contains a high proportion of sugar. Use only regular mayonnaise (not a low-fat variety) at all Insulin-Balancing Meals and Snacks. If regular mayonnaise is an inappropriate choice, select a different recipe or dressing.*

PEPPER STEAK
3 or 4 servings

An old favorite that never loses its appeal.

> 3 tablespoons olive oil*
> 1 pound chuck fillet,* cut in 1x2-inch
>   strips
> 1 garlic clove, minced
> 2 cups julienne onions
> 3 green peppers, seeded and cut in
>   strips
> 3 stalks celery, cut in small strips
> ½ cup beef broth
> 2 tablespoons teriyaki sauce
> ½ teaspoon salt
> 2 tablespoons cornstarch
> 1 tomato, cut into wedges

In a large skillet, heat the oil and add the beef and minced garlic. Brown, uncovered, for 3 minutes. Remove the meat and set aside. Add the onions, green peppers, and celery to the skillet. Cover and steam for 5 minutes.

Return the meat to the pan, add the broth, teriyaki sauce and salt, and continue cooking, uncovered, for 10 minutes.

Mix the cornstarch with ¼ cup cold water and stir into the pan liquid until it thickens. Add the tomato wedges and cook 1 additional minute.

Serve warm over rice or pasta.

Choose low-fat varieties or alternatives and/or low-salt varieties, as appropriate.

**Egg substitutes cannot be used in this recipe. If fat content is inappropriate, select a more appropriate recipe.*

†Low-fat mayonnaise often contains a high proportion of sugar. Use only regular mayonnaise (not a low-fat variety) at all Insulin-Balancing Meals and Snacks. If regular mayonnaise is an inappropriate choice, select a different recipe or dressing.*

MEDITERRANEAN VEAL CHOPS‡

4 to 6 servings

Easy to prepare but hard to forget.

4 tablespoons (1/2 stick) butter*
4 thick loin veal chops*
1 tablespoon onion, chopped
1 garlic clove, chopped
1/2 cup ham,* finely diced
1 teaspoon teriyaki sauce
2 cups green olives,* pitted and
    chopped

Heat the butter in a large skillet, add the chops, and brown both sides over medium heat. Add the onion, garlic, ham, and teriyaki sauce and stir over medium heat until the onion is transparent.

Turn the chops, cover, and cook over low heat for 20 minutes. Remove to a platter and keep warm.

Add the olives to the skillet and heat for 1 minute. Pour the contents of the skillet over the chops and serve at once.

ROAST LOIN OF PORK

6 to 8 servings

A rich, hearty main course. Marinate overnight, then cook and enjoy.

1/4 cup honey
2 tablespoons white vinegar
1 tablespoon fresh gingerroot, chopped
1/2 cup pineapple, chopped
1/4 cup teriyaki sauce
2-pound lean pork loin*

Preheat the oven to 325 degrees.

‡*This recipe contains ingredients that are particularly high in fat content. If fat content makes this an inappropriate recipe for your youngster, serve only on occasion, as a special treat as recommended by your child's physician, or choose a more appropriate recipe.*

In a large bowl, combine the honey, vinegar, ginger, pineapple, and teriyaki sauce for the marinade. Cover and marinate the pork loin in the refrigerator overnight.

Two hours before cooking, remove the marinated pork from the refrigerator and allow it to reach room temperature.

Place pork on a large piece of heavy-duty foil, turn up all sides of the foil, and pour on approximately 1 cup of the marinade. (Set aside the remainder of marinade.) Seal the foil securely around the pork and place the wrapped meat in a roasting pan. Place pan into oven and roast for 2½ hours.

Remove the roast from the oven and open the foil carefully. Add the remaining marinade, be sure all foil edges are turned up to contain the juices, and roast uncovered, for an additional 30 minutes, basting frequently.

Remove the roast from the oven and let stand for 15 to 20 minutes before slicing and serving, using any remaining marinade and drippings as a sauce, if you wish.

SWEET AND PUNGENT PORK
4 servings

Oriental cuisine is always a favorite because of wonderful contrasts in flavors.

> 1 pound lean pork,* cut in 1-inch cubes
> ¼ cup teriyaki sauce
> 1 garlic clove, quartered
> ¼ cup sugar
> ¼ cup cornstarch
> ½ cup white vinegar
> ⅓ cup heavy syrup from canned
>   apricots
> ½ teaspoon ground black pepper
> ½ cup canned apricot halves

Choose low-fat varieties or alternatives and/or low-salt varieties, as appropriate.

**Egg substitutes cannot be used in this recipe. If fat content is inappropriate, select a more appropriate recipe.*

In a large saucepan combine the pork with 1½ cups water, the teriyaki sauce, and garlic. Bring to a boil, reduce heat, cover, and simmer gently for 50 to 60 minutes. Remove the garlic and discard. Remove the meat to a plate and reserve the cooking broth.

In a clean saucepan, blend the sugar and cornstarch thoroughly; add the vinegar, apricot syrup, and pepper until well mixed. Add the reserved pork broth and cook, stirring over medium heat until the sauce becomes semiclear and thick. Add the pork cubes and apricots, stir well, and heat through.

Serve over wild rice or noodles.

BROILED LAMB CHOPS
4 to 6 servings

Prepare a few hours ahead to allow time for marinating.

>   4 double lamb chops*
>   3 tablespoons olive oil*
>   1 garlic clove, sliced
>   Salt
>   Ground black pepper, to taste
>   Butter*
>   Herbs of your choice (parsley, dill, or
>   basil)
>   Fresh lemon juice (optional)

Preheat the broiler.

Put the lamb, olive oil, and garlic in a large bowl, and marinate for 1 to 2 hours.

Arrange the lamb chops on a rack in a broiler pan and broil about 2 inches from the heat source, turning once. For rare, broil 5 minutes per side; for medium, 6 to 7 minutes per side; and for well done, 10 minutes per side.

Transfer the chops to a warm platter, sprinkle with salt and pepper to taste, and place a pat of butter on each chop.

Sprinkle with your choice of herbs. If you like, sprinkle each chop with lemon juice.

†*Low-fat mayonnaise often contains a high proportion of sugar. Use only regular mayonnaise (not a low-fat variety) at all Insulin-Balancing Meals and Snacks. If regular mayonnaise is an inappropriate choice, select a different recipe or dressing.*

ROAST LEG OF LAMB
4 to 6 servings

A delectable, tender, and satisfying dish.

> 1 leg of lamb,* 3 pounds, trimmed
> 1 garlic clove, slivered
> 1 teaspoon dried rosemary
> Fresh lemon juice
> Sesame oil*
> Salt
> Ground black pepper

Preheat the oven to 300 degrees. Cut small slits in the surface of the lamb and insert slivers of garlic. Rub the surface of the meat with rosemary, lemon juice, and oil. Add salt and pepper to taste. Insert a meat thermometer into the center of the roast.

Place a rack in a roasting pan, set the lamb on the rack, and roast until desired temperature is reached: for rare, 140 degrees for about 1 hour; for medium, 160 degrees for about 1¼ hour; for well done, 175 degrees for about 1½ hours.

Remove the meat and set on a warming tray for 20 minutes. Carve and serve with pan gravy.

Choose low-fat varieties or alternatives and/or low-salt varieties, as appropriate.

**Egg substitutes cannot be used in this recipe. If fat content is inappropriate, select a more appropriate recipe.*

CHICKEN KIEV‡

4 to 6 servings

A delight to look at and a special treat.

>4 large skinless, boneless chicken
>   breast halves
>½ cup (1 stick) chilled butter*
>Salt
>Ground black pepper
>2 tablespoons chives, chopped
>Flour for dredging
>2 eggs,* lightly beaten
>⅔ cup fresh bread crumbs
>Olive oil* for deep-frying

Place the chicken breast halves between sheets of waxed paper and pound with a mallet until thin. (Avoid tearing the flesh.)

Cut the butter into 4 finger-shaped pieces. Set 1 piece of butter in the center of each breast, add salt and pepper to taste, sprinkle ½ tablespoon chives on each breast, and roll up like a jelly roll from the short side, letting the sides overlap (no fasteners are necessary; the flesh will adhere).

Lightly dredge each roll in flour, dip into eggs, and roll in bread crumbs. Refrigerate for 1 hour.

Fill a fryer or deep skillet with enough olive oil to cover breasts. Heat the oil to 360 degrees. Add the breasts one by one and cook, turning if necessary, until brown on all sides. Drain on absorbent paper and serve warm, perhaps with rice to absorb the delicious chive-flavored butter.

---

†*Low-fat mayonnaise often contains a high proportion of sugar. Use only regular mayonnaise (not a low-fat variety) at all Insulin-Balancing Meals and Snacks. If regular mayonnaise is an inappropriate choice, select a different recipe or dressing.*

‡*This recipe contains ingredients that are particularly high in fat content. If fat content makes this an inappropriate recipe for your youngster, serve only on occasion, as a special treat as recommended by your child's physician, or choose a more appropriate recipe.*

STUFFED CHICKEN BREASTS‡

4 to 6 servings

Something exquisite but simple and quick to prepare.

> 4 large skinless, boneless chicken
>   breast halves
> 6 tablespoons (³⁄₄ stick) butter*
> 4 thin slices Virginia ham*
> 4 thin slices imported Swiss cheese*
> ¹⁄₂ cup shallots, minced
> 8 medium mushroom caps
> 1 cup tomato, chopped
> ¹⁄₄ cup heavy cream*
> ¹⁄₄ cup parsley, chopped

Rinse the chicken breasts, pat dry, and beat with mallet or cleaver between sheets of waxed paper until very thin.

In a large skillet, heat the butter until hot but not browning. One at a time, move the chicken pieces around in the hot butter until they are no longer pink (2 or 3 minutes), and immediately place them on a large, flat dish. Set aside the skillet with its drippings.

On one half of each breast place a slice of ham and a slice of cheese. Fold the other half over to cover.

To the drippings in the skillet add the shallots and mushrooms and sauté about 3 minutes. Add the tomato and simmer for 3 more minutes, then add cream.

Add the stuffed chicken breasts to the skillet and simmer without boiling for 3 minutes, turning the pieces once or twice. Sprinkle with parsley and serve immediately, ladling sauce over the breasts.

Choose low-fat varieties or alternatives and/or low-salt varieties, as appropriate.

**Egg substitutes cannot be used in this recipe. If fat content is inappropriate, select a more appropriate recipe.*

HERBED CHICKEN IN CREAM SAUCE‡
4 to 6 servings

Easy enough for every day; special enough for company.

8 chicken legs (drumsticks)
²/₃ of a lemon, squeezed for juice
2 carrots, sliced
2 celery stalks, sliced
1¹/₂ scallions, sliced
¹/₂ cup onion, chopped
2 sprigs parsley
¹/₂ teaspoon dried tarragon
1 bay leaf
8 whole peppercorns
Salt
4 tablespoons (¹/₂ stick) butter*
¹/₄ cup flour
1 ¹/₃ cups heavy cream*

Rinse the drumsticks, pat them dry, and place them in a medium bowl. Add the lemon juice, covering each piece with juice, and let stand for 15 minutes.

Put the drumsticks in a heavy saucepan with enough cold water to cover. Add the carrots, celery, scallions, onion, parsley, tarragon, bay leaf, peppercorns, and salt to taste.

Bring to a slow boil and let simmer for about 25 to 30 minutes. Remove the chicken drumsticks and keep warm.

Over high heat, cook the stock down at a vigorous boil for another 15 to 20 minutes. Strain, and measure 3 cups stock. Discard the contents of the strainer after pressing on them to extract their juice.

---

†*Low-fat mayonnaise often contains a high proportion of sugar. Use only regular mayonnaise (not a low-fat variety) at all Insulin-Balancing Meals and Snacks. If regular mayonnaise is an inappropriate choice, select a different recipe or dressing.*

‡*This recipe contains ingredients that are particularly high in fat content. If fat content makes this an inappropriate recipe for your youngster, serve only on occasion, as a special treat as recommended by your child's physician, or choose a more appropriate recipe.*

In a medium saucepan, melt ½ of the butter and add the flour. Blend well, and slowly add the vegetable stock. Stir and cook for 15 minutes. Pour heavy cream into the thickened sauce and slowly bring to a boil.

Remove from the heat and add the remaining butter. Arrange the chicken drumsticks on a serving platter and top with sauce.

HAWAIIAN CHICKEN
3 or 4 servings

A satisfying dish for the hearty and light eater alike.

> 1 tablespoon cornstarch
> ½ teaspoon salt
> 1 teaspoon teriyaki sauce
> 1 pound skinless, boneless chicken
>   breasts, cut into age-appropriate
>   bite-sized strips
> 1 large onion, cut in thin strips
> 2 ribs celery, cut diagonally
> 10 water chestnuts, sliced
> ¼ cup olive oil*
> 1 (6-ounce) can pineapple, sliced, with
>   juice

In a large bowl, mix the cornstarch, salt, 2 teaspoons cold water, and teriyaki sauce. Use this mixture to dredge chicken pieces. Reserve the liquid for the sauce.

In a saucepan, sauté the onion, celery, and water chestnuts in 2 tablespoons of the oil for 5 minutes. Remove and set aside.

Use the remaining 2 tablespoons of oil to sauté the dredged chicken pieces, turning them until brown on all sides, 8 to 10 minutes.

Add the sautéed vegetables and stir. Cut 4 slices of the pineapple into wedges and add. Mix the pineapple juice with the reserved dredging liquid, add, and simmer until heated through.

Serve over a bed of steamed rice or noodles.

Choose low-fat varieties or alternatives and/or low-salt varieties, as appropriate.

ROASTED CHICKEN
6 to 8 servings

An old favorite that deserves a visit every now and then. Delicious cold, and the leftovers make good pickings for Insulin-Balancing Meals and Snacks.

> 1 chicken (2–3 pounds)
> 1 tablespoon olive oil*
> Salt
> Ground black pepper
> Paprika
> 2½ cups dry stuffing cubes

Preheat the oven to 350 degrees.

Place the chicken on a rack in an open roasting pan, breast side down. Brush it with oil and sprinkle with salt, pepper, and paprika to taste.

In a medium bowl, combine the stuffing, ⅔ teaspoon paprika, and ⅓ cup water. Mix well and stuff into chicken.

Roast for 1 hour, then turn the bird breast side up and finish roasting until browned and tender, basting frequently with the pan drippings.

Remove from the oven, remove stuffing to a serving bowl and keep warm, and let the chicken rest for 15 minutes before carving and serving.

**Egg substitutes cannot be used in this recipe. If fat content is inappropriate, select a more appropriate recipe.*

†Low-fat mayonnaise often contains a high proportion of sugar. Use only regular mayonnaise (not a low-fat variety) at all Insulin-Balancing Meals and Snacks. If regular mayonnaise is an inappropriate choice, select a different recipe or dressing.

SHRIMP DELIGHT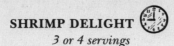
3 or 4 servings

Kids love this special treat.

> ¼ cup olive oil*
> 1½ pounds large shrimp, shelled,
>   deveined, washed, and dried
> Salt
> Black pepper, to taste
> 2 garlic cloves, chopped
> ¼ cup Italian parsley, chopped

In a large skillet, heat the oil over high heat and sauté the shrimp for 3 or 4 minutes, just until they are fully cooked. Do not overcook or the shrimp will be dry and tough. Add salt and pepper to taste and remove the shrimp to a serving platter.

Over high heat, quickly sauté the garlic in the remaining oil in the skillet.

Drizzle the garlic oil over the shrimp, sprinkle with parsley, and serve piping hot.

Choose low-fat varieties or alternatives and/or low-salt varieties, as appropriate.

**Egg substitutes cannot be used in this recipe. If fat content is inappropriate, select a more appropriate recipe.*

BROILED LOBSTER TAILS
4 servings

The best part of the lobster is the tail. Here is one simple way to enjoy this seafood delicacy.

> 4 medium-large lobster tails
> 1/4 cup fresh lime juice
> 1/2 cup olive oil*
> 1 teaspoon mild paprika
> 1 teaspoon salt
> 1 garlic clove, minced
> 1 teaspoon dried tarragon
> 1 teaspoon dried sweet basil
> Softened butter*

Preheat the broiler.

Using strong scissors, carefully cut along both sides of the undercover of the lobster tails and remove.

In a large shallow dish, combine the lime juice, olive oil, paprika, salt, garlic, tarragon, and basil. Mix well and marinate the lobster tails for 3 hours.

Remove the tails from marinade, slightly crack their upper shells with a cleaver, and bend the sides up so that tails will lie flat. Lightly coat the exposed meat with butter. Broil 5 minutes to a side.

Place on plates and serve with melted butter and any desired side dishes.

---

†Low-fat mayonnaise often contains a high proportion of sugar. Use only regular mayonnaise (not a low-fat variety) at all Insulin-Balancing Meals and Snacks. If regular mayonnaise is an inappropriate choice, select a different recipe or dressing.

FILLETS OF SOLE WITH HERBS
3 or 4 servings

This sweet and delicate fish makes a wonderful entrée.

½ cup (1 stick) butter*
2 medium fillets of sole, cut in half
2 tablespoons fresh lime juice
1 tablespoon dried tarragon
½ teaspoon garlic, minced
2 tablespoons chives, chopped
Salt
Paprika
Parsley sprigs (optional)

Preheat the oven to 350 degrees.

In a small skillet, melt the butter and use half of it to brush the fish fillets. Sprinkle the sole with lime juice.

Grease a large baking dish and arrange the fillets in it. Cover and bake until the fish flakes at the touch of fork tines, 18 to 20 minutes. Remove the fish carefully and place the fillets on a serving platter.

Add the rest of the butter to the melted butter in the skillet, add the tarragon, garlic, chives, and salt and paprika to taste. Heat contents slightly and drizzle over fish. Garnish with parsley sprigs if desired and serve at once.

*Choose low-fat varieties or alternatives and/or low-salt varieties, as appropriate.

**Egg substitutes cannot be used in this recipe. If fat content is inappropriate, select a more appropriate recipe.

BREADED FISH FILLETS

6 to 8 servings

Better than the frozen variety and almost as easy.

> 2 pounds fish fillets (such as halibut,
>   flounder, or cod)
> ½ cup seasoned bread crumbs
> 1 egg*
> 2 tablespoons olive oil*
> Parsley sprigs
> 6 to 8 lemon wedges

Rinse the fillets, pat dry on paper towels, and cut into serving-sized pieces.

Spread bread crumbs on a large dish or platter.

In a small dish, beat the egg with a fork. Dip fish pieces in egg, moistening both sides, and then into crumbs, coating both sides well.

In a large skillet heat the oil until hot. Add enough fish pieces to cover the bottom of the skillet. (Do not crowd the pan.) Reduce the heat to medium and sauté the fish until golden brown, 4 to 5 minutes. Turn the fish and sauté the other side for 4 to 5 minutes. Repeat, if necessary, with any remaining fish.

Remove the fish to the serving platter, garnish with parsley and lemon wedges, and serve, adding a favorite relish or sauce.

---

†*Low-fat mayonnaise often contains a high proportion of sugar. Use only regular mayonnaise (not a low-fat variety) at all Insulin-Balancing Meals and Snacks. If regular mayonnaise is an inappropriate choice, select a different recipe or dressing.*

BLACK PEPPERCORN TUNA
4 to 6 servings

This fantastic peppery dish will wake up everyone's taste buds.

1 tablespoon crushed black pepper

2 tablespoons teriyaki sauce

2 tablespoons fresh lemon or lime juice

4 medium tuna steaks

4 teaspoons olive oil

¼ cup chicken broth

4 thin lemon slices

Preheat the broiler.

In a small bowl, combine the crushed pepper, teriyaki sauce, and juice. Mix and set aside.

Coat both sides of each steak thinly with olive oil, place the steaks on a broiling tray, and broil each side for 5 or 6 minutes. Turn off heat but leave the tuna in the oven.

In a large skillet over medium-high heat, combine crushed pepper mixture and broth. Stirring constantly, cook over high heat until the sauce is light brown. Reduce the heat to low, remove the tuna from the oven, lay the steaks in the skillet, and sauté 1 minute on each side.

Place fish steaks on a serving platter. Pour remaining sauce over the tuna and garnish with lemon slices.

*Choose low-fat varieties or alternatives and/or low-salt varieties, as appropriate.

**Egg substitutes cannot be used in this recipe. If fat content is inappropriate, select a more appropriate recipe.

Vegetarian Style: Nonmeat Alternatives

These exciting meat-free recipes can be included in any Combo Meal or Snack.

As always, keep Combo Meals in balance with salad, protein, and vegetables and never include Combo recipes in your youngster's Insulin-Balancing Meals or Snacks.

VEGETARIAN LASAGNE

4 to 6 servings

Save this snappy dish for a once-in-a-while treat.

> ³/₄ tablespoon olive oil*
> 1 small onion, chopped
> 1 small garlic clove, minced
> ³/₄ pound ricotta cheese*
> 2 ounces Romano cheese,* grated
> ¹/₂ pound spinach, washed well and
> coarsely chopped
> 1 egg,** lightly beaten
> Salt
> Ground black pepper
> 1¹/₄ tablespoon fresh parsley, chopped
> ¹/₂ pound lasagne noodles
> 1 tablespoon butter*
> ¹/₄ pound mozzarella cheese,* coarsely
> grated
> 1¹/₂ pints tomato sauce, commercial or
> homemade

---

†*Low-fat mayonnaise often contains a high proportion of sugar. Use only regular mayonnaise (not a low-fat variety) at all Insulin-Balancing Meals and Snacks. If regular mayonnaise is an inappropriate choice, select a different recipe or dressing.*

Preheat the oven to 350 degrees.

Warm the olive oil in a medium skillet over medium heat. Add the onion and garlic to the skillet and sauté lightly.

Combine the ricotta, Romano, spinach, sautéed onion and garlic, and beaten egg in a bowl and mix well. Season the mixture with a little salt, plenty of ground black pepper, and some chopped parsley.

Cook the lasagne noodles in abundant lightly salted water until they are just al dente. Drain.

Butter a large, oblong baking dish. Arrange one-third of the cooked lasagne noodles on the bottom, spread on a layer of the ricotta mixture, sprinkle with mozzarella, and cover with tomato sauce. Repeat layers twice more, ending with sauce on top.

Cover the baking pan with aluminum foil, crimping the edges tightly. Bake the lasagne for 40 minutes, remove foil, and bake 10 to 15 minutes longer, uncovered. Serve warm.

GREEN FETTUCCINE AND "SAUSAGE"‡
3 or 4 servings

A colorful recipe that will ignite any child's taste buds.

> 4 tablespoons (½ stick) plus 2
>   teaspoons butter*
> 6 ounces vegetarian "sausage links,"
>   chopped
> ¼ teaspoon salt
> 4 ounces fresh or packaged fettuccine
> 1 teaspoon flour
> ½ cup heavy cream*
> 3 avocados
> 4 heaping tablespoons Parmesan
>   cheese,* grated
> Ground black pepper

*Choose low-fat varieties or alternatives and/or low-salt varieties, as appropriate.

**Egg substitutes cannot be used in this recipe. If fat content is inappropriate, select a more appropriate recipe.

†Low-fat mayonnaise often contains a high proportion of sugar. Use only regular mayonnaise (not a low-fat variety) at all Insulin-Balancing Meals and Snacks. If regular mayonnaise is an inappropriate choice, select a different recipe or dressing.

In a medium skillet over medium heat, melt 1 teaspoon of the butter, add the chopped "sausage," and cook until golden, 4 to 5 minutes. Set aside.

Heat 1 quart of salted water to a brisk boil in a medium pot. Add the fettuccine and cook until al dente. Drain and cover the pot to keep the pasta hot.

In a small saucepan over medium heat, melt the remaining butter. Add the flour and stir to mix thoroughly. Add cream and stir constantly while cooking for 5 minutes.

Briefly reheat the chopped "sausage" in the skillet. Meanwhile, chop 2 of the avocados and slice the third.

Place the pasta in a serving bowl. Pour the cream sauce over the pasta. Add the chopped avocado, ¾ of the "sausage," ¾ of the Parmesan cheese, and pepper to taste. Garnish with the sliced avocado and the remaining "sausage" and serve with the remaining grated cheese.

"BURGER" GOULASH
3 or 4 servings

A tasty, tempting entrée that will warm and satisfy.

2 tablespoons butter*

1 medium onion, chopped

1 garlic clove, minced

6 vegetarian "burgers," cubed

¼ cup flour

1 ½ cups tomatoes, chopped

6 small new potatoes or 2 large baking
    potatoes, cubed

Paprika

Salt

Ground black pepper

½ cup sour cream*

---

‡*This recipe contains ingredients that are particularly high in fat content. If fat content makes this an inappropriate recipe for your youngster, serve only on occasion, as a special treat as recommended by your child's physician, or choose a more appropriate recipe.*

Put the butter in a large skillet and set over medium-low heat. Add the onion and garlic and sauté for 4 or 5 minutes.

Coat the "burger" cubes with flour, add to the skillet, and brown gently for 2 or 3 minutes. Add the tomatoes, potatoes, and paprika, salt and pepper to taste.

Cover the pan and simmer for 25 minutes.

Immediately before serving, stir in the sour cream and garnish with additional paprika. Serve over rice or noodles.

TROPICAL ISLAND "CHICKEN"
3 or 4 servings

A Polynesian pleasure for any vegetarian menu.

1 pound vegetarian "chicken"
½ cup flour
2 teaspoons teriyaki sauce
¼ cup olive oil*
1 cup fresh orange juice (or ½ orange
    juice and ½ pineapple juice)
2 tablespoons fresh lemon juice
1 tablespoon cornstarch
½ cup brown sugar
1 cup papaya, cubed
1 cup fresh or canned pineapple,
    drained and diced
2 cups banana, sliced
1 cup water chestnuts, sliced

Preheat the oven to 350 degrees.

In a large plastic bag, combine serving-sized pieces of "chicken," flour, and 1 teaspoon teriyaki sauce. Shake until "chicken" is thoroughly coated.

Grease a shallow baking pan with 1 tablespoon of the butter, and arrange a single layer of coated "chicken" pieces in the bottom.

Melt the remaining butter and pour it over the "chicken." Place the pan in the oven and bake for 45 to 50 minutes.

*Choose low-fat varieties or alternatives and/or low-salt varieties, as appropriate.

In the meantime, combine the orange juice, lemon juice, cornstarch, brown sugar, and remaining teriyaki sauce in a large saucepan, whisking until the cornstarch is dissolved. Heat over medium heat, stirring constantly until sauce becomes thick and clear. Add the papaya, pineapple, banana, and water chestnuts and mix thoroughly. Set aside.

When the "chicken" is cooked, pour the fruit sauce over "chicken" and bake 10 minutes longer. Serve plain or over a bed of white or brown rice.

VEGETARIAN "CHICKEN" AND BEANS
3 or 4 servings

The beans must be soaked overnight, but plan ahead; it's worth it.

> 1 cup small dried white beans
> 1 medium onion, sliced
> 2 garlic cloves, minced
> 2 tablespoons olive oil*
> 6 vegetarian "chicken" slices
> 1 teaspoon salt
> 1/4 teaspoon ground black pepper
> 1/4 teaspoon paprika

In a large saucepan, combine the beans with 6 cups of water. Soak overnight.

Drain the beans and add fresh water to just cover them. Add the onion and garlic and cook over medium heat 1½ hours.

Warm the olive oil in a medium skillet over medium heat and sauté "chicken" slices until golden brown. Add salt, pepper, and paprika.

Cut the "chicken" slices into quarters and mix with the warm bean mixture. Serve warm.

**Egg substitutes cannot be used in this recipe. If fat content is inappropriate, select a more appropriate recipe.

†Low-fat mayonnaise often contains a high proportion of sugar. Use only regular mayonnaise (not a low-fat variety) at all Insulin-Balancing Meals and Snacks. If regular mayonnaise is an inappropriate choice, select a different recipe or dressing.

SEAFOOD-VEGETABLE MIX
3 or 4 servings

A delicious combination of tomato stew, with fish and shellfish. Nourishing and tasty.

    1 tablespoon olive oil*
    1 large carrot, chopped
    1 large celery stalk, diced
    1 large green pepper, chopped
    1 large red pepper, chopped
    1 large onion, chopped
    2 large garlic cloves, chopped
    2 cups canned, drained whole tomatoes
    2 small zucchini, peeled and sliced
    1 bay leaf
    1 teaspoon hot sauce
    $1/2$ teaspoon oregano, dried
    2 dozen littleneck clams, scrubbed, or
      vegetarian alternative
    8 green olives, pitted
    8 black olives, pitted
    $1/2$ pound shrimp, peeled and deveined,
      or vegetarian alternative
    $1/4$ cup parsley, chopped
    Ground black pepper

Coat a large, deep skillet with the oil and heat over medium-low heat.

Combine the carrots, celery, green pepper, red pepper, and onion. Sauté until the onion is soft, 4 or 5 minutes. Add the garlic, tomatoes, zucchini, bay leaf, hot sauce, and oregano. Mix well, raise the heat, and cook until small bubbles appear. Reduce the heat and simmer 15 minutes.

Choose low-fat varieties or alternatives and/or low-salt varieties, as appropriate.

**Egg substitutes cannot be used in this recipe. If fat content is inappropriate, select a more appropriate recipe.*

Add the clams, green olives, and black olives. Cover and simmer, gently shaking pan from time to time, until the clams have been steamed open, 3 or 4 minutes. Add shrimp and/or fish alternative and cook until done, an additional 3 or 4 minutes. Stir in the parsley and pepper to taste. Discard the bay leaf and any unopened clams. Serve immediately.

SILLY DILLY EGGS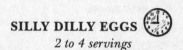
2 to 4 servings

A quick, flavorful treat.

> 4 hard-boiled eggs**
> 3 tablespoons sour cream*
> 3 tablespoons fresh dill, chopped
> Salt
> Ground black pepper

Peel the eggs, slice them lengthwise, and empty the yolks into a small bowl. Add sour cream, 2 tablespoons of the dill, and salt and pepper to taste. Combine thoroughly.

Spoon the yolk mixture back into the whites and sprinkle with the remaining dill. Serve chilled.

---

†*Low-fat mayonnaise often contains a high proportion of sugar. Use only regular mayonnaise (not a low-fat variety) at all Insulin-Balancing Meals and Snacks. If regular mayonnaise is an inappropriate choice, select a different recipe or dressing.*

EGGPLANT AND POTATOES
3 to 5 servings

A tasty combination of nature's best.

Salt
2 medium eggplant, peeled and sliced
   to $\frac{1}{2}$-inch thickness
3 large russet potatoes
2 bell peppers
$\frac{1}{2}$ cup (1 stick) butter*
$\frac{1}{2}$ teaspoon cayenne pepper
$\frac{1}{2}$ teaspoon ground cinnamon
1 teaspoon ground ginger
1 teaspoon turmeric
$\frac{1}{2}$ teaspoon ground coriander
1 teaspoon mustard seeds
1 teaspoon cumin seeds
2 garlic cloves, minced
5 firm red tomatoes, cut into small
   wedges

Salt the eggplant well and let stand in a colander for 30 to 40 minutes, pressing out the excess water at the end. Cut the slices into large cubes.

Peel and cube the potatoes, and cut up the cored, seeded bell peppers into $\frac{1}{2}$-inch squares.

In a very large skillet, melt the butter. Add the cayenne, cinnamon, ginger, turmeric, coriander, mustard seeds, cumin seeds, and garlic. Sauté the spices in the butter for several minutes, then add the eggplant, potatoes, and green peppers. Toss until the vegetables are evenly coated with spices.

Add $2\frac{1}{2}$ cups water, cover the pan, and let the vegetables simmer for about 20 to 25 minutes, stirring occasionally. Remove the cover and cook over a low flame for an additional 15 minutes, gently stirring often. Add the tomatoes and heat through. Serve immediately.

Choose low-fat varieties or alternatives and/or low-salt varieties, as appropriate.

CAULIFLOWER AND HERBS
3 or 4 servings

A great cold vegetable dish, prepared the day before, with lots of new tastes.

> 1 head of cauliflower
> ³/₄ cup olive oil*
> ¹/₂-¹/₄ cup cider vinegar
> ¹/₂ cup fresh lemon juice
> ³/₄ teaspoon dried fennel seed
> ¹/₂ teaspoon dried chervil
> ¹/₂ teaspoon dried thyme
> 1 small bay leaf
> ³/₄ teaspoon ground coriander
> 1 stalk celery, sliced
> 2 garlic cloves, minced

Wash the cauliflower and remove its green leaves. Break or cut the cauliflower into small florets.

Put 2 cups water in a large pot, add the florets and all the remaining ingredients, bring to a boil, and simmer 10 to 15 minutes. Remove from the heat and allow to cool.

Empty everything into a bowl, remove the bay leaf, and chill for 24 hours.

Drain in a colander and let the florets rest so that all excess oil drips off.

Serve on a platter as an appetizer or a salad.

**Egg substitutes cannot be used in this recipe. If fat content is inappropriate, select a more appropriate recipe.

†Low-fat mayonnaise often contains a high proportion of sugar. Use only regular mayonnaise (not a low-fat variety) at all Insulin-Balancing Meals and Snacks. If regular mayonnaise is an inappropriate choice, select a different recipe or dressing.

TROPICAL CITRUS SQUASH
4 servings

A special dish that is a pleasure to prepare and fun to eat.

> 2 small acorn squash
> 1 tablespoon melted butter*
> 1/3 cup orange marmalade
> 2/3 tablespoon candied ginger, diced
> 2/3 tablespoon fresh lemon juice
> Pinch of nutmeg

Preheat the oven to 350 degrees. Cut the squash lengthwise, remove the seeds and fibers, brush the cut sides with butter, and place cut sides down on a greased pan.

Bake 35 to 40 minutes. Turn the squash cut side up. Leave the oven on.

In a medium bowl, combine the marmalade, diced ginger, lemon juice, and nutmeg. Spoon the mixture into the squash cavities and bake 15 minutes longer. Serve warm.

Choose low-fat varieties or alternatives and/or low-salt varieties, as appropriate.

**Egg substitutes cannot be used in this recipe. If fat content is inappropriate, select a more appropriate recipe.*

VEGETARIAN "BEEF-SAUSAGE" LOAF
3 or 4 servings

An unusual meat loaf for the vegetarian or a change of pace for the carnivore.

> 1 ½ teaspoons olive oil*
> 1 medium green pepper, chopped
> 2 garlic cloves, chopped
> 1 medium tomato, chopped, with juice
> ⅓ cup fresh basil, chopped
> ½ teaspoon dried oregano
> 1 small zucchini, chopped
> ½ pound vegetarian "beef," broken up
> ½ pound vegetarian "sausage," diced
> ¼ cup rolled oats
> 3 tablespoons oat bran
> 2 large egg whites, beaten
> Salt
> Coarsely ground black pepper
> Hot sauce

Preheat the oven to 350 degrees. Coat a loaf pan with ½ teaspoon of the olive oil. Set aside.

In a saucepan over medium-low heat, combine the remaining olive oil with the green pepper and garlic. Cook for 3 minutes, stirring several times during cooking. Add the tomatoes with juice, 2 tablespoons of the basil and the oregano. Simmer for 10 minutes, stirring occasionally.

In a large bowl, combine the contents of the saucepan with the zucchini, hot sauce, "beef," "sausage," rolled oats, oat bran, egg whites, and salt, pepper, and hot sauce to taste. Mix thoroughly, transfer to the loaf pan, and spread uniformly.

Bake until golden brown on top, 1 hour. Serve warm or cold.

---

†*Low-fat mayonnaise often contains a high proportion of sugar. Use only regular mayonnaise (not a low-fat variety) at all Insulin-Balancing Meals and Snacks. If regular mayonnaise is an inappropriate choice, select a different recipe or dressing.*

COTTAGE CHEESE PANCAKES

3 or 4 servings

A light and airy little treat.

> 6 eggs,** separated
> 2 cups small-curd cottage cheese*
> 2/3 cup flour
> 2 tablespoons sugar
> Salt
> Cinnamon
> 1/8 teaspoon cream of tartar
> 2 tablespoons butter*

In a medium bowl, combine the egg yolks, cottage cheese, flour, sugar, and salt and cinnamon to taste.

In another bowl beat the egg whites with cream of tartar until stiff but not dry. Gently fold the beaten whites into the cheese mixture.

Use the butter to grease a griddle or skillet and heat on medium-high. Drop large spoonfuls of batter on the hot surface and cook the pancakes until golden brown on both sides. Serve at once with honey, ground walnuts, preserves, sour cream,* or powdered sugar.

Choose low-fat varieties or alternatives and/or low-salt varieties, as appropriate.

**Egg substitutes cannot be used in this recipe. If fat content is inappropriate, select a more appropriate recipe.*

Soups

Delicious starters for Combo Meals.

CHICKEN NOODLE SOUP
3 or 4 servings

A solid, fast-fix standby.

> 3½ cups canned or homemade chicken
>   broth
> 1 small onion, chopped
> 2 stalks celery, chopped
> 1 carrot, chopped
> 1 tablespoon teriyaki sauce
> 1 teaspoon dried parsley flakes
> 1½ cups cooked noodles
> Cheese,* grated

In a medium saucepan, combine the broth, onion, celery, carrot, teriyaki sauce, and parsley. Bring to a boil and simmer 30 minutes, or until the vegetables are soft. Skim out the vegetables, add the noodles, and cook briefly until the noodles are hot. Serve with grated cheese of choice sprinkled on top.

---

†*Low-fat mayonnaise often contains a high proportion of sugar. Use only regular mayonnaise (not a low-fat variety) at all Insulin-Balancing Meals and Snacks. If regular mayonnaise is an inappropriate choice, select a different recipe or dressing.*

CREAM OF CAULIFLOWER SOUP
3 or 4 servings

Unusually good and hearty.

> 2 cups cauliflower florets
> 3 tablespoons butter*
> ½ cup onion, sliced
> 1 large celery stalk with leaves,
>   chopped
> 3 cups canned or homemade chicken
>   broth
> 1 cup heavy cream*
> 2 tablespoons parsley, chopped
> Coarsely ground black pepper

In a medium pot of boiling water, cook the cauliflower until soft, about 10 minutes. Drain the florets and set the pot aside.

Mash the cauliflower in a medium bowl and set aside.

In the pot used to cook the cauliflower, melt the butter over medium heat, and add the onion and celery. Cook until the onion is soft, 4 or 5 minutes. Add the broth and cauliflower florets and heat to boiling. Reduce the heat and add the cream. Stir constantly for 5 minutes without allowing the soup to boil. Turn off heat, cool slightly, and serve garnished with parsley and black pepper to taste.

Choose low-fat varieties or alternatives and/or low-salt varieties, as appropriate.

**Egg substitutes cannot be used in this recipe. If fat content is inappropriate, select a more appropriate recipe.*

CREAM OF TOMATO SOUP

3 or 4 servings

This smooth soup is best served on a cold winter's night but it's great at any time of the year.

> 2½ tablespoons butter*
> 2½ tablespoons flour
> Salt
> 1 ½ cups milk*
> 6 ounces tomato paste
> 2 cups canned peeled tomatoes,
>   puréed
> ⅛ teaspoon pepper
> 1 bay leaf
> ⅓ teaspoon cloves
> ⅔ tablespoon onion, minced

In a small saucepan over medium heat, melt the butter. Stir in the flour and salt to taste until blended and then add the milk, stirring constantly. Cook until the mixture boils and thickens. Set aside.

In a soup pot, combine the tomato paste, puréed tomatoes, pepper, bay leaf, clove, and onion. Bring the mixture to a boil. Reduce heat the and simmer 10 minutes.

Set the thickened milk mixture over medium heat, add the tomato mixture, and heat, stirring constantly until well blended and hot. Pour the mixture into soup, stirring constantly. Remove the bay leaf and serve warm.

---

†*Low-fat mayonnaise often contains a high proportion of sugar. Use only regular mayonnaise (not a low-fat variety) at all Insulin-Balancing Meals and Snacks. If regular mayonnaise is an inappropriate choice, select a different recipe or dressing.*

FRUIT-LOOP SOUP
3 or 4 servings

This delightful soup is best served cold.

    1 ⅓ apples, peeled and cored
    1⅓ cups cherries, pitted
    4 plums, skinned and pitted
    ⅛ teaspoon salt
    ⅓ cup sugar
    1 tablespoon cornstarch
    Sour cream* or plain yogurt*

In a medium pot, combine the apples, cherries, plums, 4 cups water, salt, and sugar. Cook for 25 to 30 minutes over medium heat.

In a cup, blend the cornstarch with a little cold water and add to the pot.

Heat and stir until the soup thickens slightly. Cook for 3 minutes.

Chill and serve each portion garnished with a tablespoon of sour cream or plain yogurt.

SPLIT PEA SOUP
3 or 4 servings

Thick and super-satisfying.

    ½ cup dried split peas
    2½ cups beef broth
    1 garlic clove
    1 cup cooked lean beef,* coarsely
       chopped
    1 small onion, chopped
    1 celery stalk, chopped
    ½ teaspoon salt
    ¼ teaspoon black pepper

Choose low-fat varieties or alternatives and/or low-salt varieties, as appropriate.

**Egg substitutes cannot be used in this recipe. If fat content is inappropriate, select a more appropriate recipe.*

In a saucepan, combine the peas, beef broth, and garlic, and cook over medium heat until peas are tender, 45 to 50 minutes.

Cool for 15 minutes, then pour the mixture into a blender. Using medium speed, blend until the mixture is smooth. Pour back into saucepan, add the beef, onion, celery, salt, and pepper, and cook until the vegetables are tender. Serve warm.

SWEET AND SOUR CABBAGE SOUP
3 to 4 servings

A new taste, a brand-new treat.

> 1 medium onion, diced
> 3 tablespoons olive oil*
> 3½ cups beef broth
> ½ pound sauerkraut*
> ½ head of cabbage, cored and coarsely
>   shredded
> 2 tablespoons raisins
> 1¾ tablespoons vinegar
> ⅛ teaspoon pepper
> 4½ ounces tomato sauce
> 2 tablespoons brown sugar
> ¼ teaspoon salt

In a small skillet over medium heat, combine the onion and olive oil and sauté until onion is golden brown.

Transfer the mixture to a large pot. Add the broth, sauerkraut, cabbage, raisins, vinegar, pepper, tomato sauce, brown sugar, and salt. Mix thoroughly. Over low heat, simmer for 45 to 50 minutes. Taste and adjust seasoning. Serve warm.

---

†*Low-fat mayonnaise often contains a high proportion of sugar. Use only regular mayonnaise (not a low-fat variety) at all Insulin-Balancing Meals and Snacks. If regular mayonnaise is an inappropriate choice, select a different recipe or dressing.*

MINESTRONE SOUP
3 to 4 servings

A robust Italian favorite that will please the entire family. Before you begin, however, the beans must be soaked overnight.

> ½ cup large white beans, dried
> ¼ pound salt pork,* chopped
> ¼ cup lentils
> 3 cups beef broth
> 1 small onion, chopped
> ½ cup tomato purée
> ¼ cup canned garbanzo beans, drained
> ½ cup carrot, diced
> 1 stalk celery, diced
> ½ small zucchini, sliced
> 1 bay leaf
> ½ cup potatoes, peeled and diced
> Salt
> Ground black pepper
> ½ cup fresh or defrosted frozen peas
> ¼ cup elbow macaroni
> Parmesan cheese*

Put the beans in a small bowl with enough water to cover and soak overnight.

Add 2 cups water and the salt pork to a large pot or kettle and heat to boiling. Reduce the heat immediately and simmer 10 to 15 minutes.

Drain the beans, add them and the lentils to the pot and simmer about 1 hour until the beans and lentils are tender to the touch of a fork. Add the broth, onion, tomato purée, garbanzos, carrot, celery, zucchini, and bay leaf. Simmer for 20 minutes. Add the potatoes and salt and pepper to taste. Simmer until the potatoes are almost tender to the touch of a fork. Add the peas and pasta and cook until the pasta is tender, 10 to 12 minutes. (Add water if the soup is too thick.) Remove the bay leaf.

Serve warm or cold, sprinkling Parmesan cheese on each serving.

Choose low-fat varieties or alternatives and/or low-salt varieties, as appropriate.

Desserts

These Combo Dessert recipes offer special treats that can top off your youngster's Combo Meal.

Remember to consider dessert part of the one-fourth carbohydrate portion.

BUNNY PUDDING
3 or 4 servings

Good for bunnies, great for kids.

> 1/2 cup carrots, roughly chopped
> 1/2 cup potatoes, roughly chopped
> 1/4 cup olive oil*
> 1/2 teaspoon cinnamon
> 1/2 teaspoon allspice
> 1/2 cup flour
> 1/2 teaspoon nutmeg
> 1/2 cup sugar
> 1/2 teaspoon salt
> 1/2 teaspoon baking soda
> 1/2 cup raisins
> 1/2 cup walnuts, chopped

Using a food grinder, combine and mince the carrots and potatoes.

In a large ovenproof bowl or casserole dish, combine the mixture thoroughly with all the remaining ingredients. Cover and place in 1 1/2 inches of water. Place in 350-degree oven and cook for 2 hours. Check water level regularly.

Serve plain or with any favorite regular or low-fat toppings.

**Egg substitutes cannot be used in this recipe. If fat content is inappropriate, select a more appropriate recipe.

†Low-fat mayonnaise often contains a high proportion of sugar. Use only regular mayonnaise (not a low-fat variety) at all Insulin-Balancing Meals and Snacks. If regular mayonnaise is an inappropriate choice, select a different recipe or dressing.

FRUITY-FRUITY COMPOTE
4 servings

Fruity dessert that your youngster may never have had before.

> 12 ounces assorted dried fruits
> 1/2 cup sugar
> 4 slices fresh citrus fruits (lemon, lime,
> or orange), peeled and seeded

Wash the dried fruit well in warm water and place in a large cooking pot. Add sugar, 2 cups water, and sliced citrus rings, and cook, covered, for 1/2 hour.

Serve chilled.

TROPICAL SWEET POTATO
3 or 4 servings

A delicious dessert with a taste of the islands.

> 4 medium sweet potatoes baked at 350
> degrees for 40 minutes
> 1-pound can pineapple chunks
> 2 bananas
> 2/3 cup brown sugar
> 2 tablespoons butter*
> 1 cup miniature marshmallows

Preheat the oven to 325 degrees.

Peel the baked sweet potatoes, slice into 1-inch-thick rounds and place in a large casserole.

Drain the pineapple and set the juice aside.

Cut the bananas diagonally in 1-inch slices and arrange on top of the sweet potato slices. Distribute the pineapple chunks evenly over the bananas, then sprinkle on the brown sugar and dot with butter. Pour a little of the pineapple juice into the casserole and cover the entire top with miniature marshmallows.

Cover and bake for about 25 to 30 minutes.

FRUITY DUMPLINGS

3 or 4 servings

A fun dessert that combines complex carbohydrates to help balance the simple sugars.

> 2 tablespoons salt
> 1 cup cooked and mashed potatoes
> 1 egg,** beaten
> 1 cup flour
> 1/2 teaspoon baking powder
> 1/2 pound freestone peaches, peeled,
>   pitted, and coarsely chopped
> 1/2 pound blueberries, washed
> 1/2 cup sugar

Fill a large pot ³⁄₄ full with water, add 1 teaspoon of the salt, and set over low-medium heat.

In a large bowl, combine the potatoes, the remaining salt, the egg, flour, and baking powder, and mix until a firm dough is formed.

Generously flour a pastry board and roll out the dough about ⅛ inch thick. Cut into 4-inch squares.

In a medium bowl combine the sliced peaches, blueberries, and sugar. Fill the center of each dough square with some of the fruit mixture. Carefully fold the dough over the fruit and tightly pinch all the seams closed. Use a little flour around the top of each dumpling to tighten and dry the dough so that the boiling water does not seep in and the juices do not seep out.

Drop the dumplings into the pot of boiling salted water; cover and cook for 8 to 10 minutes. The dumplings will float to the surface. Remove one by one with a slotted spoon.

Fruit-filled dumplings are especially good coated with a mixture of ground walnuts and a dollop of yogurt or sour cream.

*Choose low-fat varieties or alternatives and/or low-salt varieties, as appropriate.

**Egg substitutes cannot be used in this recipe. If fat content is inappropriate, select a more appropriate recipe.

†Low-fat mayonnaise often contains a high proportion of sugar. Use only regular mayonnaise (not a low-fat variety) at all Insulin-Balancing Meals and Snacks. If regular mayonnaise is an inappropriate choice, select a different recipe or dressing.

FRIED APPLES
3 to 4 servings

A scrumptious dessert that Adam would find hard to resist.

>2 eggs**
>1/4 cup sugar
>2 teaspoons flour
>6 large apples, peeled and sliced
>2 tablespoons butter* or
>   polyunsaturated oil*
>Sugar

In a medium bowl, combine the eggs, sugar, and flour. Cover the apple slices with the egg mixture.

Melt the butter in a medium skillet over medium-high heat, and fry the apples until golden brown. Sprinkle with sugar to taste and serve warm.

NATURE'S HARVEST
3 or 4 servings

A delightful combination that takes advantage of the "fruits" of nature.

>2 oranges, peeled, sectioned, and cut
>   into chunks
>2 cups pineapple chunks, drained
>2 bananas, peeled and sliced
>2 peaches, peeled, pitted, and sliced
>1 cup fresh strawberries
>2 pieces candied ginger, thinly sliced
>1/2 cup coconut, coarsely grated
>1/4 cup honey
>1/4 cup fresh lemon juice

*Choose low-fat varieties or alternatives and/or low-salt varieties, as appropriate.

**Egg substitutes cannot be used in this recipe. If fat content is inappropriate, select a more appropriate recipe.

In a large bowl, combine the orange pieces, pineapple chunks, bananas, peaches, ginger, and coconut. Toss lightly. Cover and put aside to chill.

In a medium bowl, combine honey and lemon juice to form dressing.

Just before serving, toss the fruit with the honey-lemon dressing.

CREAMY PLUM TARTS‡
3 to 4 servings

A luscious, creamy dessert that can be saved for rare and special occasions.

> ½ cup (1 stick) butter*
> ½ cup plum jelly
> 2 eggs**
> ½ cup sugar
> 1 tablespoon vanilla extract
> Salt
> 8 tart shells
> 1 cup heavy cream,* whipped, or low-fat
>   alternative

Preheat the oven to 350 degrees.

In a double boiler over high heat, melt the butter and jelly, then allow to cool.

Beat eggs and sugar until the mixture forms a ribbon; add to the melted and cooled jelly. Add the vanilla and salt to taste and mix well.

Pour the mixture into the prepared tart shells and bake for 30 to 35 minutes, or until the pastry browns.

Remove, allow to cool, and serve with whipped cream or low-fat alternative.

†*Low-fat mayonnaise often contains a high proportion of sugar. Use only regular mayonnaise (not a low-fat variety) at all Insulin-Balancing Meals and Snacks. If regular mayonnaise is an inappropriate choice, select a different recipe or dressing.*

‡*This recipe contains ingredients that are particularly high in fat content. If fat content makes this an inappropriate recipe for your youngster, serve only on occasion, as a special treat as recommended by your child's physician, or choose a more appropriate recipe.*

APPLE TARTS‡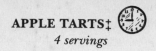
4 servings

So simple and so satisfying.

> 4 medium-sized baking apples
> 6 tablespoons butter*
> 4 thin slices white bread
> ¼ cup brown sugar

Preheat the oven to 350 degrees. Core and peel the apples.

With 1 tablespoon of butter, grease the bottom of a baking dish, arrange the bread slices in the bottom of the dish, and put an apple on each slice. Fill half of each apple hollow with ½ tablespoon butter and the rest with ½ tablespoon sugar. Bake 45 to 60 minutes.

In a small skillet, melt the remaining butter and combine with the remaining sugar. Spoon a little of the mixture over the apples from time to time.

When the apples are tender, remove from the oven and serve warm with the juice from the bottom of the pan.

*Choose low-fat varieties or alternatives and/or low-salt varieties, as appropriate.

**Egg substitutes cannot be used in this recipe. If fat content is inappropriate, select a more appropriate recipe.

STRAWBERRY SURPRISE‡

3 to 4 servings

Sweet and satisfying finish for Combo Meals.

> ½ cup olive oil*
> 1½ cups flour
> 2 eggs,** separated
> 1 teaspoon cinnamon
> ½ teaspoon salt
> ¾ cup milk*
> 12 whole ripe strawberries, large
>   and very firm
> Powdered sugar

Pour the oil into a deep skillet and heat to 375 degrees.

Put the flour in a large bowl and make a well in the center. Place the egg yolks, cinnamon, and salt in the well and work into the flour until all the ingredients are thoroughly combined. Add the milk gradually and stir until the mixture is smooth.

Beat the egg whites stiff and fold gently into the batter.

Dip each strawberry into the batter and fry 3 to 5 minutes. Drain on paper towels. Discard remaining oil. Sprinkle with powdered sugar and serve.

†*Low-fat mayonnaise often contains a high proportion of sugar. Use only regular mayonnaise (not a low-fat variety) at all Insulin-Balancing Meals and Snacks. If regular mayonnaise is an inappropriate choice, select a different recipe or dressing.*

‡*This recipe contains ingredients that are particularly high in fat content. If fat content makes this an inappropriate recipe for your youngster, serve only on occasion, as a special treat as recommended by your child's physician, or choose a more appropriate recipe.*

Low-Fat and Other Health Agency Dietary Recommendations[1]

Important Note: The recommendations that follow have been established for the adult population at large. There is still some debate regarding recommendations for children, although some of the *current recommendations indicate that children under two years of age should* never *be given a low-fat eating program.* Before incorporating any dietary guidelines, including those that follow, into your youngster's eating program, you should consult his or her physician. Only your youngster's physician can determine which recommendations are appropriate to your youngster's individual health needs.

Health Agency Recommendation #1

Eat a variety of foods.

To Incorporate Recommendation #1 into Your Youngster's Program

Provide a variety of Insulin-Balancing Foods so that your youngster can choose from an assortment of salad items, vegetables,

---

[1]Adapted from the U.S. Surgeon General's *Report on Nutrition and Health;* the U.S. Department of Agriculture and the Department of Health and Human Services' *Report on Dietary Guidelines for Americans;* the American Heart Association's Diet, *Eating Plan for Healthy Americans,* and the American Cancer Society's *Eat to Live.*

and regular or low-fat proteins and dairy items for Add-On Food Choices or Insulin-Balancing Meals (depending on your youngster's choice of plans). In addition to Insulin-Balancing Foods, your youngster's Combo Meals should contain a wide variety of Carbohydrate-Rich Foods, including whole-grain breads and other grain products, pasta, rice, and other starches, dairy choices, fruits and fruit and vegetable juices, and "healthy" desserts. Remember to keep Combo Meals balanced and never include carbos in Insulin-Balancing Meals.

Health Agency Recommendation #2

Reduce consumption of fat* (especially saturated fat) and cholesterol.

To Incorporate Recommendation #2 into Your Youngster's Program

When appropriate, and as directed by your youngster's physician, eggs can be replaced by egg substitutes, and low-cholesterol margarine and cooking sprays can be used instead of butter. In place of higher-fat varieties, your youngster may choose low-fat or skim milk; low-fat or low-cholesterol cheeses; and sour cream, cream cheese, and whipped cream substitutes. In place of higher-fat meats, select chicken or turkey without skin, fish, or very lean cuts of meat, trimmed of all fat. For additional low-fat choices, substitute turkey for the typical pork and beef usually found in burgers and sausage. When possible, use pans and sprays that eliminate the need for cooking oils. When cooking oils are needed or desired, however, olive oil appears to be better than heavy tropical or other saturated oils. However, olive oil may not be appropriate when cooking foods at high heat. So if high heat is required, the next best choice appears to be polyunsaturated oils.

---

*Low-fat diets are generally not recommended for children under two years of age and for all children and teens only as per physician recommendations.

Health Agency Recommendation #3

Add foods rich in vitamins A and C.

To Incorporate Recommendation #3 into Your Youngster's Program

Whenever possible (depending on your youngster's likes and dislikes), encourage your child or teen to include dark green leafy vegetables as well as cruciferous vegetables (from the cabbage family) in as many meals and snacks as possible. Keep some of the following foods on hand and, in keeping with the Program's guidelines, try adding them to your youngster's appropriate meals and snacks whenever possible: bok choy, broccoli, brussels sprouts, cabbage, cauliflower, collards, kale, kohlrabi, mustard greens, rutabagas, and turnips and their greens.

At Combo Meals, in keeping with the Program's guidelines, encourage your youngster to choose a balanced portion of Carbohydrate-Rich Foods that, in addition to grain products and Carbohydrate-Rich Vegetables, include citrus fruits and juices, cantaloupe, and strawberries, and tomatoes.

Health Agency Recommendation #4

Achieve and maintain a desirable body weight.

To Incorporate Recommendation #4 into Your Youngster's Program

By making The Carbohydrate Addict's Program for Children and Teens available to your youngster, you may well have provided him or her with guidelines that are needed to reach and maintain an ideal weight level for life and, in doing so, to reduce many of the health risks often associated with excess weight in adulthood.

Health Agency Recommendation #5

Increase consumption of complex carbohydrates and fiber by choosing whole-grain foods and cereal products, vegetables, and fruits. Avoid too much sugar.

To Incorporate Recommendation #5 into Your Youngster's Program

At your Combo Meals, your youngster should be encouraged to select whole-grain breads, cereal products, rice, pasta, potatoes and other starchy vegetables, and fresh fruits as the needed Carbohydrate-Rich Foods. At all meals, include lots of fiber-rich Insulin-Balancing Vegetables.

At Combo Meals, you can help keep your youngster's intake of sugar low by making available desserts that are made of complex carbohydrates, like whole-grain breads, popcorn, pretzels, and low-fat whole-grain snacks instead of cookies, cakes, and candy. Swap Choices will automatically help guide your youngster in trading high-sugar foods for complex carbo treats.

Health Agency Recommendation #6

Limit the amount of salt-cured, smoked, and nitrate-cured foods.

To Incorporate Recommendation #6 into Your Youngster's Program

Choose ham, bacon, hot dogs, sausages, pastrami, corned beef, salami, and other cold cuts only on rare and special occasions rather than as a regular part of your youngster's eating program. A good rule of thumb: Packaged foods almost always contain a great deal more salt than home-cooked varieties made from scratch.

Health Agency Recommendation #7

Reduce intake of sodium by choosing foods relatively low in sodium and by limiting the amount of salt added in food preparation and at the table.

To Incorporate Recommendation #7 into Your Youngster's Program

Remember to consult your physician before decreasing your youngster's salt intake. If a reduction is recommended, you may choose to limit the amount of salt you add while cooking, or encourage your child to use less salt at the table, or both. If a low-salt diet is recommended at all meals, serve low-salt varieties of canned and packaged foods, as well as low-salt cheese and other dairy products. At restaurants, encourage the use of low-salt alternatives. When possible, avoid smoked and salted products.

Health Agency Recommendation #8

Health Agency Recommendation #8 relates to the moderate consumption of alcoholic beverages and therefore is not relevant to youngsters' eating programs.

Health Agency Recommendation #9

Women should increase consumption of foods high in calcium, including low-fat dairy products, and those of child-bearing age should consume foods that are good sources of iron.

To Incorporate Recommendation #9 into Your Youngster's Program

If your youngster's physician recommends the inclusion of food sources high in calcium, feel free (at any meal) to encourage your youngster to eat calcium-rich canned fish (such as mackerel, salmon, sardines, and water-packed tuna), as well as spinach and greens, oysters, tofu, and low-fat cheeses, and iron-rich foods, such as lamb, chicken, turkey, green beans, and mushrooms. At Combo Meals, your youngster can choose to include Carbohydrate-Rich Foods such as iron-rich popcorn, potatoes, pasta, rice, and fresh fruits.

If you are including fruit as part of the Carbohydrate-Rich Foods of your youngster's Combo Meals, consider the fruit's proportion to the meal along with any other Carbohydrate-Rich Foods and balance it with equal portions of protein and Insulin-Balancing Vegetables.

APPENDIX II

Selected Bibliography

Abraham, S., and M. Nordsieck. "Relationship of Excess Weight in Children and Adults." *Public Health Reports* 25 (1960): 263–273.

Anderson, R. A. "Nutritional Role of Chromium." *Science of the Total Environment* 17 (1981): 13–29.

Anderson, R. A. "Chromium Metabolism and Its Role in Disease Processes in Man." *Clinical Physiology and Biochemistry* 4 (1986): 31–41.

Anderson, R. A. "Selenium, Chromium, and Manganese: (B) Chromium." In *Modern Nutrition in Health and Disease,* 7th ed., edited by M. E. Shils and V. R. Young, 268–273. Philadelphia: Lea & Febiger, 1988.

Anderson, R. A. "Essentiality of Chromium in Humans." *Science of the Total Environment* 86, no. 1–2 (1989): 75–81.

Anderson, R. A., N. A. Bryden, M. M. Polansky, and S. Reisner. "Urinary Chromium Excretion and Insulinogenic Properties of Carbohydrates." *American Journal of Clinical Nutrition* 51, no. 5 (1990): 864–868.

Anderson R. A., M. M. Polansky, N. A. Bryden, S. J. Bhathena, and J. J. Canary. "Effects of Supplemental Chromium on Patients with Symptoms of Reactive Hypoglycemia." *Metabolism* 36, no. 4 (1987): 351–355.

Anderson R. A., M. M. Polansky, N. A. Bryden, and H. N. Guttman. "Strenuous Exercise May Increase Dietary Needs for Chromium and Zinc." In *Sports, Health and Nutrition,* vol. 2, edited by F. I. Katch, 83–88. Champaign, IL: Human Kinetics, 1986.

Anderson, R. A., M. M. Polansky, N. A. Bryden, E. E. Roginski, K. Y. Patterson, and D. C. Reamer. "Effect of Exercise (Running) on Serum Glucose, Insulin, Glucagon, and Chromium Excretion." *Diabetes* 31 (1982): 212–216.

Armstrong, T. *The Myth of the A.D.D. Child.* New York: Dutton, 1995.

Bantle, J. P., D. C. Laine, G. W. Castle, J. W. Thomas, et al. "Postprandial Glucose and Insulin Responses to Meals Containing Different Carbohydrates in Normal and Diabetic Subjects." *New England Journal of Medicine* 309 (1983): 7–12.

Barkely, R. A. *Attention Deficit Hyepractivity Disorder: A Handbook for Diagnosis and Treatment.* New York: Guilford, 1990.

Barrett-Connor, L. "Obesity, Atherosclerosis, and Coronary Heart Disease." *Annals of Internal Medicine* 103, no. 6, pt. 2 (1985): 1010–1019.

Beck-Nielsen, H., O. H. Nielsen, P. Damsbo, A. Vaag, A. Handberg, and J. R. Henriksen. "Impairment of Glucose Tolerance: Mechanism of Action and Impact on the Cardiovascular System." *American Journal of Obstetrics and Gynecology* 163, no. 1, pt. 2 (1990): 292–295.

Berne, C. "Insulin in Hypertension—A Relationship with Consequences?" *Journal of Internal Medicine Supplement* 735 (1991): 65–73.

Beverly, C. "Sugary Foods May Be Hazardous for Those Who Have Breast Cancer." *Natural Healing Newsletter* 3, no. 1G (1991): 5.

Bjorntorp, P. "Obesity and Adipose Tissue Distribution As a Risk Factor for the Development of Disease: A Review." *Infusionstherapie* 17, no. 1 (1990): 24–27.

Black, H. R. "The Coronary Artery Disease Paradox: The Role of Hyperinsulinemia and Insulin Resistance and Its Implications for Therapy." *Journal of Cardiovascular Pharmacology* 15, suppl. 5 (1990): S26-S38.

Blackburn, G. L. "Medical Treatment of Obesity." In *Treatment of Obesity: A Multidisciplinary Approach,* conference compendium edited by G. L. Blackburn, P. N. Benotti, and E. A. Mascioli. Boston: Harvard Medical School, 1991.

Blackburn, G. L., P. N. Benotti, and E. A. Mascioli, eds. *Treatment of Obesity: A Multidisciplinary Approach* (conference compendium). Boston: Harvard Medical School, 1991.

Blessing, P. "Childhood Obesity: A NICHD Workshop Report." *Children Today,* September-October 1986, 26–29.

Boston Women's Health Book Collective. *The New Our Bodies, Ourselves—Updated and Expanded for the '90s.* New York: Touchstone/Simon & Schuster, 1992.

Bottermann, P., and M. Classen. "Diabetes Mellitus and Arterial Hypertension: In Search of the Connecting Link." *Zeitschrift fur die Gesamte Innere Medizin und Ihre Grengebiete* 46, no. 15 (1991): 558–562.

Bougneres, P. F., E. Artavia-Loria, S. Henry, A. Basdevant, and L. Castano. "Increased Basal Glucose Production and Utilization in Children with Recent Obesity Versus Adults with Long Term Obesity." *Diabetes* 38, no. 4 (1989): 477–483.

Brands, M. W., and J. E. Hall. "Insulin Resistance, Hyperinsulinemia, and Obesity-Associated Hypertension." *Journal of American Society of Nephrology* 3, no. 5 (1992): 1064–1077.

Brazelton, T. B. "Food Fights: How to Cope with Picky, Messy, Sneaky Eaters." *Family Circle,* April 2, 1991, 54–56.

Brindley, D. N., and Y. Rolland. "Possible Connections Between Stress, Diabetes, Obesity, Hypertension and Altered Lipoprotein Metabolism That May Result in Atherosclerosis." *Clinical Science* 77, no. 5 (1989): 453–461.

Brody, J. E. *Jane Brody's Nutrition Book.* New York: Norton, 1981.

Brody, J. E. *Jane Brody's The New York Times Guide to Personal Health.* New York: Times Books/New York Times Book Company, 1982.

Brooks, C. G. "Consequences of Childhood Obesity." *World Medical Journal* 3 (1972): 45.

Bruning, P. F., J. M. Bonfrer, P. A. van Noord, A. A. Hart, M. de Jong-Bakker, and W. J. Nooijen. "Insulin Resistance and Breast Cancer Risk." *International Journal of Cancer* 52, no. 4 (1992): 511–516.

Chiumello, G., M. J. Del Guercio, M. Carnelutti, and G. Bidone. "The Relationship between Obesity, Chemical Diabetes, and Pancreatic Function in Children." *Diabetes* 18, no. 4 (1969): 238–243.

Conn, H. L., Jr., E. A. DeFelice, and P. T. Kuo. *Health and Obesity.* New York: Raven Press, 1983.

Conway, G. S., P. M. Clark, and D. Wong. "Hyperinsulinemia in the Polycystic Ovary Syndrome Confirmed with a Specific Immunoradiometric Assay for Insulin." *Clinical Endocrinology* (Oxford) 38, no. 2 (1993): 219–222.

Coulston, A. M., C. B. Hollenbeck, A. L. M. Swislocki, Y. D. I. Chen, and G. Reaven. "Deleterious Metabolic Effects of High-Carbohydrate, Sucrose-Containing Diets in Patients with Non-Insulin-Dependent Diabetes Mellitus." *American Journal of Medicine* 82 (February 1987): 213–220.

Coulston, A. M., G. C. Liu, and G. M. Reaven. "Plasma Glucose, Insulin and Lipid Responses to High-Carbohydrate Low-Fat Diets in Normal Humans." *Metabolism* 32, no. 1 (1983): 52–56.

Davis, A. *Let's Have Healthy Children.* New York: Signet/Penguin USA, 1972.

DeFronzo, R. A., and E. Ferrannini. "Insulin Resistance: A Multifaceted Syndrome Responsible for NIDDM, Obesity, Hypertension, Dys lipidemia, and Atherosclerotic Cardiovascular Disease." *Diabetes-Care* 14, no. 3 (1991): 173–194.

Del Prato, S. "Hyperinsulinemia: Causes and Mechanisms." *La Presse Medicale: Edizione Italiana* 21, no. 28 (1992): 1312–1317.

de Parscau, L., and P. Guibaud. "Etiologic Diagnosis of Hypoglycemia in Children." *Pediartie* 45, no. 3 (1990): 165–171.

Devlin, J. T., and E. S. Horton. "Hormone and Nutrient Interactions." In *Modern Nutrition in Health and Disease,* 7th ed., edited by M. E. Shils and V. R. Young, 570–584. Philadelphia: Lea & Febiger, 1988.

Drash, A. "Relationship Between Diabetes Mellitus and Obesity in the Child." *Metabolism* 22, no. 2 (1973): 337–344.

Eaton, S. B., and M. J. Konner. "Stone Age Nutrition: Implications for Today." *ASDC Journal of Dentistry for Children* 53, no. 4 (1986): 300–303.

Eaton, S. B., M. J. Konner, and M. Shostak. "Stone Agers in the Fast Lane: Chronic Degenerative Diseases in Evolutionary Perspective." *American Journal of Medicine* 84, no. 4 (1988): 739–749.

Eden, A. N. *Growing Up Thin.* New York: McKay, 1975.

Ellison, R. C., J. W. Newburger, and D. M. Gross. "Pediatric Aspects of Essential Hypertension." *Journal of the American Dietetic Association* 80 (1982): 21–25.

Farquhar, J. W., A. Frank, R. C. Gross, and G. M. Reaven. "Glucose, Insulin, and Triglyceride Responses to High and Low Carbohydrate Diets in Man." *The Journal of Clinical Investigation* 45, no. 10 (1966): 1648–1656.

Feingold, B. F. *Why Your Child Is Hyperactive.* New York: Random House, 1975.

Felker, D. W. "Relationship Between the Self-Concept, Body Building, and Perception of Father's Interest in Sports in Boys." *Research Quarterly* 39 (1968): 513–517.

Feraille, E., M. Krempf, B. Chabonnel, J. B. Bouhour, and G. Nicolas. "Arterial Hypertension in Patients with Obesity: Role of Hyperinsulinism and Insulin Resistance." *Revue de Mediecine Interne* 11, no. 4 (1990): 293–296.

Ferrari, P., P. Weidmann, S. Shaw, D. Giachino, W. Riesen, Y. Allemann, and G. Heynen. "Altered Insulin Sensitivity, Hyperinsulinemia, and Dyslipidemia in Individuals with a Hypertensive Parent." *American Journal of Medicine* 91, no. 6 (1991): 589–596.

Fisher, J. A. *The Chromium Program.* New York: Harper & Row, 1990.

Flodin, N. W. "Atherosclerosis: An Insulin-Dependent Disease?" *Journal of the American College of Nutrition* 5 (1986): 417–427.

Fontbonne, A., M. A. Charles, N. Thibult, J. L. Richard, J. R. Claude, J. M. Warnet, G. E. Rosselin, and E. Eschwege. "Hyperinsulinemia As a Predictor of Coronary Heart Disease Mortality in a Healthy Population: The Paris Prospective Study, 15-Year Follow-Up." *Diabetologia* 34, no. 5 (1991): 356–361.

Fontbonne, A., and E. Eschwege. "Diabetes, Hyperglycemia, Hyperinsulinemia and Atherosclerosis: Epidemiological Data." *Diabetes and Metabolism* 13, no. 3, pt. 2 (1987): 350–353.

Garg, A., S. M. Grundy, and R. H. Unger. "Comparison of Effects of High and Low Carbohydrate Diets on Plasma Lipoproteins and

Insulin Sensitivity in Patients with Mild NIDDM." *Diabetes* 41, no. 10 (1992): 1278–1285.

Garg, A., J. H. Helderman, M. Koffler, R. Ayuso, J. Rosenstock, and P. Raskin. "Relationship Between Lipoprotein Levels in Vivo Insulin Action in Normal Young White Men." *Metabolism* 37, no. 10 (1988): 982–987.

Geiselman, P. J. "Sugar-Induced Hyperphagia: Is Hyperinsulinemia, Hypoglycemia, or Any Other Factor a 'Necessary' Condition?" *Appetite* 11, suppl. 1 (1988): 26–34.

Geiselman, P. J., and D. Novin. "The Role of Carbohydrates in Appetite, Hunger and Obesity." *Appetite* 3 (1982): 203–223.

Gschwend S., C. Ryan, J. Atchison, S. Arslania, and D. Becker. "Effects of Acute Hyperglycemia on Mental Efficiency and Counterregulatory Hormones in Adolescents with Insulin-Dependent Diabetes Mellitus." *Journal of Pediatrics* 126 (1995): 178–184.

Ginsberg, H., J. M. Olefsky, G. Kimmerling, P. Crapo, and G. M. Reaven. "Induction of Hypertriglyceridemia by a Low-Fat Diet." *Journal of Clinical Endocrinology and Metabolism* 42 (1976): 729–735.

Gong, E. J., and F. P. Heald. "Diet, Nutrition, and Adolescence." In *Modern Nutrition in Health and Disease*, 7th ed., edited by M. E. Shils and V. R. Young, 969–981. Philadelphia: Lea & Febiger, 1988.

Gortmaker, S. L., A. Must, J. M. Perrin, A. M. Sobol, and W. H. Dietz. "Social and Economic Consequences of Overweight in Adolescence and Young Adulthood." *New England Journal of Medicine* 329 (1993): 1008–1012.

Grimaldi, A., C. Sachon, F. Bosquet, and R. Doumith. "Intolerance to Carbohydrates: The Seven Questions." *Revista de Medicina Interna* 11, no. 4 (1990): 297–307.

Hallfrisch, J. "Metabolic Effects of Dietary Fructose." *FASEB Journal* 4, no. 9 (1990): 2652–2660.

Haust, M. D. "The Genesis of Atherosclerosis in Pediatric Age-Group." *Pediatric Pathology* 10, no. 1–2 (1990): 253–271.

Heaton, K. W., S. N. Marcus, P. M. Emmett, and C. H. Bolton. "Particle Size of Wheat, Maize, and Oat Test Meals: Effects on Plasma Glucose and Insulin Responses and on the Rate of Starch Digestion in the Liver." *American Journal of Clinical Nutrition* 47, no. 4 (1988): 675–682.

Heller, R. F., and R. F. Heller. "Dietary Carbohydrates: The Frequency Factor." Paper presented at the annual meeting of the American Institute of Nutrition, New Orleans, LA, April 30, 1993.

Heller, R. F., and R. F. Heller. "Hunger and Cravings in the Overweight: A Physical Cause." Paper presented at the annual meetings of the American Institute of Nutrition, April 27, 1994.

Heller, R. F., and R. F. Heller. "Hunger and Cravings in the Over-weight: Correcting a Physical Cause." Paper presented at the annual meeting of the American Institute of Nutrition, Anaheim, CA, April 27, 1994.

Heller, R. F., and R. F. Heller. "Hyperinsulinemic Obesity and Carbohy-drate Addiction: The Missing Link Is the Carbohydrate Frequency." *Medical Hypotheses* 42 (1994): 307–312.

Heller, R. F., and R. F. Heller. "Hypertension in the Normal-Weight and Overweight: Correcting a Physical Cause." Paper presented at the annual meeting of the American Institute of Nutrition, Atlanta GA, April 13, 1995.

Heller, R. F., and R. F. Heller. "Hypertriglyceridemia in the Normal-Weight and Overweight: Correcting a Physical Cause." Paper pre-sented at the annual meeting of the American Institute of Nutrition, Atlanta, GA, April 13, 1995.

Heller, R. F., and R. F. Heller. "Profactor-H (Elevated Circulating Insulin): The Link to Health Risk Factors and Diseases of Civiliza-tion." *Medical Hypotheses,* 45, no. 4 (October 1995): 325–330.

Hilts, P. J. "U.S. Dietary Guide Sets Fat and Alcohol Limits: Diets for Children Are Also Included for the First Time." *New York Times,* November 6, 1990, C1.

Hollis, J. *Fat Is a Family Affair—A Hope-Filled Guide for Those Who Suffer from Eating Disorder and Those Who Love Them.* San Francisco: Harper/Hazeldon, 1985.

Hubner, G., H. H. von Dorsche, and H. Zuhlke. "Morphological Studies of the Effect of Chromium-III-Chloride on the Islet Cell Organ in Rats Under the Conditions of High and Low Fat Diets." *Anatomischer Anzeiger* 167, no. 5 (1988): 389–391.

Johnston, F. E. "Health Implications of Childhood Obesity." *Annals of Internal Medicine* 103, no. 6, pt. 2 (1985): 1068–1072.

Jones, T. W., et al. "Enhanced Adrenomedullary Response and Increased Susceptibility to Neuroglycopenia: Mechanisms Underlying the Adverse Effects of Sugar Ingestion in Healthy Children." *Journal of Pediatrics* 126, no. 2 (1995): 171–177.

Kakar, F., S. D. Hursting, M. M. Henderson, and M. D. Thorquist. "Dietary Sugar and Breast Cancer: Epidemiologic Evidence." *Clinical Nutrition* 9 (1990): 68–71, 1990.

Kaker, F., M. D. Thornquist, M. M. Henderson, R. D. Klein, S. M. Kozawa, G. A. Santisteben, S. D. Hursting, and N. D. Urban. "The Effect of Dietary Sugar and Dietary Antioxidants on Mammary Tumor Growth and Lethality in BALB/c Mice." *Clinical Nutrition* 9 (1990): 62–67.

Kaplan, N. M. "The Deadly Quartet." *Archives of Internal Medicine* 149 (1989): 1514–1520.

Kazumi, T., G. Yoshino, K. Matsuba, M. Iwai, I. Iwatani, M. Matsushita, T. Kasama, T. Hosokawa, F. Numano, and S. Baba. "Effects of Dietary Glucose or Fructose on the Secretion Rate and Particle Size of Triglyceride-Rich Lipoproteins in Zucker Fatty Rats." *Metabolism* 40, no. 9 (1991): 962–966.

Kinderlehrer, J. "Wake Up Your Life with a Healthy Breakfast." *Prevention*, February 1984, 50.

Kirschenbaum, D. S., W. G. Johnson, and P. M. Stalonas, Jr. *Treating Childhood and Adolescent Obesity. Psychological Practitioner Guidebooks.* New York: Pergamon Press, 1987.

Kneebone, G. M. "Childhood Obesity: The Diagnosis and Management." *Australian Family Physician* 19, no. 3 (1990): 367–370.

Kohlhoff, R., and G. Dorner. "Perinatal Hyperinsulinism and Perinatal Obesity Are Risk Factors for Hyperinsulinaemia in Later Life." *Experimental and Clinical Endocrinology* 96, no. 1 (1990): 105–108.

Koop, C. E. *The Surgeon General's Report on Nutrition and Health.* Publication No. 88–50210. Washington, D.C.: U.S. Department Health and Human Services, 1988.

Kozlovsky, A. S., P. B. Moser, S. Reisner, and R. A. Anderson. "Effects of Diets High in Simple Sugars on Urinary Chromium Losses." *Metabolism* 35, no. 6 (1986): 515–518.

Kumpulainen, J. T., W. R. Wolf, C. Veillon, and W. Mertz. "Determination of Chromium in Selected United States Diets." *Journal of Agriculture and Food Chemistry* 27, no. 3 (1979): 490–494.

Kusekova, M., and M. Sasinka. "Hyperinsulinism—A New Pathogenic Cause of Cardiovascular Diseases." *Cesko Slovenska Pediatrie* 48, no. 3 (1993): 136–140.

Kwiterovich, P. O. "Pediatric Aspects of Hyperlipoproteinemia." In *Hyperlipemia: Diagnosis and Therapy*, edited by B. M. Rifkind and R. I. Levy, 249–279. New York: Grune & Stratton, 1977.

Lambert, N. M., J. Sandoval, and D. Sassone. "Prevalence of Hyperactivity in Elementary School Children as a Function of Social System Definers." *American Journal of Orthopsychiatry* 48 (1978): 446–63.

Lauer, R. M., W. E. Conner, P. E. Leaverton, M. A. Reiter, and W. R. Clark. "Coronary Heart Disease Risk Factors in School Children." *Journal of Pediatrics* 86 (1975): 697–706.

Lawson, C. "3,813 Pounds Down, 6,187 or So to Go." *New York Times*, July 18, 1991, C1.

LeBow, M. D. *Child Obesity—A New Frontier of Behavior Therapy.* New York, NY: Springer, 1984.

Lefebvre, P. J., and A. J. Scheen. "Hypoglycemia." In *Diabetes Mellitus,* 4th ed., edited by H. Rifkin and D. Porte, Jr. New York: Elsevier, 1990.

Linder, C. M., ed. *Nutritional Biochemistry and Metabolism—With Clinical Applications.* New York: Elsevier, 1985.

Liu, G., A. Coulston, C. Hollenbeck, and G. Reaven. "The Effect of Sucrose Content in High and Low Carbohydrate Diets on Plasma Glucose, Insulin, and Lipid Responses in Hypertriglyceridemic Humans." *Journal of Clinical Endocrinology and Metabolism* 59, no. 4 (1984): 636–642.

MacDonald, I. "Carbohydrates." In *Modern Nutrition in Health and Disease,* 7th ed., edited by M. E. Shils and V. R. Young, 38–51. Philadelphia: Lea & Febiger, 1988.

Mahan, L. K. "Family-Focused Behavioral Approach to Weight Control in Children." *Pediatric Clin N Am* 34, no. 4 (1987): 983–996.

Margalit, M. "Diagnostic Application of the Conners Abbreviated Symptom Questionnaire." *Journal of Clinical Child Psychology* 12, no. 3 (1983): 355–357.

Mendelson, B. K., and D. R. White. "Development of Self-Body Esteem in Overweight Youngsters." *Developmental Psychology* 21 (1985): 90–96.

Molnar, D. "Insulin Secretion and Carbohydrate Tolerance in Childhood Obesity." *Klinische Paediatre* 202 (1980): 131–135.

Molnar, D., and J. Porszasz. "The Effect of Fasting Hyperinsulinaemia on Physical Fitness in Obese Children." *European Journal of Pediatrics* 149, no. 8 (1990): 570–573.

Morgan, D. L. G. *Nutrition Prescription—Strategies for Preventing and Treating 50 Common Diseases.* New York: Crown, 1987.

Morriss, R. *Children with Attention Disorders in School: A Descriptive Guide for Parents and Teachers.* ERIC Document ED 329 061/EC 300 055.

New York Times. "Despite Better Diets, Adults in Their 20s Are Weighing More." March 18, 1994, C4.

Nobels, F., and D. Dewailly. "Puberty and Polycystic Ovarian Syndrome: The Insulin/Insulin-Like Growth Factor I Hypothesis." *Fertility and Sterility* 58, no. 4 (1992): 655–666.

O'Dea, K. "Westernization, Insulin Resistance and Diabetes in Australian Aborigines." *Medical Journal of Australia* 155, no. 4 (1991): 258–264.

O'Dea, K. "Westernization and Non-Insulin-Dependent Diabetes in Australian Aborigines." *Ethnicity and Disease* 1, no. 2 (1991): 171–187.

Powers, P. S. *Obesity: The Regulation of Weight.* Baltimore: Williams & Wilkins, 1980.

Ravussin, E. "Energy Metabolism in Obesity: Studies in the Pima Indians." *Diabetes Care* 16, no. 1 (1993): 232–238.

Ravussin, E., and C. Bogardus. "Energy Expenditure in the Obese: Is There a Thrifty Gene?" *Infusionstherapie* 17 (1990): 108–112.

Reaven, G. M. "Role of Insulin Resistance in Human Disease." *Diabetes* 37 (1988): 1595–1607.

Reaven, G. M. "Insulin Resistance and Compensatory Hyperinsulinemia: Role in Hypertension, Dyslipidemia, and Coronary Heart Disease." *American Heart Journal* 121, no. 4, pt. 2 (1991): 1283–1288.

Reaven, G. M. "Insulin Resistance, Hyperinsulinemia, and Hypertriglyceridemia in the Etiology and Clinical Course of Hypertension." *American Journal of Medicine* 90, no. 2A (1991): 7S–11S.

Reaven, G. M. "Relationship Between Insulin Resistance and Hypertension." *Diabetes Care* 14, suppl. 4 (1991): 33–38.

Reaven, G. M. "Role of Insulin Resistance in Human Disease." *Diabetes* 37 (1991): 1595–1607.

Reaven, G. M., and B. B. Hoffman. "Hypertension As a Disease of Carbohydrate and Lipoprotein Metabolism." *American Journal of Medicine* 87, no. 6A (1989): 2S–6S.

Reed, R., and A. Schauss. *Food, Teens and Behavior.* Manitowoc, Wis.: Natural Press, 1983.

Reiser, S., M. C. Bickard, J. Hallfrisch, O. E. Michaelis IV, and E. S. Prather. "Blood Lipids and Their Distribution in Lipoproteins in Hyperinsulinemic Subjects Fed Three Different Levels of Sucrose." *Journal of Nutrition* 111 (1981): 1045–1057.

Reiser, S., A. S. Powell, D. J. Scholfield, P. Panda, K. C. Ellwood, and J. J. Canary. "Blood Lipids, Lipoproteins, Apoproteins, and Uric Acid in Men Fed Diets Containing Fructose or High-Amylose Cornstarch." *American Journal of Clinical Nutrition* 49, no. 5 (1989): 832–839.

Roberts, S. B., J. Savage, W. A. Coward, B. Chew, et al. "Energy Expenditure and Intake in Infants Born to Lean and Overweight Mothers" *New England Journal of Medicine* 318, no. 8 (1988): 461–466.

Rocchini A. P. "Adolescent Obesity and Hypertension." *Pediatric Clinics of North America* 40, no. 1 (1993): 81–89.

Rodale Press. *The Prevention Total Health System—Understanding Vitamins and Minerals.* Emmaus, PA,: Rodale Press, 1984.

Rodin, J. "Insulin Levels, Hunger, and Food Intake: An Example of Feedback Loops in Body Weight Regulation." *Health Psychology* 4 (1985): 1–18.

Schauss, A., and S. Schoenthaler. *Diet, Crime and Delinquency.* Berkeley, Calif.: Parker House, 1981.

Schroeder, H. A. "The Role of Chromium in Mammalian Nutrition." *American Journal of Clinical Nutrition* 21, no. 6 (1968): 230–244.

Sharma, A. M., K. Ruland, K. P. Spies, and A. Distler. "Salt Sensitivity in Young Normotensive Subjects Is Associated with a Hyperinsulinemic

Response to Oral Glucose." *Journal of Hypertension* 9, no. 4 (1991): 329–335.

Shils, M. E., and V. R. Young, eds. *Modern Nutrition in Health and Disease,* 7th ed. Philadelphia: Lea & Febiger, 1988.

Silberstein, W. P., and L. Galton. *Helping Your Child Grow Slim—Safe Dieting for Overweight Children and Adolescents.* New York: Simon & Schuster, 1982.

Simonson, D. C. "Hyperinsulinemia and Its Sequelae." *Hormone and Metabolic Research Supplement* 22 (1990): 17–25.

Simopoulos, A. P. "Characteristics of Obesity: An Overview." *Annals of the New York Academy of Science* 499 (1987): 4–13.

Singer, P., and R. Baumann. "Glucose-Induced or Postprandial Hyperinsulinemia in Mild Essential Hypertension—An Underestimated Biochemical Risk Factor." *Medical Hypotheses* 34, no. 2 (1991): 157–164.

Smith, L. *Feeding Your Kids Right.* New York: McGraw-Hill, 1979.

Smith, L. *Diet Plan for Teenagers.* New York: McGraw-Hill, 1986.

Spring, B., J. Chiodo, M. Harden, M. J. Bourgeois, J. D. Mason, and L. Lutherer. "Psychobiological Effects of Carbohydrates." *Journal of Clinical Psychiatry* 50, no. 5, suppl. (1989): 27–33.

Storlien, L. H., E. W. Kraegen, A. B. Jenkins, and D. J. Chisholm. "Effects of Sucrose vs. Starch Diets on in Vivo Insulin Action, Thermogenesis, and Obesity in Rats." *American Journal of Clinical Nutrition* 47, no. 3 (1988): 420–427.

Stout, R. W. "Overview of the Association Between Insulin and Atherosclerosis." *Metabolism* 34, no. 12 (1985): 7–12.

Stout, R. W. "Insulin and Atheroma. 20-Year Perspective." *Diabetes Care* 13, no. 6 (1990): 631–654.

Stout, R. W. "Insulin and Atherogenesis." *European Journal of Epidemiology* 8, suppl. 1 (1992): 134–135.

Taber's Cyclopedic Medical Dictionary, 18th ed., edited by Thomas Clayton. Philadelphia: F. A. Davis, 1997.

Taylor, E., and S. Sandberg. "Hyperactive Behavior in English Schoolchildren: A Questionnaire Survey." *Journal of Abnormal Child Psychology* 12, no. 1 (1984): 143–55.

Toepfer, E. W., W. Mertz, E. E. Roginski, and M. M. Polansky. "Chromium in Foods in Relation to Biological Activity." *Journal of Agriculture and Food Chemistry* 21, no. 1 (1973): 69–73.

Tufts University. "Little Ones Should Eat for Health, Too." *Tufts University Diet and Nutrition Letter* 9, no. 4 (1991): 1.

Tufts University. "When Growing Pains Hurt Too Much: Teens at Risk." *Tufts University Diet and Nutrition Letter* 9, no. 4 (1991): 3–6.

Tufts University. "Teen Obesity: A Heavy Burden Even in Adulthood." *Tufts University Diet and Nutrition Letter* 10, no. 11 (1993): 1–2.

Tufts University. "Warning: Keep Dieting Out of Reach of Children." *Tufts University Diet and Nutrition Letter* 11, no. 10 (1993): 3–6.

Weihang, B., S. R. Srinivasan, and G. S. Berenson. "Persistent Elevation of Plasma Insulin Levels Is Associated with Increased Cardiovascular Risk in Children and Young Adults: The Bogalusa Heart Study." *Circulation* 93 (1996): 54–59.

Wervach, M. R. *Nutritional Influences on Illness—A Sourcebook of Clinical Research.* Tarzana, CA: Third Line Press, 1987.

Wolff, J. M., and D. Lipe. *Help for the Overweight Child.* New York, NY: Penguin, 1980.

Wunderlich, R., and D. K. Kalita. *Nourishing Your Child: A Bioecologic Approach.* New Canaan, Conn.: Keats, 1984.

Yam, D., A. Fink, I. Nir, and P. Budowski. "Insulin-Tumor Interrelationships in Thymoma Bearing Mice: Effects of Dietary Glucose and Fructose." *British Journmal of Cancer* 64, no. 6 (1991): 1043–1046.

Zavaroni, I., E. Bonora, M. Pagliara, E. Dall'Aglio, L. Luchetti, G. Buonanno, P. A. Bonati, M. Bergonzani, L. Gnudi, M. Passeri, and G. Reaven. "Risk Factors for Coronary Artery Disease in Healthy Persons with Hyperinsulinemia and Normal Glucose Tolerance." *New England Journal of Medicine* 320, no. 11 (1989): 702–706.

Zinner, S. H., P. Levy, and E. H. Kass. "Familial Aggregation of Blood Pressure in Children." *New England Journal of Medicine* 283 (1971): 401–408.

STANDARD HEIGHT AND WEIGHT
CHARTS FOR CHILDREN AND TEENS

It is important to keep in mind that youngsters grow at different rates at different times. Often children and teens appear to be overweight when, in a little while, a growth spurt results in several inches added to their height, returning them to a normal weight level.

This chart has been included for those familiar with this manner of measurement. While the Body Mass Index (BMI) that follows on page 435 is the preferred method of evaluating height and weight relationships, this chart is easier to read and can give you a baseline, an average weight and height level, for the "average" youngster. This chart is not meant to recommend or prescribe weights appropriate for your child or teen but rather to help you visualize where, in the statistical curve that your physician most likely uses, your youngster fits. If you see differences that are of concern, always check with your youngster's physician.

PHYSICAL GROWTH TABLE*
(2 TO 18 YEARS)

AGE (IN YEARS)	AVERAGE HEIGHT (ROUNDED TO NEAREST INCH)		AVERAGE WEIGHT (ROUNDED TO NEAREST POUND)	
GIRLS/BOYS	GIRLS	BOYS	GIRLS	BOYS
2	34	34	26	28
3	37	37	31	32
4	40	41	35	37
5	43	43	40	41
6	45	46	43	45
7	47	48	48	52
8	50	50	55	55
9	52	52	63	62
10	54	54	72	70
11	57	56	81	78
12	60	59	94	88
13	62	62	101	99
14	63	64	110	112
15	64	67	118	125
16	64	68	123	137
17	64	69	125	146
18	64	70	125	152

*Adapted from data from the National Center for Health Statistics. "Average" weight and height based on fiftieth percentile.

BODY MASS INDEX

The Body Mass Index (BMI) is the preferred method of evaluating height and weight relationships and is often used by researchers. The calculations may be unfamiliar and the results less easily visualized, however, than typical height/weight charts you will find on page 434. This chart is not meant to recommend or prescribe weights appropriate for your child or teen; for those recommendations, check with your youngster's physician.

Body mass index (BMI = weight in kilograms divided by height in meters squared) for persons 2–19 years of age.

MALE			FEMALE		
Age in years	Mean BMI	50th Pecentile	Age in years	Mean BMI	50th Pecentile
2	16.3	16.3	2	16.1	16.0
3	15.9	15.8	3	15.6	15.4
4	15.8	15.6	4	15.5	15.3
5	15.6	15.4	5	15.6	15.3
6	16.0	15.3	6	15.7	15.3
7	16.0	15.7	7	16.1	15.7
8	16.6	16.2	8	16.4	15.9
9	16.8	16.4	9	17.5	16.5
10	18.0	17.3	10	17.8	17.0
11	18.7	17.5	11	18.9	18.1
12	18.8	18.0	12	19.4	18.8
13	19.6	18.9	13	20.1	19.3
14	20.2	19.6	14	21.1	20.4
15	20.8	20.5	15	20.6	19.9
16	22.1	21.6	16	21.8	21.0
17	21.7	21.3	17	22.3	21.4
18	22.7	22.1	18	22.3	21.6
19	23.0	22.6	19	22.5	21.6

*Adapted from U.S. Department of Health and Human Services,
Data from the National Health Survey, Series 11, No. 238.

APPENDIX IV

WEIGHT CHART*

Record your youngster's weight every day. To see if your youngster is losing weight, compare weekly averages only.

(To get your youngster's weekly average, add up all the weights in that week, then divide by the number of weighings that week. For details, see page 248.)

Week Start (date)	Mon Weight	Tues Weight	Wed Weight	Thurs Weight	Fri Weight	Sat Weight	Sun Weight	Average Weight for Week

* Your youngster's physician's approval, advice, and monitoring are essential.

SUBJECT INDEX

RECIPE INDEX

Using the Recipe Index:

The Recipe Index that follows contains entries for recipes in Part IV (pages 291–415). For other information, *see* the Subject Index (pages 437–444).

In the entries that follow:

(IB) indicates that this recipe can be included in Insulin-Balancing Meals and Snacks Recipes.

(COMBO) indicates that this recipe can be included in Combo Meals and Snacks.

(SWAP) indicates recipe may be used as a Swap Choice.

Many recipes may be included in more than one meal:

(IB/COMBO) indicates that a specific recipe may be included in either Insulin-Balancing or Combo Meals, for instance.

About the Authors

RICHARD F. HELLER, M.S., PH.D. and
RACHAEL F. HELLER, M.A., M.PH., PH.D.

For more than a decade, the Drs. Heller each held two professorial appointments and conducted research, at Mount Sinai School of Medicine in New York City and in the Department of Biomedical Sciences in the Graduate Center of the City University of New York. Richard holds a third appointment as Professor Emeritus at the City University of New York. Together, they are the authors of the bestselling books *Healthy for Life* and *The Carbohydrate Addict's Diet*, as well as *The Carbohydrate Addict's Lifespan Program*, *The Carbohydrate Addict's Program for Success*, and *The Carbohydrate Addict's Gram Counter*.